I0047056

Basic Human Anatomy & Physiology

Subcourses
MD0006, MD0007

Edition 100

Basic Human
Anatomy & Physiology

Subcourses
MD0006, MD0007

Edition 100

Basic Human Anatomy & Physiology: Subcourses MD0006, MD0007; Edition 100

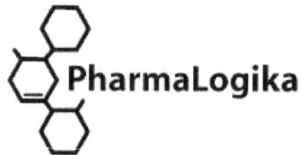

PharmaLogika

PharmaLogika, Inc.
PO Box 461
Willow Springs, NC 27592

www.pharmalogika.com

Author / Editor: Mindy J. Allport-Settle

Published by PharmaLogika, Inc.

Printed in the United States of America.

ISBN 0-9830719-6-9
ISBN-13 978-0-9830719-6-9

Contents

LIST OF ILLUSTRATIONS

LIST OF TABLES

Basic Human Physiology

13. The Special Senses

LIST OF FIGURES

LIST OF TABLES

Overview

About this Book

The United States Army is recognized internationally as the standard for complete, efficient and effective adult education. The Army has a tradition of pioneering training systems (including computer-based training) that then transition into the corporate sector. This manual has been continuously tested and updated to successfully educate every member of the modern United States Army. The needs of the instructor, the student, and the Army are perfectly balanced. This is the model all educators strive to follow when developing and delivering training programs.

Included Documents and Features

Basic Human Anatomy

1. Introduction to Basic Human Anatomy

2. Tissues of the Body

3. The Human Integumentary and Fascial Systems

4. The Human Skeletal System

5. The Human Muscular System

6. The Human Digestive System

7. The Human Respiratory System and Breathing

8. The Human Urogenital Systems

9. The Human Cardiovascular and Lymphatic Systems

10. The Human Endocrine System

11. The Human Nervous System

Basic Human Physiology

1. Introduction to Basic Human Physiology

2. Physiology of Cells and Miscellaneous Tissues

Orientation

Human Anatomy

The human body consists of biological systems. Biological systems consist of organs. Organs consist of tissues. Tissues consist of cells and connective tissue. Human anatomy is primarily the scientific study of the morphology of the human body.[1] Anatomy is subdivided into gross anatomy and microscopic anatomy. Gross anatomy (also called topographical anatomy, regional anatomy, or anthropotomy) is the study of anatomical structures that can be seen by unaided vision. Microscopic anatomy is the study of minute anatomical structures assisted with microscopes, which includes histology (the study of the organization of tissues), and cytology (the study of cells). Anatomy, physiology (the study of function) and biochemistry (the study of the chemistry of living structures) are complementary basic medical sciences when applied to the human body. As such, these subjects are usually taught together (or in tandem) to students in the medical sciences.

In some of its facets human anatomy is closely related to embryology, comparative anatomy and comparative embryology, through common roots in evolution; for example, much of the human body maintains the ancient segmental pattern that is present in all vertebrates with basic units being repeated, which is particularly obvious in the vertebral column and in the ribcage, and can be traced from very early embryos.

The history of anatomy has been characterized, over a long period of time, by a continually developing understanding of the functions of organs and structures in the body. Methods have also advanced dramatically, advancing from examination of animals through dissection of preserved cadavers (dead human bodies) to technologically complex techniques developed in the 20th century.

History of anatomy

The development of anatomy as a science extends from the earliest examinations of sacrificial victims to the sophisticated analyses of the body performed by modern scientists. It has been characterized, over time, by a

---

[1] "Introduction page, "Anatomy of the Human Body." Henry Gray. 20th edition. 1918."
http://www.bartleby.com/107/1.html.

continually developing understanding of the functions of organs and structures in the body. The field of Human Anatomy has a prestigious history, and is considered to be the most prominent of the biological sciences of the 19th and early 20th centuries. Methods have also improved dramatically, advancing from examination of animals through dissection of cadavers to technologically complex techniques developed in the 20th century.[2]

Anatomy is one of the cornerstones of a medical professional's education. Despite being a persistent portion of teaching from at least the renaissance, the format and the amount of information being taught has evolved and changed along with the demands of the profession. What is being taught today may differ in content significantly from the past but the methods used to teach this have not really changed that much. For example all the famous public dissections of the Middle Ages and early renaissance were in fact prosections. In a dissection, students learn by doing; in a prosection, students learn by either observing a dissection being performed by an experienced anatomist or examining a specimen that has already been dissected by an experienced anatomist.[3] Prosection is the direction in which many current medical schools are heading in order to aid the teaching of anatomy and some argue that dissection is better. However looking at results of post graduate exams, medical schools (specifically Birmingham) that use prosection as opposed to dissection do very well in these examinations.[4] This would suggest that prosection can fit very well into the structure of modern medical training.

Human Physiology

Physiology is the study of the function of living systems. This includes how organisms, organ systems, organs, cells and biomolecules carry out the chemical or physical functions that exist in a living system.

Systems

Traditionally, the academic discipline of physiology views the body as a collection of interacting systems, each with its own combination of functions

---

[2] Hakim Syed Zillur Rahman. Tarikh llm Tashrih [An extensive Book in Urdu on History of anatomy] (1967), Tibbi Academy, Delhi, Second revised edition 2009 (ISBN 978-81-906070-), Ibn Sina Academy of Medieval Medicine and Sciences, Aligarh.

[3] "Prosection." In Dorland's Illustrated Medical Dictionary. 30th ed. Douglas Anderson, ed. Philadelphia, Pa.: Saunders, 2007.

[4] Skelton, J. 2008. CAWC (Curriculum and Welfare Committee) Meet the Dean Q&A session- year 2 students. Birmingham Medical School, 25 February 2008. Available at: http://medsoc.bham.ac.uk/cawc/index.php?option=com_content&view=article&id=71:2ndyrQ&Asession&catid=42:feedbackQAdean&Itemid=61

---

and purposes. The traditional divisions by system are somewhat arbitrary. Many body parts participate in more than one system, and systems might be organized by function, by embryological origin, or other categorizations.

Systems

Nervous System	Consists of the central nervous system (which is the brain and spinal cord) and peripheral nervous system. The brain is the organ of thought, emotion, and sensory processing, and serves many aspects of communication and control of various other systems and functions. The special senses consist of vision, hearing, taste, and smell. The eyes, ears, tongue, and nose gather information about the body's environment.
Musculoskeletal System	Consists of the human skeleton (which includes bones, ligaments, tendons, and cartilage) and attached muscles. It gives the body basic structure and the ability for movement. In addition to their structural role, the larger bones in the body contain bone marrow, the site of production of blood cells. Also, all bones are major storage sites for calcium and phosphate.
Circulatory System	Consists of the heart and blood vessels (arteries, veins, capillaries). The heart propels the circulation of the blood, which serves as a "transportation system" to transfer oxygen, fuel, nutrients, waste products, immune cells, and signalling molecules (i.e., hormones) from one part of the body to another. The blood consists of fluid that carries cells in the circulation, including some that move from tissue to blood vessels and back, as well as the spleen and bone marrow.
Respiratory System	Consists of the nose, nasopharynx, trachea, and lungs. It brings oxygen from the air and excretes carbon dioxide and water back into the air.
Gastrointestinal System	Consists of the mouth, esophagus, stomach, gut (small and large intestines), and rectum, as well as the liver, pancreas, gallbladder, and salivary glands. It converts food into small, nutritional, non-toxic molecules for distribution by the circulation to all tissues of the body, and excretes the unused residue.

Systems

Integumentary System
Consists of the covering of the body (the skin), including hair and nails as well as other functionally important structures such as the sweat glands and sebaceous glands. The skin provides containment, structure, and protection for other organs, but it also serves as a major sensory interface with the outside world.

Urinary System
Consists of the kidneys, ureters, bladder, and urethra. It removes water from the blood to produce urine, which carries a variety of waste molecules and excess ions and water out of the body.

Reproductive System
Consists of the gonads and the internal and external sex organs. The reproductive system produces gametes in each sex, a mechanism for their combination, and a nurturing environment for the first 9 months of development of the offspring.

Immune System
Consists of the white blood cells, the thymus, lymph nodes and lymph channels, which are also part of the lymphatic system. The immune system provides a mechanism for the body to distinguish its own cells and tissues from alien cells and substances and to neutralize or destroy the latter by using specialized proteins such as antibodies, cytokines, and toll-like receptors, among many others.

Endocrine System
Consists of the principal endocrine glands: the pituitary, thyroid, adrenals, pancreas, parathyroids, and gonads, but nearly all organs and tissues produce specific endocrine hormones as well. The endocrine hormones serve as signals from one body system to another regarding an enormous array of conditions, and resulting in variety of changes of function.

Army Medical Command

The U.S. Army Medical Command (MEDCOM) is a major command of the U.S. Army that provides command and control of the Army's fixed-facility medical, dental, and veterinary treatment facilities, providing preventive care, medical research and development and training institutions.

Structure and Subordinate Commands

MEDCOM is divided into Regional Medical Commands that oversee day-to-day operations in military treatment facilities, exercising command and control over the medical treatment facilities in their regions. There are currently five of these regional commands:

- Europe Regional Medical Command

- Southern Regional Medical Command

- Northern Regional Medical Command

- Pacific Regional Medical Command

- Western Regional Medical Command.

Additional subordinate commands of MEDCOM include:

- Army Medical Department Center & School (AMEDDC&S)

- U.S. Army Public Health Command (Provisional), (known as the U.S. Army Center for Health Promotion & Preventive Medicine prior to 1 October 2009 {USACHPPM or CHPPM})

- U.S. Army Medical Research and Materiel Command (USAMRMC)

- Warrior Transition Command (WTC)

- U.S. Army Dental Command (DENCOM)

Operations

In Garrison (Peacetime)

MEDCOM maintains day-to-day health care for soldiers, retired soldiers and the families of both. Despite the wide range of responsibilities involved in providing health care in traditional settings as well as on the battlefield, the Army Medical Department's quality of care compares very favorably with that of civilian health organizations, when measured by civilian standards. Many Army medical facilities report on their own quality-of-care standards on their individual Internet sites.

Deployments

When Army field hospitals deploy, most clinical professional and support personnel come from MEDCOM's fixed facilities. In addition to support of combat operations, deployments can be for humanitarian assistance, peacekeeping, and other stability and support operations. Under the Professional Officer Filler System (PROFIS), up to 26 percent of MEDCOM physicians and 43 percent of MEDCOM nurses are sent to field units during a full deployment. To replace PROFIS losses, Reserve units and Individual Mobilization Augmentees (non-unit reservists) are mobilized to work in medical treatment facilities. The department also provides trained medical specialists to the Army's combat medical units, which are assigned directly to combatant commanders.

Many Army Reserve and Army National Guard units deploy in support of the Army Medical Department. The Army depends heavily on its Reserve component for medical support—about 63 percent of the Army's medical forces are in the Reserve component.

Army Medical Department

The Army Medical Department of the U.S. Army (AMEDD) comprises the Army's six medical Special Branches (or "Corps") of officers and medical enlisted soldiers. It was established as the "Army Hospital" in July 1775 to coordinate the medical care required by the Continental Army during the Revolutionary War. The AMEDD is led by the Surgeon General of the U.S. Army, a lieutenant general.

The AMEDD is the U.S. Army's healthcare organization, not a U.S. Army command. The AMEDD is found in all three components of the Army: the Active Army, the U.S. Army Reserve, and the Army National Guard. Its headquarters are at Fort Sam Houston, San Antonio, Texas, which hosts the AMEDD Center and School. Equal numbers of AMEDD senior leaders can be found in Washington D.C., divided between the Pentagon and the Walter Reed Army Medical Center (WRAMC).

The Academy of Health Sciences, under the Army Medical Department Center & School, provides training to the officers and enlisted soldiers of the AMEDD. As a result of BRAC 2005, enlisted medical training was transferred to the new Medical Education and Training Campus, consolidating most military enlisted medical training at Fort Sam Houston.[5]

Medical Special Branches

- Medical Corps (MC)

- Nurse Corps (AN)

- Dental Corps (DC)

- Veterinary Corps (VC)

- Medical Service Corps (MS)

- Medical Specialist Corps (AMSC)

United States Army Training and Doctrine Command

Established 1 July 1973, the United States Army Training and Doctrine Command (TRADOC) is an army command of the United States Army headquartered at Fort Monroe, Virginia. It is charged with overseeing training of Army forces, the development of operational doctrine, and the development and procurement of new weapons systems. TRADOC operates 33 schools and centers at 16 Army installations. TRADOC schools conduct 2,734 courses (81 directly in support of mobilization) and 373 language courses. The 2,734 courses include 503,164 seats for 434,424 soldiers; 34,675 other-service personnel; 7,824 international soldiers; and 26,241 civilians.[6]

TRADOC MissionThe official mission statement for TRADOC states:

> TRADOC develops the Army's Soldiers and Civilian leaders and designs, develops and integrates capabilities, concepts and doctrine in order to build a campaign-capable, expeditionary Army in support of joint warfighting capability through Army Force Generation (ARFORGEN).[7]

---

[5] U.S. Army Medical Department AMEDD Center and School Portal available on the Internet at: http://www.cs.amedd.army.mil/. Additional information specific to the Fort Sam Houston consolidation is available n the Internet at: http://www.aetc.af.mil/shared/media/document/AFD-071026-035.pdf

[6] TRADOC fact sheet available at: http://www.tradoc.army.mil/about.htm

[7] TRADOC commander on ARFORGEN, and the US Army available at: http://www.tradoc.army.mil/about.htm

TRADOC is the official command component that is responsible for training and developing the United States Army.

TRADOC History

TRADOC was established as a major U.S. Army command on 1 July 1973. The new command, along with the U.S. Army Forces Command (FORSCOM), was created from the Continental Army Command (CONARC) located at Fort Monroe, VA. That action was the major innovation in the Army's post-Vietnam reorganization, in the face of realization that CONARC's obligations and span of control were too broad for efficient focus. The new organization functionally realigned the major Army commands in the continental United States. CONARC, and Headquarters, U.S. Army Combat Developments Command (CDC), situated at Fort Belvoir, VA, were discontinued, with TRADOC and FORSCOM at Fort Belvoir assuming the realigned missions. TRADOC assumed the combat developments mission from CDC, took over the individual training mission formerly the responsibility of CONARC, and assumed command from CONARC of the major Army installations in the United States housing Army training center and Army branch schools. FORSCOM assumed CONARC's operational responsibility for the command and readiness of all divisions and corps in the continental U.S. and for the installations where they were based.

Joined under TRADOC, the major Army missions of individual training and combat developments each had its own lineage. The individual training responsibility had belonged, during World War II, to Headquarters Army Ground Forces (AGF). In 1946 numbered Army areas were established in the U.S. under AGF command. At that time, the AGF moved from Washington, D.C. to Fort Monroe, VA. In March 1948, the AGR was replaced at Fort Monroe with the new Office, Chief of Army Field Forces (OCAFF). OCAFF, however, did not command the training establishment. That function was exercised by Headquarters, Department of the Army through the numbered Armies to the corps, division, and Army Training Centers. In February 1955, HQ Continental Army Command (CONARC) replaced OCAFF, assuming its missions as well as the training missions from DA. In January, HQ CONARC was redesignated U.S. Continental Army Command. Combat developments emerged as a formal Army mission in the early 1950s, and OCAFF assumed that role in 1952. In 1955, CONARC assumed the mission. In 1962, HQ U.S. Army Combat Development Command (CDC) was established to bring the combat developments function under one major Army command.[8]

---

[8] TRADOC history available at: http://www.tradoc.army.mil/about.htm

TRADOC Priorities

1. Leader Development

2. Initial Military Training

3. Concepts and Capabilities Integration

4. Human Capital Enterprise

5. Army Training and Learning Concept

6. Doctrine

This page intentionally left blank.

Basic Human Anatomy

Subcourse MD0006

This page intentionally left blank.

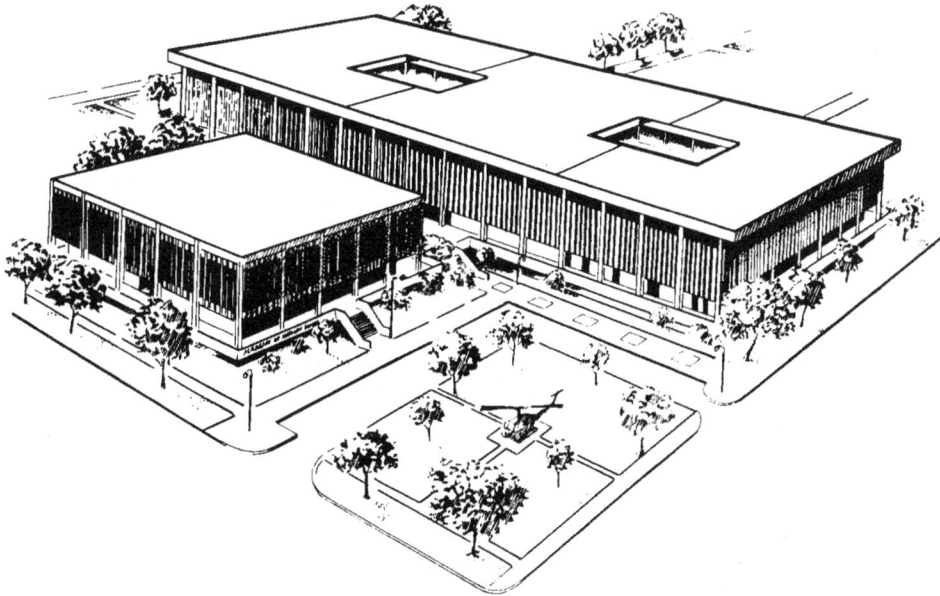

MD0006

BASIC HUMAN ANATOMY

EDITION 100

DEVELOPMENT

This subcourse reflects the current thought of the Academy of Health Sciences and conforms to printed Department of the Army doctrine as closely as currently possible. Development and progress render such doctrine continuously subject to change.

When used in this publication, words such as "he," "him," "his," and "men" are intended to include both the masculine and feminine genders, unless specifically stated otherwise or when obvious in context.

ADMINISTRATION

Students who desire credit hours for this correspondence subcourse must meet eligibility requirements and must enroll through the Nonresident Instruction Branch of the U.S. Army Medical Department Center and School (AMEDDC&S).

Application for enrollment should be made at the Internet website: http://www.atrrs.army.mil. You can access the course catalog in the upper right corner. Enter School Code 555 for medical correspondence courses. Copy down the course number and title. To apply for enrollment, return to the main ATRRS screen and scroll down the right side for ATRRS Channels. Click on SELF DEVELOPMENT to open the application and then follow the on screen instructions.

In general, eligible personnel include enlisted personnel of all components of the U.S. Army who hold an AMEDD MOS or MOS 18D. Officer personnel, members of other branches of the Armed Forces, and civilian employees will be considered eligible based upon their AOC, NEC, AFSC or Job Series which will verify job relevance. Applicants who wish to be considered for a waiver should submit justification to the Nonresident Instruction Branch at e-mail address: accp@amedd.army.mil.

For comments or questions regarding enrollment, student records, or shipments, contact the Nonresident Instruction Branch at DSN 471-5877, commercial (210) 221-5877, toll-free 1-800-344-2380; fax: 210-221-4012 or DSN 471-4012, e-mail accp@amedd.army.mil, or write to:

NONRESIDENT INSTRUCTION BRANCH
AMEDDC&S
ATTN: MCCS-HSN
2105 11TH STREET SUITE 4191
FORT SAM HOUSTON TX 78234-5064

TABLE OF CONTENTS

LIST OF ILLUSTRATIONS

LIST OF TABLES

CORRESPONDENCE COURSE OF THE
U.S. ARMY MEDICAL DEPARTMENT CENTER AND SCHOOL

SUBCOURSE MD0006

BASIC HUMAN ANATOMY

INTRODUCTION

In this subcourse, you will study basic human anatomy. Anatomy is the study of body structure. Physiology is the study of body functions. Anatomy and physiology are two subject matter areas that are vitally important to most medical MOSs. Do your best to achieve the objectives of this subcourse. As a result, you will be better able to perform your job or medical MOS.

Subcourse Components:

This subcourse consists of 11 lessons and an examination. The lessons are:

Lesson 1, Introduction to Basic Human Anatomy.

Lesson 2, Tissues of the Body.

Lesson 3, The Human Integumentary and Fascial Systems.

Lesson 4, The Human Skeletal System.

Lesson 5, The Human Muscular System.

Lesson 6, The Human Digestive System.

Lesson 7, The Human Respiratory System and Breathing.

Lesson 8, The Human Urogenital Systems.

Lesson 9, The Human Cardiovascular and Lymphatic Systems.

Lesson 10, The Human Endocrine System.

Lesson 11, The Human Nervous System.

Credit Awarded:

Upon successful completion of this subcourse, you will be awarded 26 credit hours.

Material Furnished:

In addition to this subcourse booklet, you are furnished an examination answer sheet and an envelope. Answer sheets are not provided for individual lessons in this subcourse because you are to grade your own lessons. Exercises and solutions for all lessons are contained in this booklet.

You must furnish a #2 pencil to be used when marking the examination answer sheet.

You may keep the subcourse.

Procedures for Subcourse completion:

You are encouraged to complete the subcourse lesson by lesson. When you have completed all of the lessons to your satisfaction, fill out the examination answer sheet and mail it to the AMEDDC&S along with the Student Comment Sheet in the envelope provided. *Be sure that your name, rank, social security number, and address is on all correspondence sent to the AMEDDC&S.* You will be notified by return mail of the examination results. Your grade on the examination will be your rating for the subcourse.

Study Suggestions:

Here are some suggestions that may be helpful to you in completing this subcourse:

Read and study each lesson assignment carefully.

After reading and studying the first lesson assignment, work the lesson exercises for the first lesson, marking your answers in the lesson booklet. Refer to the text material as needed.

When you have completed the exercises to your satisfaction, compare your answers with the solution sheet located at the end of the lesson. Reread the referenced material for any questions answered incorrectly.

After you have successfully completed one lesson, go to the next lesson and repeat the above procedures.

When you have completed all of the lessons, complete the examination. Reread the subcourse material as needed. We suggest that you mark your answers in the subcourse booklet. When you have completed the examination items to your satisfaction, transfer your responses to the examination answer sheet.

Student Comment Sheet:

Provide us with your suggestions and comments by filling out the Student Comment Sheet found at the back of this booklet and returning it to us with your examination answer sheet.

LESSON 1	Introduction to Basic Human Anatomy.
TEXT ASSIGNMENT	Paragraphs 1-1 through 1-15.
LESSON OBJECTIVES	After completing this lesson, you should be able to:

1-1. Define anatomy.

1-2. Characterize individuals according to body type and state clinical significance.

1-3. Identify kinds of anatomical studies.

1-4. Trace the organization of the human body into cells, tissues, organs, organ systems, and the total organism.

1-5. List the parts of an upper member and the parts of a lower member.

1-6. Identify a reason for studying terminology.

1-7. Define the anatomical position.

1-8. Given drawings illustrating planes and directions, name the planes and directions.

1-9. Define the cell and match names of major components with drawings representing them.

SUGGESTION After completing the assignment, complete the exercises at the end of this lesson. These exercises will help you to achieve the lesson objectives.

LESSON 1

INTRODUCTION TO BASIC HUMAN ANATOMY

Section I. GENERAL

1-1. DEFINITIONS

a. <u>Anatomy</u> is the study of the structure of the body. Often, you may be more interested in functions of the body. Functions include digestion, respiration, circulation, and reproduction. <u>Physiology</u> is the study of the functions of the body.

b. The body is a chemical and physical machine. As such, it is subject to certain laws. These are sometimes called natural laws. Each part of the body is engineered to do a particular job. These jobs are functions. For each job or body function, there is a particular structure engineered to do it.

c. In the laboratory, anatomy is studied by dissection (SECT = cut, DIS = apart).

1-2. BODY TYPES

No two human beings are built exactly alike, but we can group individuals into three major categories. These groups represent basic body shapes.

MORPH = body, body form

ECTO = all energy is outgoing

ENDO = all energy is stored inside

MESO = between, in the middle

ECTOMORPH = slim individual

ENDOMORPH = broad individual

MESOMORPH = body type between the two others, "muscular" type

Ectomorphs, slim persons, are more susceptible to lung infections. Endomorphs are more susceptible to heart disease.

1-3. NOTE ON TERMINOLOGY

a. Each profession and each science has its own language. Lawyers have legal terminology. Physicians and other medical professions and occupations have medical terminology. Accountants have debits, credits, and balance sheets. Physicists have quantums and quarks. Mathematicians have integrals and differentials. Mechanics have carburetors and alternators. Educators have objectives, domains, and curricula.

b. To work in a legal field, you should know the meaning of <u>quid pro quo</u>. To work in a medical field, you should know the meanings of terms such as <u>proximal</u>, <u>distal</u>, <u>sagittal</u>, <u>femur</u>, <u>humerus</u>, <u>thorax</u>, and <u>cerebellum</u>.

1-4. KINDS OF ANATOMICAL STUDIES

a. <u>Microscopic anatomy</u> is the study of structures that cannot be seen with the unaided eye. You need a microscope.

b. <u>Gross anatomy by systems</u> is the study of organ systems, such as the respiratory system or the digestive system.

c. <u>Gross anatomy by regions</u> considers anatomy in terms of regions such as the trunk, upper member, or lower member.

d. <u>Neuroanatomy</u> studies the nervous system.

e. <u>Functional anatomy</u> is the study of relationships between functions and structures.

1-5. ORGANIZATION OF THE HUMAN BODY

The human body is organized into cells, tissues, organs, organ systems, and the total organism.

a. <u>Cells</u> are the smallest living unit of body construction.

b. A <u>tissue</u> is a grouping of like cells working together. Examples are muscle tissue and nervous tissue.

c. An <u>organ</u> is a structure composed of several different tissues performing a particular function. Examples include the lungs and the heart.

d. <u>Organ systems</u> are groups of organs which together perform an overall function. Examples are the respiratory system and the digestive system.

e. <u>The total organism</u> is the individual human being. You are a total organism.

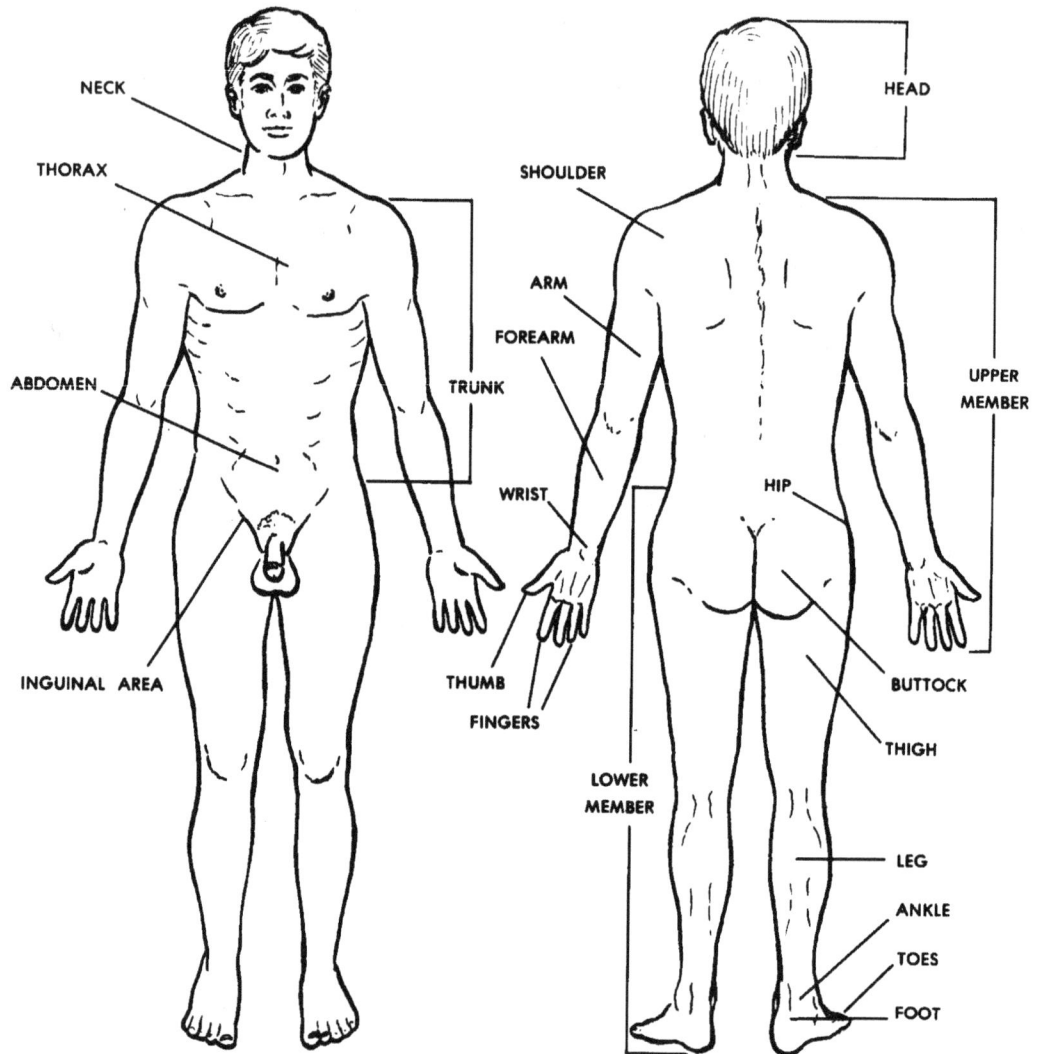

Figure 1-1. Regions of the human body.

1-6. REGIONS OF THE HUMAN BODY (FIGURE 1-1)

The human body is a single, total composite. Everything works together. Each part acts in association with ALL other parts. Yet, it is also a series of regions. Each region is responsible for certain body activities. These regions are:

a. **Back and Trunk**. The torso includes the back and trunk. The trunk includes the thorax (chest) and abdomen. At the lower end of the trunk is the pelvis. The perineum is the portion of the body forming the floor of the pelvis. The lungs, the heart, and the digestive system are found in the trunk.

b. **Head and Neck**. The brain, eyes, ears, mouth, pharynx, and larynx are found in this region.

c. **Members**.

(1) Each <u>upper member</u> includes a shoulder, arm, forearm, wrist, and hand.

(2) Each <u>lower member</u> includes a hip, thigh, leg, ankle, and foot.

Section II. ANATOMICAL TERMINOLOGY

1-7. ANATOMICAL TERMINOLOGY

a. As mentioned earlier, you must know the language of a particular field to be successful in it. Each field has specific names for specific structures and functions. Unless you know the names and their meanings, you will have trouble saying what you mean. You will have trouble understanding what others are saying. You will not be able to communicate well.

b. What is a <u>scientific term</u>? It is a word that names or gives special information about a structure or process. Some scientific terms have two or three different parts. These parts are known as a PREFIX, a ROOT (or base), and a SUFFIX. An example is the word <u>subcutaneous</u>.

SUB = below <u>prefix</u>

CUTIS = skin <u>root</u>

SUBCUTANEOUS = below the skin

A second example is the word <u>myocardium</u>.

MYO = muscle <u>prefix</u>

CARDIUM = heart <u>root</u>

MYOCARDIUM = muscular wall of the heart

A third example is the word <u>tonsillitis</u>.

TONSIL = tonsil (a specific organ) <u>root</u>

ITIS = inflammation <u>suffix</u>

TONSILLITIS = an inflammation of the tonsils

1-8. THE ANATOMICAL POSITION

<u>The anatomical position</u> is an artificial posture of the human body (see figure 1-2). This position is used as a standard reference throughout the medical profession. We always speak of the parts of the body as if the body were in the anatomical position. This is true regardless of what position the body is actually in. The anatomical position is described as follows:

a. The body stands erect, with heels together.

b. Upper members are along the sides, with the palms of the hands facing forward.

c. The head faces forward.

1-9. PLANES OF THE BODY

See figures 1-3A through 1-3C for the imaginary planes used to describe the body.

a. <u>Sagittal planes</u> are vertical planes that pass through the body from front to back. The <u>median</u> or <u>midsagittal plane</u> is the vertical plane that divides the body into right and left halves.

b. <u>Horizontal (transverse) planes</u> are parallel to the floor. They are perpendicular to both the sagittal and frontal planes.

c. <u>Frontal (coronal) planes</u> are vertical planes which pass through the body from side to side. They are perpendicular to the sagittal plane.

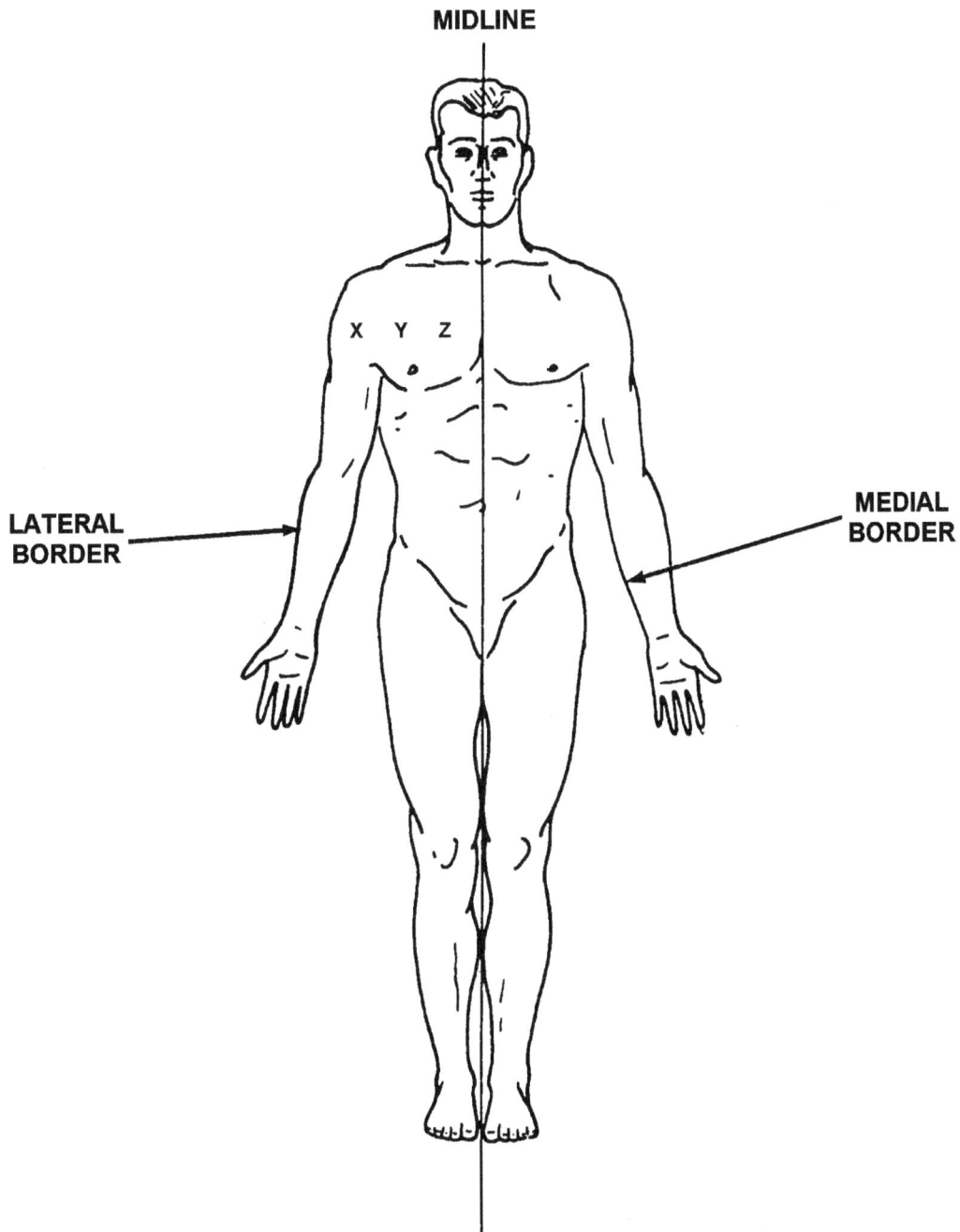

MIDLINE

LATERAL BORDER

MEDIAL BORDER

X Y Z

X is lateral to Y and Z; Y is medial to X and lateral to Z
In the example shown, the body is in the normal anatomical position.

Figure 1-2. Anatomical position and medial-lateral relationships.

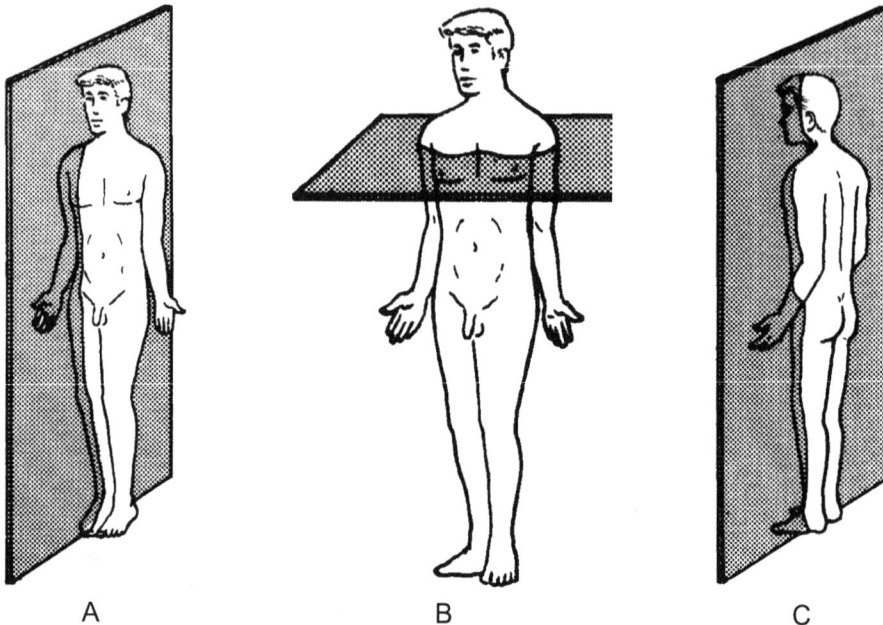

Figure 1-3, A. The sagittal plane. B. The horizontal plane. C. The frontal plane.

1-10. DIRECTIONS

a. **Superior, Inferior**. Superior means above. Inferior means below.

b. **Anterior, Posterior**.

(1) Anterior (or ventral) refers to the front of the body.

(2) Posterior (or dorsal) refers to the back of the body.

c. **Medial, Lateral**. Medial means toward or nearer the midline of the body. Lateral means away from the midline or toward the side of the body.

d. **Superficial, Deep**. Superficial means closer to the surface of the body. Deep means toward the center of the body or body part.

e. **Proximal, Distal**. Proximal and distal are terms applied specifically to the limbs. Proximal means nearer to the shoulder joint or the hip joint. Distal means further away from the shoulder joint or the hip joint. Sometimes proximal and distal are used to identify the "beginning" and "end" of the gut tract--that portion closer to the stomach being proximal while that further away being distal.

1-11. NAMES

a. Names are chosen to describe the structure or process as much as possible. An international nomenclature was adopted for anatomy in Paris in 1955. It does not use the names of people for structures. (The single exception is the Achilles tendon at the back of the foot and ankle.)

b. Names are chosen to identify structures properly. Names identify structures according to shape, size, color, function, and/or location. Some examples are:

TRAPEZIUS MUSCLE

TRAPEZIUS = trapezoid (shape)

ADDUCTOR MAGNUS MUSCLE

AD = toward

DUCT = to carry   (function)

MAGNUS = very large   (size)

ERYTHROCYTE

ERYTHRO = red   (color)

CYTE = cell

BICEPS BRACHII MUSCLE

BI = two

CEPS = head   (shape)

BRACHII = of the arm   (location)

Section III. CELLS

1-12. INTRODUCTION

A <u>cell</u> is the microscopic unit of body organization. The "typical animal cell" is illustrated in figure 1-4. A typical animal cell includes a cell membrane, a nucleus, a nuclear membrane, cytoplasm, ribosomes, endoplasmic reticulum, mitochondria, Golgi apparatus, centrioles, and lysosomes.

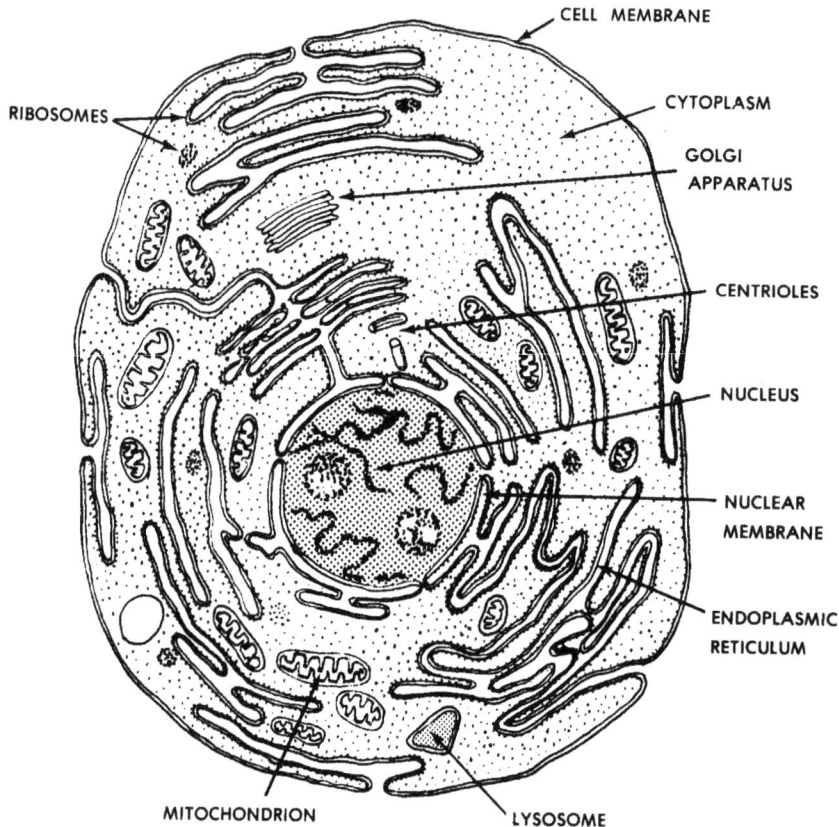

Figure 1-4. A "typical" animal cell (as seen in an electron microscope).

1-13. MAJOR COMPONENTS OF A "TYPICAL" ANIMAL CELL

a. **Nucleus**. The nucleus plays a central role in the cell. Information is stored in the nucleus and distributed to guide the life processes of the cell. This information is in a chemical form called nucleic acids. Two types of structures found in the nucleus are chromosomes and nucleoli. Chromosomes can be seen clearly only during cell divisions. Chromosomes are composed of both nucleic acid and protein. Chromosomes contain genes. Genes are the basic units of heredity which are passed from parents to their children. Genes guide the activities of each individual cell.

b. **Cell Membrane**. The cell membrane surrounds and separates the cell from its environment. The cell membrane allows certain materials to pass through it as they enter or leave the cell.

c. **Cytoplasm**. The semifluid found inside the cell, but outside the nucleus, is called the cytoplasm.

d. **Mitochondria (Plural)**. Mitochondria are the "powerhouses" of the cell. The mitochondria provide the energy wherever it is needed for carrying on the cellular functions.

e. **Endoplasmic Reticulum**. The endoplasmic reticulum is a network of membranes, cavities, and canals. The endoplasmic reticulum helps in the transfer of materials from one part of the cell to the other.

f. **Ribosomes**. Ribosomes are "protein factories" in the cell. They are composed mainly of nucleic acids which help make proteins according to instructions provided by the genes.

g. **Centrioles**. Centrioles help in the process of cell division.

h. **Lysosomes**. Lysosomes are membrane bound spheres which contain enzymes that can digest intracellular structures or bacteria.

1-14. CELL MULTIPLICATION (MITOSIS)

Individual cells have fairly specific life spans. Some types of cells have longer life spans than others. During the processes of growth and repair, new cells are being formed. The usual process of cell multiplication is called mitosis. There are two important factors to consider:

a. From one cell, we get two new cells.

b. The genes of the new cells are identical (for all practical purposes) to the genes of the original cell.

1-15. HYPERTROPHY/HYPERPLASIA

Hypertrophy and hyperplasia are two ways by which the cell mass of the body increases.

a. With HYPERTROPHY, there is an increase in the size of the individual cells. No new cells are formed. An example is the enlargement of muscles due to exercise by the increased diameter of the individual striated muscle fibers.

b. With HYPERPLASIA, there is an increase in the total number of cells. An example of abnormal hyperplasia is cancer.

c. ATROPHY is seen when there is a loss of cellular mass.

Continue with Exercises

EXERCISES, LESSON 1

REQUIREMENT. The following exercises are to be answered by completing the incomplete statement or by writing the answer in the space provided at the end of the question. After you have completed all the exercises, turn to "Solutions to Exercises," at the end of the lesson and check your answers.

1.   What is anatomy?

2.   What is the body type for each of the following individuals?

A broad individual: _____.

A slim individual: _____.

A person with average build: _____.

3.   What kind of anatomical study is described by each of the items below?

Study of structures that cannot be seen with the unaided eye:

_____.

Study of relationships between functions and structures:

_____.

Study of the nervous system: _____.

Study of organ systems: _____.

4.   What are the five levels or systems into which the body is organized, in ascending order?

_____

_____

_____

_____

_____

5. What is a cell?

6. What is a tissue?

7. What is an organ?

8. What is an organ system?

9. What is the total organism?

10. What are the parts of the upper member? _____, _____,
_____, _____, and _____.

11. What are the parts of the lower member? _____, _____,
_____, _____, and _____.

12. What is one reason for studying terminology?

13. Describe the anatomical position.

    a. The body stands _____ with _____ together.

    b. The upper members are along the _____ with palms
facing _____.

    c. The head faces _____.

14.   Each plane in figure 1-5 is marked by a letter a, b, c, or d. Write the name of each plane in the appropriate space below.

a.   _____ plane.

b.   _____ plane.

c.   _____ plane.

d.   _____ plane.

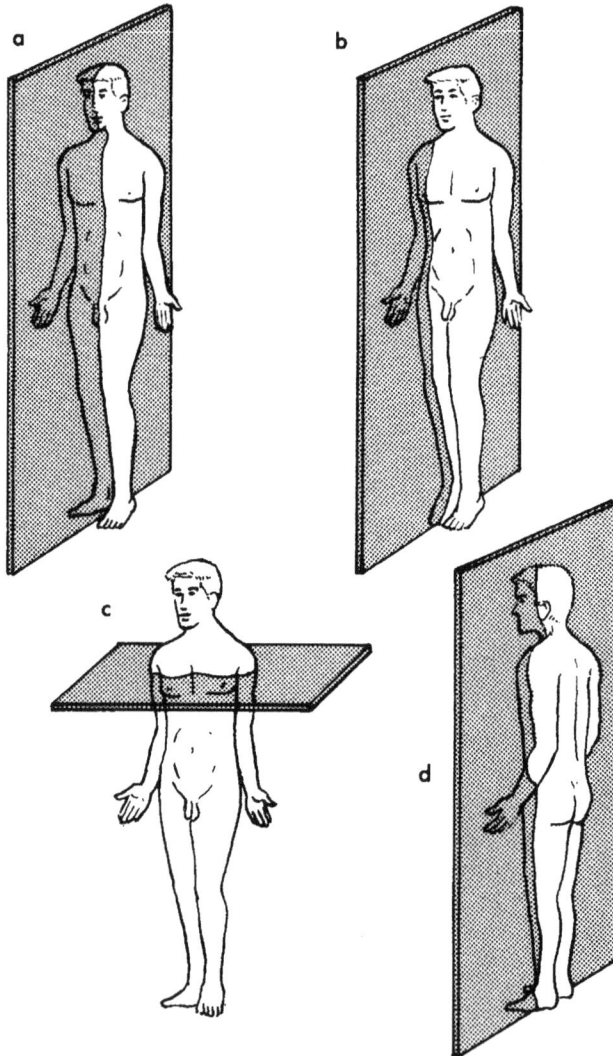

Figure 1-5. Planes of the body (exercise 14).

15. In figure 1-6, three points are labeled a, b, and c, and two borders are labeled d and e. It is correct to say that a is _____ to b and c, b is _____ to a and _____ to c, and c is _____ to a and b. We speak of d as the _____ border. We speak of e as the _____ border.

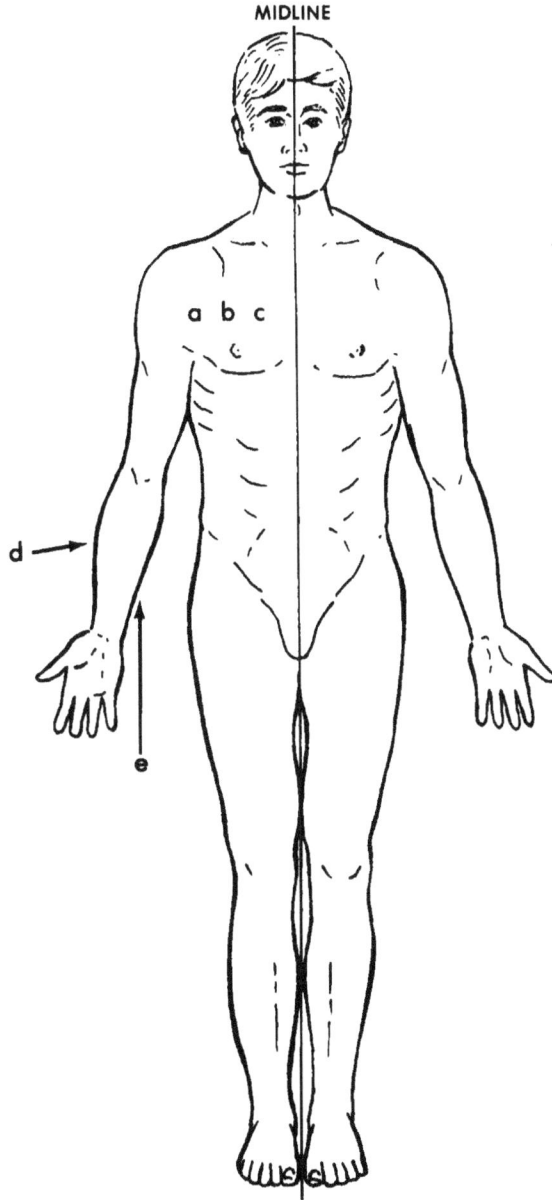

Figure 1-6. Directions (exercise 15).

16.   In figure 1-7, three portions of the arm are marked a, b, and c. The two ends of the arm are marked d and e. The portion marked a is the _____ third. The portion marked c is the _____ third. The end marked d is the _____ end. The end marked e is the _____ end.

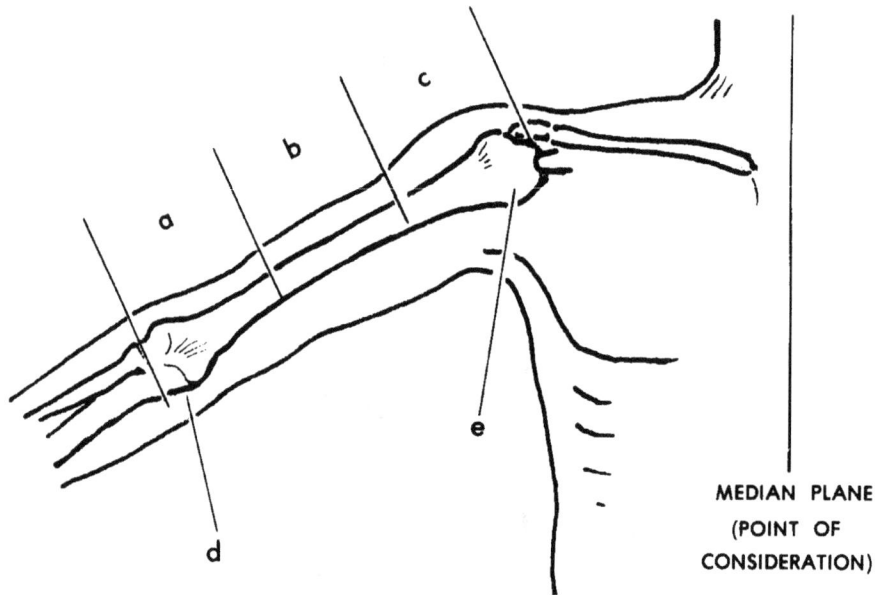

Figure 1-7. Directions upon members (exercise 16).

17.   A cell is the _____ unit of body organization.

18. In figure 1-8, parts of a "typical animal cell" are marked with the letters a through g. In the spaces below, provide the name of each structure.

a. _____   e. _____

b. _____   f. _____

c. _____   g. _____

d. _____

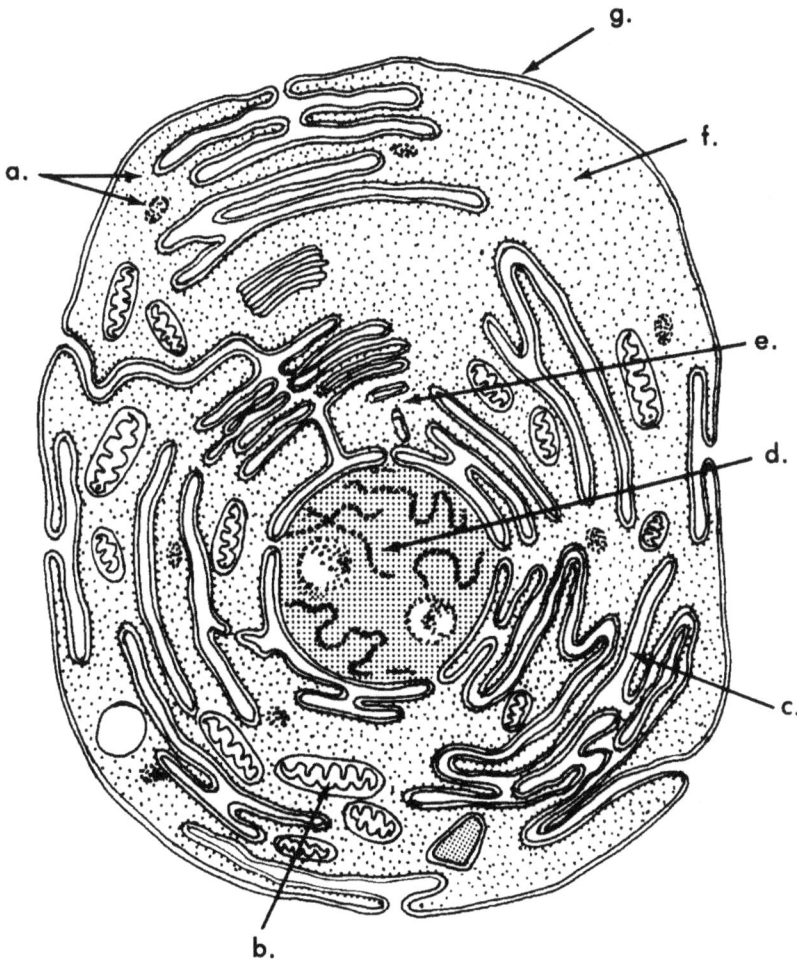

Figure 1-8. A "typical" animal cell (exercise 18).

Check Your Answers on Next Page

SOLUTIONS TO EXERCISES, LESSON 1

1. Anatomy is <u>the study of the structure of the body</u>. (para 1-1a)

2. A broad individual: <u>endomorph</u>.
    A slim individual: <u>ectomorph</u>.
    A person with average build: <u>mesomorph</u>. (para 1-2)

3. Study of structures that cannot be seen with the unaided eye: <u>microscopic anatomy</u>.
    Study of relationships between functions and structures: <u>functional anatomy</u>.
    Study of the nervous system: <u>neuroanatomy</u>.
    Study of organ systems: <u>gross anatomy by systems</u>. (para 1-4)

4. The body is organized into <u>cells, tissues, organs, organ systems, and the total organism</u>. (para 1-5)

5. A cell is <u>the smallest discrete living unit of the body construction</u>. (para 1-5a)

6. A tissue is a <u>grouping of like cells working together</u>. (para 1-5b)

7. An organ is <u>a structure composed of several different tissues performing a particular function</u>. (para 1-5c)

8. An organ system is <u>a group of organs performing an overall function together</u>. (para 1-5d)

9. The total organism is <u>the individual human being</u>. (para 1-5e)

10. The parts of the upper member are the <u>shoulder</u>, <u>arm</u>, <u>forearm</u>, <u>wrist</u>, and <u>hand</u>. (para 1-6c(1))

11. The parts of the lower member are the <u>hip</u>, <u>thigh</u>, <u>leg</u>, <u>ankle</u>, and <u>foot</u>. (para 1-6c(2))

12. One reason for studying terminology is <u>to be successful</u> in a medical field. Another reason is to be able <u>to communicate well</u>. (para 1-7a)

13. The anatomical position is described as follows:

    a. The body stands <u>erect</u>, with <u>heels</u> together.
    b. The upper members are along the <u>sides</u>, with palms facing <u>forward</u>.
    c. The head faces <u>forward</u>. (para 1-8)

14. a.   Midsagittal or median plane.
    b.   Sagittal plane.
    c.   Horizontal or transverse plane.
    d.   Frontal or coronal plane. (para 1-9)

15. It is correct to say that a is lateral to b and c, b is medial to a and lateral to c, and c is medial to a and b. We speak of d as the lateral border. We speak of e as the medial border. (para 1-10c)

16. The portion marked a is the distal third. The portion marked c is the proximal third. The end marked d is the distal end. The end marked e is the proximal end. (para 1-10e)

17. A cell is the microscopic unit of body organization. (para 1-12)

18. a.   Ribosomes.
    b.   Mitochondrion.
    c.   Endoplasmic reticulum.
    d.   Nucleus.
    e.   Centrioles.
    f.   Cytoplasm.
    g.   Cell membrane. (fig 1-4)

End of Lesson 1

LESSON ASSIGNMENT

LESSON 2   Tissues of the Body.

TEXT ASSIGNMENT   Paragraphs 2-1 through 2-17.

LESSON OBJECTIVES   After completing this lesson, you should be
                          able to:

          2-1. Define <u>tissue</u>.

          2-2. Name four major types of tissues.

          2-3. Define <u>epithelial tissue</u>, <u>connective tissue</u>,
                          <u>muscle tissue</u>, and <u>nervous tissue</u>.

          2-4. Given a description of epithelial tissue, matrix,
                          fibrous connective tissue, cartilage connective
                          tissue, bone connective tissue, fat connective
                          tissue, smooth muscle tissue, striated muscle
                          tissue, cardiac muscle tissue, nervous tissue,
                          neuron, or glia, name it.

          2-5. Name four major types of connective tissue
                          (CT); name the characteristic cells of fibrous CT,
                          cartilage CT, and bone CT; and describe the
                          matrix of fibrous CT, cartilage CT, and fat CT.

SUGGESTION   After completing the assignment, complete the
                          exercises at the end of this lesson. These exercises
                          will help you to achieve the lesson objectives.

LESSON 2

TISSUES OF THE BODY

Section I. GENERAL

2-1. DEFINITION

A <u>tissue</u> is a grouping of like cells working together.

2-2. TYPES OF TISSUES

There are several major types of tissues. The most common types are epithelial, connective, muscle, and nervous tissues. Later, this lesson will discuss each type.

2-3. TISSUES AND ORGANS

a. Tissues make up organs. An <u>organ</u> is a structure performing a particular function. An organ is composed of several different tissues. Examples of organs are the lungs and the heart.

b. In some cases, a term may be used to describe both a type of tissue and a kind of organ. For example, we speak of bone tissue and of bones. We speak of muscle tissue and of muscles.

Section II. EPITHELIAL TISSUES

2-4. DEFINITION

<u>Epithelial tissue</u> is tissue that covers surfaces and lines cavities. Here, it may protect, absorb, and/or secrete. Epithelial tissue covers the outer surface of the body. It lines the intestines, the lungs, and other hollow organs.

2-5. TYPES OF EPITHELIAL CELLS (BY SHAPE)

Figure 2-1 illustrates the basic types of epithelial cells by shape. The three basic shapes are <u>squamous</u> (flat), <u>cuboidal</u> (cubes), and <u>columnar</u> (columns).

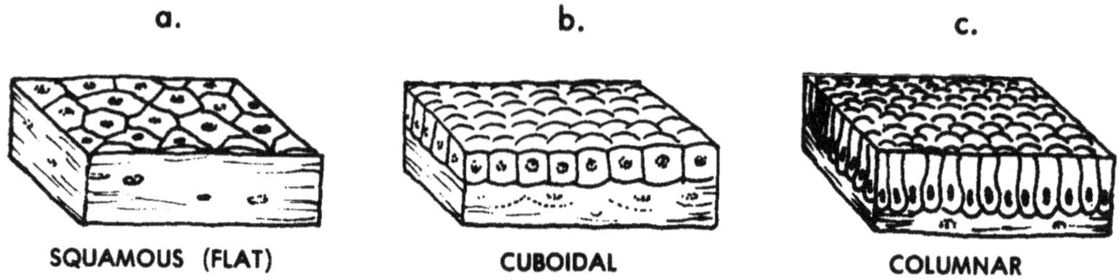

Figure 2-1. Epithelial cells.

2-6. TYPES OF EPITHELIAL TISSUES

a. **Layers**. In epithelial tissues, the cells are in single or multiple layers. If there is only one layer, the tissue is called a simple epithelium. If there is more than one layer, the tissue is called a stratified epithelium. See figure 2-2.

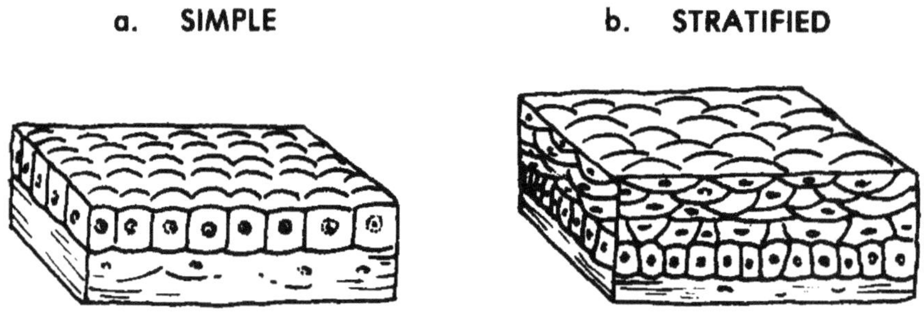

Figure 2-2. Types of epithelial tissues.

b. **Naming**. Epithelial tissues are named by the number of layers and the type of cell in its outermost layer. For example, if there are several layers and if the outermost layer consists of squamous (flat) cells, then the tissue is called a stratified squamous epithelium.

c. **Examples of Epithelial Tissues**.

(1) A simple squamous epithelium called endothelium lines the heart and blood vessels.

(2) As serous membranes, simple squamous epithelial tissue lines the cavities of the abdomen (peritoneal lining) and the chest (pleural lining). Serous membranes are membranes which secrete a lubricating fluid.

(3) Epithelial tissue forms the secretory part of glands and also parts of the various sense organs.

d. **Functions**. According to its location, epithelial tissue has different functions. As the skin, epithelial tissue protects the tissues beneath. In the small intestines, the epithelial tissue absorbs. In the lungs, epithelial tissue is a membrane through which the gases pass easily. In the glands, epithelial tissue secretes.

Section III. CONNECTIVE TISSUES

2-7. DEFINITION

a. <u>Connective tissue</u> is tissue that supports other tissues, holds tissues together, or fills spaces.

b. Among and outside the cells of the connective tissues, there is a material called <u>matrix</u>. The matrix is manufactured by the connective tissue cells. Each type of connective tissue has its own particular type of matrix.

2-8. TYPES OF CONNECTIVE TISSUE

There are several major types of connective tissue (CT). These include fibrous CT (FCT), cartilage CT, bone CT, and fat CT. Blood is sometimes considered an additional type of CT.

2-9. FIBROUS CONNECTIVE TISSUE (FCT)

a. **Fibroblasts**. The characteristic cells of FCT are fibroblasts. Fibroblasts are able to form elongated fibers.

b. **Matrix**. These fibers make up the matrix of FCT.

c. **Fibers**. The fibers are either white or yellow.

(1) White fibers are made from a protein called collagen. White fibers tend to have a fixed length. White fibers are not very easily stretched.

(2) Yellow fibers are made from a protein called elastin. Yellow fibers are elastic. They can be stretched and then they can snap back (like a rubber band).

d. **Types of FCT**. The types of FCT are recognized by the arrangement of their fibers. These types include:

(1) <u>Loose areolar FCT</u>. Loose areolar FCT has an open irregular arrangement of its fibers.

AREOLAR = airy

Loose areolar FCT is found widely throughout the body. An example is the superficial fascia (subcutaneous layer). The superficial fascia is the connective tissue which lies beneath the skin. Loose areolar FCT is the filling substance around most organs and tissues of the body.

(2) Dense FCT. The fibers of dense FCT are closely packed and parallel. There are no significant spaces between the fibers. Examples of dense FCT are ligaments and tendons. A ligament is a band of dense FCT that holds the bones together at a joint. A tendon attaches a muscle to a bone.

2-10. CARTILAGE CONNECTIVE TISSUE

a. **Cartilage Cells**. Cartilage cells are also called chondroblasts. Cartilage cells are clustered in microscopic pockets within the cartilage matrix. The cartilage cells produce the material of the matrix.

b. **Matrix**. The matrix produced by the cartilage cells appears homogeneous (the same throughout). The matrix also appears amorphous (shapeless).

c. **Types of Cartilage CT**.

(1) Hyaline cartilage CT. Hyaline cartilage CT appears homogeneous and clear.

HYALINE = clear

This type of cartilage helps to cover bone surfaces at joints. Hyaline cartilage is found as incomplete rings which keep the trachea (windpipe) open.

(2) Fibrous cartilage CT. Fibrous cartilage CT includes dense masses of fibers (of FCT). It is more rigid than hyaline cartilage. The auricle of the external ear is stiffened with fibrous cartilage.

(3) Calcified cartilage CT. Calcified cartilage CT is cartilage that has been stiffened by the addition of calcium salts. This is not the same as bone tissue. An example is the cartilages of the larynx (the voice box) which become calcified with age.

2-11. BONE CONNECTIVE TISSUE

a. **Osteoblasts/Osteoclasts**. Osteoblasts are cells that make and repair bone. Osteoclasts are cells which tear down and remove bone. Bone is continually being remodeled as a person lives. Remodeling is in direct response to the stresses placed on the bone.

b. **Types of Bone Tissues**. There are two major types of bone tissue. One is compact bone CT, which is dense. The other is cancellous bone CT, which is spongy. Compact bone CT forms the hard outer layers of bones as organs. Cancellous bone CT forms the inner, lighter portion of bones.

2-12. FAT CONNECTIVE TISSUE

a. **Fat Cells**. A large fraction of the volume of a fat cell is occupied by a droplet of fat. This droplet has its own membrane, in addition to the outer membrane of the cell. The remaining components of the fat cell, including the nucleus, are found in an outer layer of cytoplasm surrounding the droplet of fat.

b. **Matrix**. Fat connective tissue has a matrix of lipid (oil or fat). There may be yellow fat CT or brown fat CT.

c. **Functions**. Fat CT acts as a packing material among the organs, nerves, and vessels. Fat CT also helps to insulate the body from both heat and cold. Some fat CT serves as a high-energy storage area.

2-13. BLOOD "CONNECTIVE TISSUE"

Some experts consider blood to be a type of connective tissue. Blood will be discussed in lesson 9.

Section IV. MUSCLE TISSUES

2-14. DEFINITION

There are muscle tissues and there are organs called muscles. Muscles are made up of muscle tissues. Muscle tissues and the muscles they make up are specialized to contract. Because of their ability to shorten (contract), muscles are able to produce motion.

2-15. TYPES OF MUSCLE TISSUES

See figure 2-3 for the three types of muscle tissue.

a. **Skeletal Muscle Tissue**. The cells (muscle fibers) of skeletal muscle tissue are long and cylindrical and have numerous nuclei. The arrangement of the cellular contents is very specific and results in a striated appearance when viewed with the microscope. This type of muscle tissue is found mainly in the skeletal muscles.

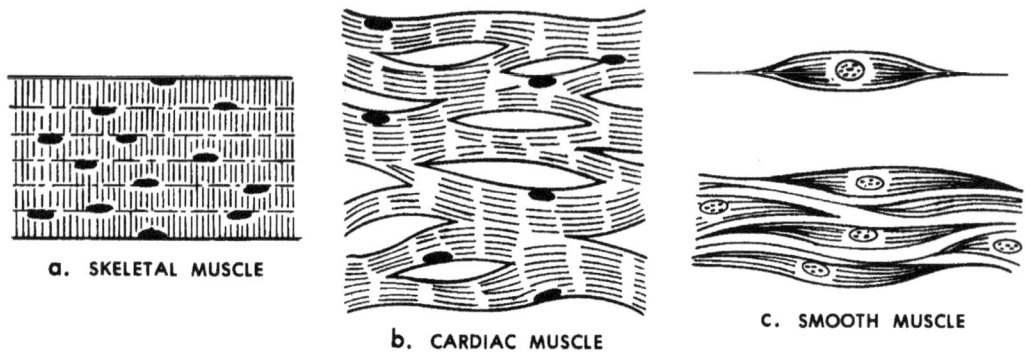

Figure 2-3. Types of muscle tissue.

b. **Cardiac Muscle Tissue**. The cells (muscle fibers) of cardiac muscle tissue are short, branched, contain one nucleus, and are striated. This tissue makes up the myocardium (wall) of the heart.

c. **Smooth Muscle Tissue**. The cells (muscle fibers) of smooth muscle tissue are spindle-shaped, contain one nucleus, and are not striated. Smooth muscle tissue is generally found in the walls of hollow organs such as the organs of the digestive and respiratory systems, the blood vessels, the ureters, urinary bladder, urethra, and reproductive ducts.

Section V. NERVOUS TISSUE

2-16. DEFINITION

Nervous tissue is a collection of cells that respond to stimuli and transmit information.

2-17. NERVOUS TISSUE CELLS

a. A neuron (figure 2-4), or nerve cell, is the cell of the nervous tissue that actually picks up and transmits a signal from one part of the body to another. A synapse (figure 2-5) is the point at which a signal passes from one neuron to the next.

b. The neuroglia (also known as glia) is made up of the supporting cells of the nervous system (glial cells).

c. The nervous tissues will be discussed in a later lesson.

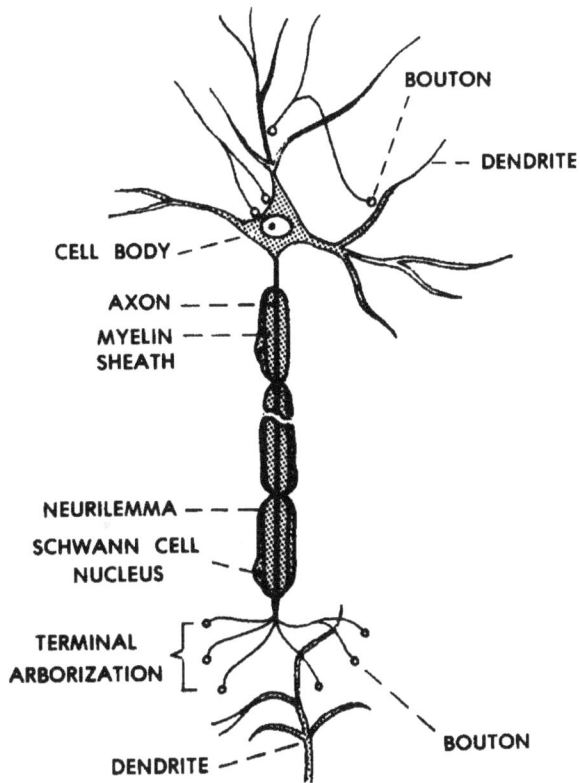

Figure 2-4. A neuron.

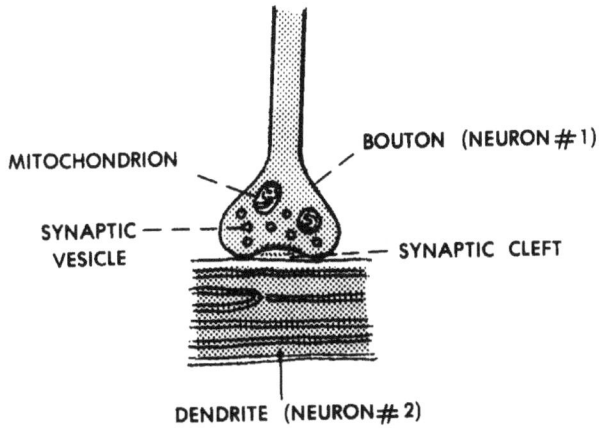

Figure 2-5. A synapse.

Continue with Exercises

EXERCISES, LESSON 2

REQUIREMENT. The following exercises are to be answered by completing the incomplete statement or by writing the answer in the space provided at the end of the question.

After you have completed all the exercises, turn to "Solutions to Exercises," at the end of the lesson and check your answers.

1.   What is a tissue?

2.   What are the most common types of tissues?

      a.   _____.

      b.   _____.

      c.   _____.

      d.   _____.

3.   What is epithelial tissue?

4.   If an outer layer of epithelial tissue consists of flat cells and if there are several layers of cells in the tissue, then what is the type of epithelial tissue?

5.   What is connective tissue?

6.   What term is used for the material found among and outside the cells of connective tissue?

7.   The four major types of connective tissue (CT) are _____CT, _____CT, _____ CT, and _____ CT.

8.   Characteristic cells of fibrous CT are _____. Cartilage cells are also called _____. Cells that make and repair bone are _____. Cells that tear down and remove bone are _____.

9.   The matrix of fibrous CT consists of _____. The matrix produced by cartilage cells appears h_____and a _____. Fat CT has a matrix of _____.

10.   Two major types of fibrous connective tissue (FCT) are _____ FCT, which is a filling substance around most organs and tissues of the body, and_____ FCT, which is found, for example, in ligaments and tendons.

11.   What type of connective tissue has an amorphous, homogeneous matrix?

12.   What type of connective tissue has a matrix of lipid (fat or oil)?

13.   What are muscle tissues?

14.   The cells of one type of muscle tissue are spindle-shaped, contain one nucleus, and are not striated. What is this tissue called?

15.   Which type of muscle tissue has cells which have one nucleus and are short, branched, and striated?

16.   Which type of muscle tissue has cells which have numerous nuclei and are long and cylindrical?

17.   What is nervous tissue?

18.   What type of tissue has cells that respond to stimuli and transmit information?

19. A nerve cell, which actually picks up and transmits a signal, is also known as a _____.

20. The supporting structure of the nervous system is known as the _____ or the _____.

Check Your Answers on Next Page

SOLUTIONS TO EXERCISES, LESSON 2

1. A tissue is <u>a grouping of like cells working together</u>. (para 2-1)

2. a. <u>Epithelial</u>.
    b. <u>Connective</u>.
    c. <u>Muscle</u>.
    d. <u>Nervous</u>. (para 2-2)

3. Epithelial tissue is <u>tissue that covers surfaces and lines cavities</u>. (para 2-4)

4. If there are several layers and if the outer layer consists of flat cells, then the tissue is called a <u>stratified squamous epithelium</u>. (para 2-6b)

5. Connective tissue is <u>tissue that supports other tissues, holds tissues together, or fills spaces</u>. (para 2-7a)

6. The term used for material found among and outside the cells of connective tissue is <u>matrix</u>. (para 2-7b)

7. The four major types of connective tissue (CT) are <u>fibrous</u> CT, <u>cartilage</u> CT, <u>bone</u> CT, and <u>fat</u> CT. (para 2-8)

8. Characteristic cells of fibrous CT are <u>fibroblasts</u>. Cartilage cells are also called <u>chondroblasts</u>. Cells that make and repair bone are <u>osteoblasts</u>. Cells that tear down and remove bone are <u>osteoclasts</u>. (paras 2-9a, 2-10a, 2-11a)

9. The matrix of fibrous CT consists of <u>fibers</u>. The matrix produced by cartilage cells appears <u>homogeneous</u> and <u>amorphous</u>. Fat CT has a matrix of <u>lipid</u>. (paras 2-9b, 2-10b, 2-12b)

10. Two major types of fibrous connective tissue (FCT) are <u>loose areolar</u> FCT, which is a filling substance around most organs and tissues of the body, and <u>dense</u> FCT, which is found, for example, in ligaments and tendons. (para 2-9d)

11. <u>Cartilage CT</u>. (para 2-10b)

12. <u>Fat CT</u>. (para 2-12b)

13. Muscle tissues <u>are tissues whose contracting elements enable muscles to produce motion</u>. (para 2-14)

14. <u>Smooth muscle tissue</u>. (para 2-15c)

15. <u>Cardiac muscle tissue</u>. (para 2-15b)

16. <u>Skeletal muscle tissue</u>. (para 2-15a)

17. Nervous tissue is <u>a collection of cells that respond to stimuli and transmit information</u>. (para 2-16)

18. <u>Nervous tissue</u>. (para 2-16)

19. A nerve cell, which actually picks up and transmits a signal, is also known as a <u>neuron</u>. (para 2-17a)

20. The supporting structure of the nervous system is known as the <u>glia</u>, or the <u>neuroglia</u>. (para 2-17b)

End of Lesson 2

LESSON ASSIGNMENT

LESSON 3   The Human Integumentary and Fascial Systems.

TEXT ASSIGNMENT   Paragraphs 3-1 through 3-14.

LESSON OBJECTIVES After completing this lesson, you should be able to:

3-1. Define <u>integumentary system</u>, <u>integument proper</u>, <u>integumentary derivatives</u>, <u>fascia</u>, <u>superficial fascia (subcutaneous layer)</u>, <u>deep fasciae</u>, and <u>investing deep fascia</u>.

3-2. Identify the three coverings, or envelopes, for the human body.

3-3. Name and describe the two layers of the skin.

3-4. Name and describe three types of integumentary derivatives--hairs, glands, and nails.

3-5. Define <u>serous cavities</u>, describe a bursa, and give examples of serous cavities in the body.

SUGGESTION   After completing the assignment, complete the exercises at the end of this lesson. These exercises will help you to achieve the lesson objectives.

LESSON 3

THE HUMAN INTEGUMENTARY AND FASCIAL SYSTEMS

Section I. GENERAL

3-1. DEFINITIONS

An <u>organ system</u> is a group of organs together performing an overall function. Portions of two organ systems, the integumentary and fascial systems, are represented in figure 3-1.

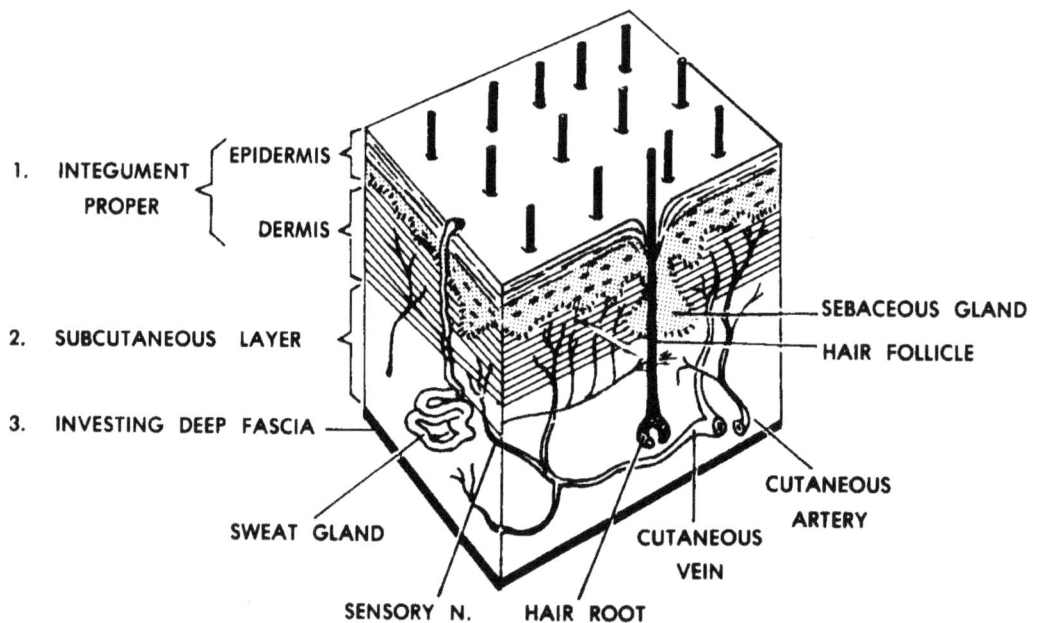

Figure 3-1. The integument and related structures.

a. **Integumentary System**. The <u>integumentary system</u> includes the <u>integument proper</u> and the <u>integumentary derivatives</u>. We know the <u>integument proper</u> as the skin. It is the outermost covering of the whole body. The <u>integumentary derivatives</u> include the hairs, nails, and various glands of the skin.

b. **Fascial System**. A <u>fascia</u> is a sheet or collection of fibrous connective tissue (FCT). The <u>superficial fascia</u> is the connective tissue which lies immediately beneath the skin and is often known as the <u>subcutaneous layer</u>. <u>Deep fasciae</u> (plural) form envelopes for muscles and other organs and fill spaces. One <u>deep fascial</u> membrane is the third envelope of the whole body, beneath the skin and the subcutaneous layer. It is known as the <u>investing deep fascia</u>.

3-2. COVERINGS OF THE HUMAN BODY

The entire body is surrounded by three layers or envelopes, one inside the other. These coverings separate the body from the external environment. These envelopes include (from outside inward)--the skin (the integument proper), the subcutaneous layer, and the investing deep fascia.

Section II. THE HUMAN INTEGUMENTARY SYSTEM

3-3. THE INTEGUMENT PROPER

The integument proper is the outermost layer of the human body. It is usually known as the skin. The skin has two layers--the superficial or outer layer called the epidermis and the deeper or inner layer called the dermis.

a. **The Epidermis**. The epidermis is a stratified squamous epithelium. This means that it is made up of several layers of cells, the outermost being flat-type epithelial cells.

(1) The outer layers of the epidermis include cells which are transparent, flattened, dead, and without nuclei. These hardened cells of the outermost layers are completely filled with keratin and are known as cornified cells. These dead flat cells in the outermost layers resemble scales. Day by day, these cells are scraped away or just fall away from the body. They are replaced by cells from the intermediate layers.

(2) In the intermediate layers of the epidermis, the cells change their shapes. As the cells move towards the surface, they gain granules, begin to manufacture a hardening material called keratin, and lose their nuclei.

(3) The innermost layer of the epidermis is especially important because it is the source of all the other layers of the epidermis. It is known as the basal or germinative layer. The cells of this layer are capable of multiplication (mitosis). Its basic structure is a single layer of columnar-type epithelial cells.

b. **The Dermis (Dermal Layer)**. The dermis is the layer of the skin lying just beneath the epidermis. It is dense FCT consisting of white and yellow fibers. This layer in animal hides is used to make leather. The dermis has finger-like projections called papillae. These papillae extend into the epidermis and keep the dermis and epidermis from sliding on each other. The dermal layer includes blood vessels, lymph vessels, nerve endings, hair follicles, and glands.

3-4. INTRODUCTION TO INTEGUMENTARY DERIVATIVES

The integumentary derivatives include the glands, hairs, and nails associated with the skin. All integumentary derivatives are formed from the tissues of the integument proper (dermis and epidermis). All are appended (attached) to the integument proper and are often known as the appendages of the skin. See figure 3-2.

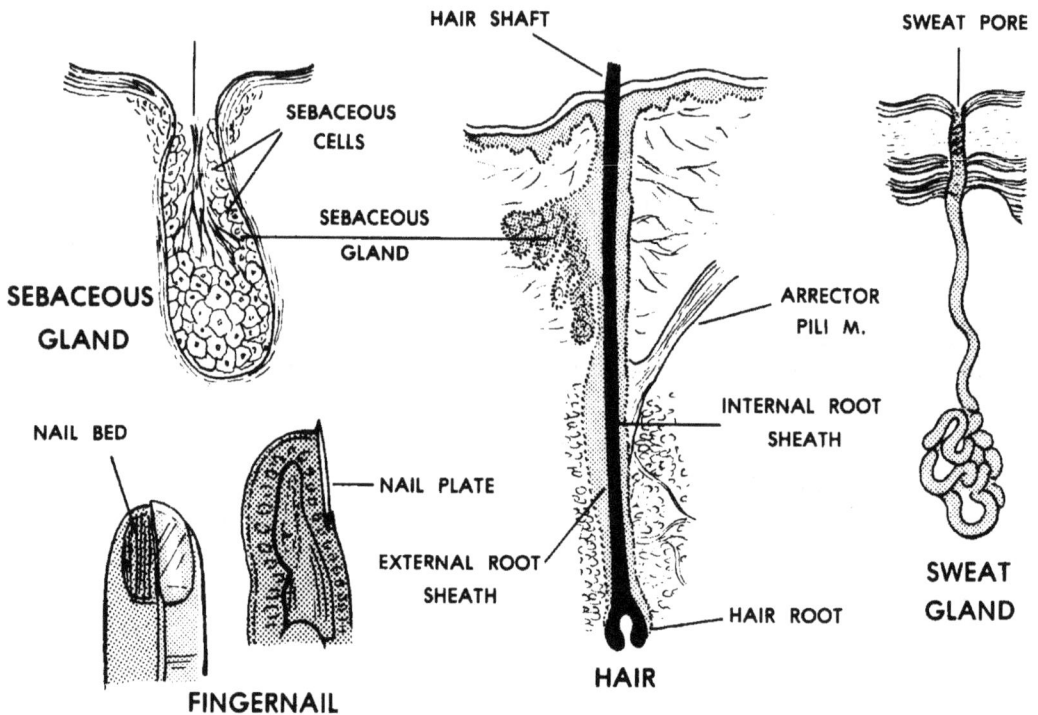

Figure 3-2. The integumentary derivatives (appendages).

3-5. HAIRS

a. A hair follicle is formed by the extension of the skin (dermis and epidermis) deeper into the surface of the body. Follicles may extend into the subcutaneous layer.

b. At the base of the hair follicle is the hair root. The hair shaft grows out from the root. The hair shaft is made of cells from the outermost layers of the epidermis.

c. Scalp and facial hairs grow continuously. Other hairs of the body grow to fixed lengths. The types and patterns of hairs are determined for each individual by genetics, including his/her sex.

3-6. GLANDS

The types of glands included are the sweat glands, the sebaceous (fat/ oil) glands, and the mammary glands (breasts). The ducts and secretory parts of these glands are made of epithelial tissues. Backup or supporting tissue is of FCT.

a. **Sweat Glands**. Sweat glands consist of a coiled secretory portion and a wavy duct which leads to the surface of the skin. The coiled secretory portion is located in the dermis or deeper. Sweat glands are found everywhere on the body in association with the skin.

b. **Sebaceous Glands**. Sebaceous glands produce an oily substance which lubricates the skin and hairs. The oil keeps the skin and hairs flexible. The sebaceous glands are usually found as a part of the walls of hair follicles and their oil flows into the follicle. In a few places without hairs, they open directly to the skin surface.

c. **Mammary Glands**. In the adult human female, the mammary gland lies in the subcutaneous layer anterior to the chest muscle (pectoralis major M.). Its function is to nourish the newborn. A nipple is located near the center of each breast. Around each nipple is a darkened area known as the areola. The tip of the nipple has many small openings to allow the passage of the milk from the milk ducts. These ducts are connected to lobes of glandular tissue located throughout the breast. Fat and fibrous CT fill in the spaces among the lobes.

3-7. NAILS

Nails are found on the ends of the digits (thumbs, fingers, and toes). Nails help to protect the ends of these digits. Each nail bed is attached to the top of the terminal phalanx (bone) of each digit. The nail itself is made up of cornified (hardened) outer cell layers of the epidermis. The nails grow continuously from their roots.

3-8. SKIN COLORATION

a. The skin includes red, black, and yellow pigments. The proportion of these pigments determine the skin color. This proportion is determined by genetics. The absence of all pigments is called albinism. In albinism, white light is reflected and a pink hue results from the color of the blood shining through the transparent skin.

b. These pigments are the source of hair color as well as the skin color.

Section III. THE FASCIAL SYSTEM OF THE HUMAN BODY

3-9. GENERAL

Most of the fibrous connective tissues (FCT) are fascial. These may occur as sheets or masses. NOT included in this definition are the tendons, ligaments, or aponeuroses (wide flat tendons). The different fasciae have varying proportions of white fibers, yellow fibers, fat, and tissue fluid. Some serve as membranes to inclose the body and its parts. Fasciae also help to support some organs and allow motions between other organs to be easier.

3-10. SUPERFICIAL FASCIA

a. The superficial fascia is the second envelope of the body. It is the layer between the skin (integument proper) and the investing deep fascial envelope. It is often called the subcutaneous layer, but it is technically not a part of the integumentary system as such.

b. The superficial fascia is made up primarily of loose areolar FCT with the spaces filled by fatty tissue and tissue fluid. It contains the superficial or cutaneous branches of nerves, arteries, veins, and lymphatics (NAVL) of the skin.

3-11. DEEP FASCIAE

a. The deep fasciae include various membranes made of consolidated or dense FCT. A deep fascia envelops the entire body as the third envelope. This third envelope is known as the investing deep fascia. It is beneath the skin and subcutaneous layer.

b. Deep fasciae also include the envelopes of the muscles and other organs. Around individual organs (for example, the kidney), it is called a capsule.

c. Another form of deep fascia is found in the collections of loose areolar FCT and fat that are found as filling among the organs. Similar deep fasciae attach organs to the body wall.

Section IV. SEROUS CAVITIES OF THE HUMAN BODY

3-12. GENERAL

The term serous refers to a watery- type fluid. Serous cavities are sacs lined with serous membranes. These cavities serve as lubricating devices. They reduce the friction during the motion between organs.

3-13. BURSA

a. A <u>bursa</u> (figure 3-3) is the simplest of serous cavities. Each bursa is a small sac located between two moving structures, usually a muscle moving over a bony surface. The bursa reduces the friction between the two structures. For example, a bursa prevents excessive friction between the skin and patella (knee cap). This bursa, called the prepatellar bursa, allows the skin to move freely over the patella. (When injured, it produces excessive amounts of the serous fluid and is known as "housemaid's knee.")

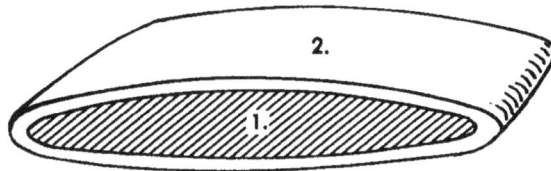

1. SEROUS (BURSAL) CAVITY:

    a. SPACE CONTAINING JUST ENOUGH SEROUS FLUID TO MOISTEN INNER SURFACE.

    b. SPACE ARTIFICIALLY WIDENED FOR DIAGRAMMATIC PURPOSES.

2. (BURSAL) CAPSULE:

    a. BAG-LIKE — SURROUNDING THE SEROUS CAVITY.

    b. FCT MEMBRANE MAIN STRUCTURAL ELEMENT.

    c. A SEROUS MEMBRANE (SIMPLE SQUAMOUS EPITHELIAL TISSUE) AS AN INNER LINING OF THE CAPSULE. THE SEROUS MEMBRANE INCLOSES THE SEROUS CAVITY AND SECRETES THE SEROUS FLUID.

Figure 3-3. A bursa--the simplest serous cavity.

b. As a fibrous sac, each bursa has a central cavity which is lined with a serous membrane. This membrane is a simple squamous epithelium. The serous membrane secretes a serous fluid into the serous cavity. The serous fluid is the lubricant, minimizing friction.

3-14. OTHER SEROUS CAVITIES OF THE BODY

a. Other important serous cavities are associated with the major hollow organs, referred to as visceral organs. Each lung is encased in a serous cavity called the <u>pleural cavity</u>. The heart lies in a serous cavity called the <u>pericardial cavity</u>. The intestines are allowed to move freely during the digestive processes within the <u>peritoneal cavity</u>.

b. Each serous cavity has an inner and an outer membrane. The inner membrane is intimately associated with the surface of the visceral organ. The outer membrane forms the outer wall of the cavity. The serous lining of the cavity secretes the serous fluid into the cavity to act as a lubricant between the membranes, allowing freer motion for the organs.

Continue with Exercises

EXERCISES, LESSON 3

REQUIREMENT. The following exercises are to be answered by completing the incomplete statement or by writing the answer in the space provided at the end of the question.

After you have completed all the exercises, turn to "Solutions to Exercises," at the end of the lesson and check your answers.

1.   What is included in the integumentary system?

2.   What is another name for the integument proper?

3.   What are three types of integumentary derivatives?

4.   What is a fascia?

5.   What is the subcutaneous layer (superficial fascia)?

6.   Where are deep fasciae found in the body?

7.   What is the investing deep fascia?

8.   What is the outer layer of the skin?

What is the inner and deeper layer of the skin?

9.   What type of tissue makes up the epidermis?

What is the basic structure of the innermost layer of the epidermis?

What are characteristics of cells found in the outermost layers of the epidermis?

10.   What type of tissue makes up the dermis?

What are papillae and what is their function?

What other structures are found in the dermis?

11.   A hair follicle is formed by the _____.
At the base of the hair follicle is the _____.
The hair shaft grows out from the _____.
The hair shaft is made of cells from the _____.

12.   Sweat glands consist of _____.

13.   Sebaceous glands produce _____.
Its function is to _____.
The sebaceous glands are usually found as a part of the walls of
_____.

14.   In mammary glands, milk ducts connect each nipple with
_____.

What types of connective tissue fill in the spaces?

15.   Nails are found on the ends of the _____.
Nails help to protect _____.
The nail itself is made up of _____.
The nails grow continuously from their _____.

16. The term serous refers to a _____.
    Serous cavities are _____.
    These cavities serve as _____.

17. Each bursa is a small sac located between _____,
usually a muscle moving over a _____. The bursa reduces the _____ between
two structures. The serous membrane lining the cavity within a bursa is a _____ and
it secretes a _____ into the serous cavity.

18. Each lung is encased in a serous cavity called the _____. The heart lies in
a serous cavity called the _____. The intestines move freely within the
_____ cavity.

Check Your Answers on Next Page

SOLUTIONS TO EXERCISES, LESSON 3

1.   The integumentary system includes the integument proper (skin) and the integumentary derivatives (hairs, nails, and glands of the skin). (para 3-1a)

2.   Another name for the integument proper is the skin. (para 3-1a)

3.   Three types of integumentary derivatives are the hair, nails, and various glands of the skin. (para 3-1a)

4.   A fascia is a sheet or collection of fibrous connective tissue (FCT). (para 3-1b)

5.   The subcutaneous layer (superficial fascia) is the connective tissue which lies immediately beneath the skin. (para 3-1b)

6.   Deep fasciae are found as envelopes for muscles and other organs and they fill spaces. (para 3-1b)

7.   The investing deep fascia is the third envelope of the whole body beneath the skin and the subcutaneous layer. (para 3-1b)

8.   The outer layer of the skin is the epidermis. The inner and deeper layer of skin is the dermis. (para 3-3)

9.   The epidermis is a stratified squamous epithelium.
     The basic structure of the innermost layer of the epidermis is a single layer of columnar-type epithelial cells.
     The cells found in the outermost layers of the epidermis are transparent, flattened, dead, cornified, and without nuclei. (para 3-3a)

10. The dermis is dense FCT consisting of white and yellow fibers.
     Papillae are finger-like projections of the dermis that extend into the epidermis.
     Papillae prevent the dermis and epidermis from sliding on each other.
     Other structures found in the dermis include blood vessels, lymph vessels, nerve endings, hair follicles, and glands. (para 3-3b)

11. A hair follicle is formed by the extension of the skin (dermis and epidermis) deeper into the surface of the body. At the base of the hair follicle is the hair root. The hair shaft grows out from the root. The hair shaft is made of cells from the outermost layers of the epidermis. (paras 3-5a, b)

12. Sweat glands consist of a coiled secretory portion and a wavy duct which leads to the surface of the skin. (para 3-6a)

13.   Sebaceous glands produce an oily substance. Its function is to lubricate the skin and hairs and to keep them flexible. The sebaceous glands are usually found as a part of the walls of hair follicles. (para 3-6b)

14.   In mammary glands, milk ducts connect each nipple with lobes of glandular tissue. Fat and fibrous CT fill in the spaces among the lobes. (para 3-6c)

15.   Nails are found on the ends of the digits. Nails help to protect the ends of these digits. The nail itself is made up of cornified (hardened) outer cell layers of the epidermis. The nails grow continuously from their roots. (para 3-7)

16.   The term serous refers to a watery-type fluid. Serous cavities are sacs lined with serous membranes. These cavities serve as lubricating devices. (para 3-12)

17.   Each bursa is a small sac located between two moving structures, usually a muscle moving over a bony surface. The bursa reduces the friction between the two structures. The serous membrane lining the cavity within a bursa is a simple squamous epithelium and it secretes a serous fluid into the serous cavity. (para 3-13)

18.   Each lung is encased in a serous cavity called the pleural cavity. The heart lies in a serous cavity called the pericardial cavity, the intestines move freely within the peritoneal cavity. (para 3-14a)

End of Lesson 3

LESSON ASSIGNMENT

LESSON 4	The Human Skeletal System.
TEXT ASSIGNMENT	Paragraphs 4-1 through 4-14.
LESSON OBJECTIVES	After completing this lesson, you should be able to:

4-1. Define skeleton.

4-2. Name four functions of the human skeleton.

4-3. Name the layers and describe the basic structure of an individual bone, name and describe the parts of an individual long bone, and describe the periosteum and the blood supply of an individual bone.

4-4. Describe the development of an individual bone.

4-5. Name four types of bones by shape.

4-6. Describe major categories used in classification of joints.

4-7. Name the major parts of a "typical" synovial joint.

4-8. Name and describe classifications of synovial joints according to the kind of motion and number of axes.

4-9. Name and define the two major subdivisions of the skeleton.

4-10. Describe a typical vertebra. Name the regions of the vertebral column and give the number of vertebrae in each region. Describe the intervertebral discs and ligaments that hold vertebrae together.

4-11. Describe the thoracic cage.

4-12. Describe the skull.

4-13. Describe the general pattern of the bones of the upper and lower members.

SUGGESTION

After completing the assignment, complete the exercises at the end of this lesson. These exercises will help you to achieve the lesson objectives.

LESSON 4

THE HUMAN SKELETAL SYSTEM

Section I. GENERAL

4-1. INTRODUCTION

The <u>skeleton</u> serves as a support or framework of the human body. It is a combination of bones joined together.

4-2. FUNCTIONS OF THE HUMAN SKELETON

The human skeleton serves the following functions:

a. **Bodily Support**. The skeletal system provides a framework for the human body.

b. **Protection**. The skeleton protects certain soft structures within the human body. An example is the skull, which surrounds the brain.

c. **Motion**. Muscles are attached to and move the bones. Bones provide leverage for motion.

d. **Formation of Blood Cells (Hematopoiesis)**. Blood cells are manufactured in the red bone marrow, mainly found in flat bones.

4-3. PRIMARY STUDY AREAS

In this text, we study the skeletal system from four different viewpoints:

a. **Bone As Tissues**. This aspect of the human skeletal system was discussed in paragraph 2-11 and will not be further discussed here.

b. **Bone As An Individual Organ**. Section II of this lesson discusses bone as an individual organ.

c. **Articulations (Joints)--Arthrology**. Section III of this lesson introduces the study of joints, or arthrology.

d. **The Human Skeleton**. Section IV of this lesson discusses the human skeleton as a whole in terms of its major subdivisions.

Section II. BONE AS AN INDIVIDUAL ORGAN

4-4. BASIC STRUCTURE OF AN INDIVIDUAL BONE

See figure 4-1 for the basic structure of an individual bone.

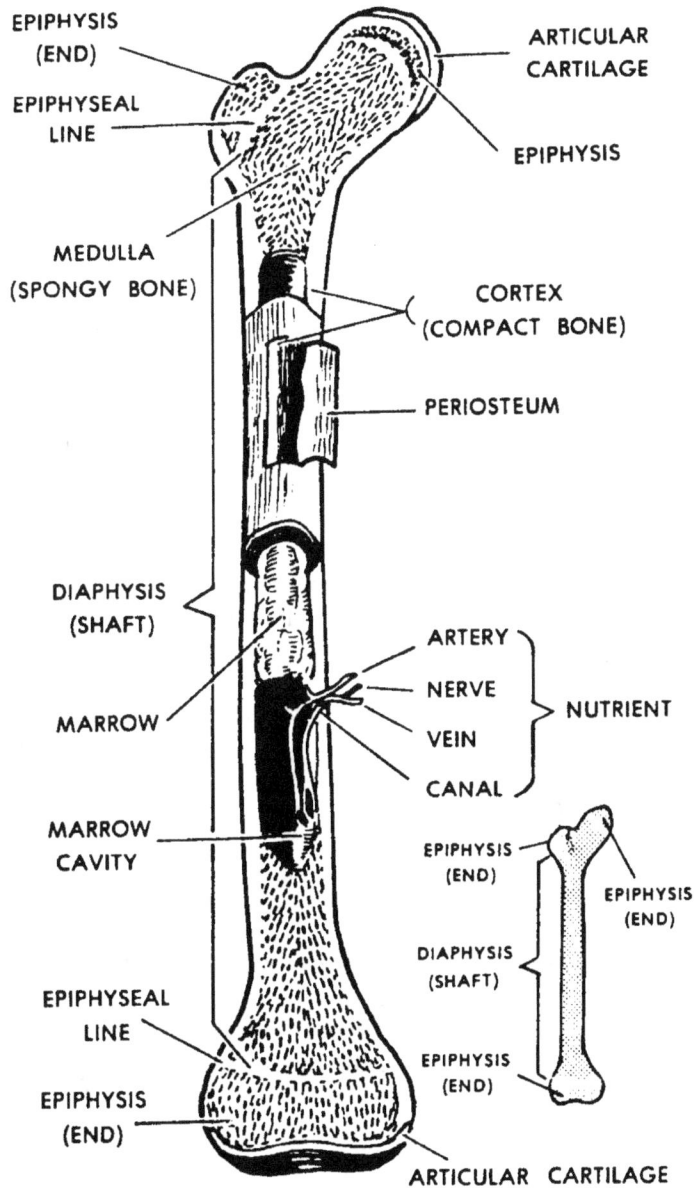

Figure 4-1. A mature long bone (femur).

a. **Use of Bony Tissues to Form an Individual Bone**.

(1) Cortex. The cortex is the outer layer of the individual bone. It is made up of compact (dense) bony tissue.

(2) Medulla. The medulla is the central portion of the individual bone. It generally consists of cancellous (spongy) bone tissue. In some bones, particularly long bones, the medulla may include a space without any bony tissue. This space is called the medullary or marrow cavity.

b. **Marrow**. Marrow serves as a filler of the inside of bones. There are two types of bone marrow--yellow bone marrow and red bone marrow. Yellow bone marrow is mostly yellow fat tissue. Red bone marrow is the only site in adults for the formation of red blood cells (hematopoiesis).

c. **Named Parts of an Individual Long Bone**.

(1) Shaft (diaphysis). The shaft is the central portion of a long bone. Here, the cortex is thickened as required by applied physical stresses.

(2) Ends (epiphyses). The ends of long bones are made up mainly of cancellous (spongy) bone tissue. An articular cartilage covers each area where a bone contacts another bone(s). This articular cartilage is made up of hyaline cartilage tissue and provides a smooth surface for motions.

d. **Periosteum**. The periosteum is a covering of the bone surface area not covered by articular cartilage. It has two layers--the innermost layer and the fibrous layer.

(1) The innermost layer, which lies against the outer surface of the bone, consists of bone-forming cells (osteoblasts). It is the osteogenic (bone-forming) layer.

(2) The outermost layer is a FCT (fibrous connective tissue) layer.

(3) The periosteum is well supplied with blood vessels and sensory-type nervous tissue.

e. **Blood Supply of an Individual Bone**. A system of blood vessels enters and spreads out through the periosteum. Additional blood vessels, called "nutrient vessels," penetrate the cortex of the bone and spread out through the marrow. The passageways for penetration of these vessels are called the nutrient canals.

4-5. DEVELOPMENT OF AN INDIVIDUAL BONE

a. **General**. The human skeleton is "preformed" in the early fetus, but the early form is not of bony material. There are two types of bones according to their preformed basis: membranous bones and cartilage bones. These are in the location and have the general shape of the adult bones they will later become.

(1) Membranous bones. The outer skull bones are an example of membranous bones. Osteoblasts invade a membrane to form a center of ossification (formation of bone). Bone-forming activity spreads out from this center until a full bone plate is formed.

(2) Cartilage bones. In the fetus, many bones, for example, long bones, exist first as models formed of cartilage.

b. **Sesamoid Bones**. Sesamoid bones are small masses of bone that develop in tendons at points where great forces are applied to the tendons. The most obvious and largest sesamoid bone is the patella, or kneecap.

c. **Ossification Centers**. An ossification center is a growing mass of actual bone within the preformed material, as noted above.

(1) Initial bone formation involves destruction of the preforming material and replacement with bony tissue.

(2) In the development of long bones, there are two types of ossification centers:

(a) Diaphyseal--in the shaft region.

(b) Epiphyseal--in the end(s).

(3) As a long bone grows in length, the preforming material grows faster than the ossification center can tear it down. Ultimately, with time, the preforming material is overcome and growth ceases.

d. **Growth in Bone Width**. A bone grows wider through the activity of the osteogenic layer of the periosteum. Remember, the periosteum covers most of the outer surface of the bone.

4-6. TYPES OF BONES

Bones of the skeleton can be grouped into the following major types: long, short, flat, and irregular. Each type has a somewhat different construction pattern.

a. **Long Bones**. The basic structure of a long bone is illustrated in figure 4-1 and discussed in paragraph 4-4. Example: femur.

b. **Short Bones**. The short bones, such as those of the wrist and feet, have a thin layer of compact bone surrounding an inner mass of spongy bone. Example: carpal bones.

c. **Flat Bones**. The flat bones are constructed with two plates of compact bone, which enclose between them a layer of spongy bone. The spongy bone is richly supplied with blood vessels and red marrow. Example: the cranial frontal bone.

d. **Irregular Bones**. The irregular bones are those that do not fit into the three categories above. Example: a vertebra.

Section III. ARTHROLOGY--THE STUDY OF JOINTS (ARTICULATIONS)

4-7. DEFINITION

A joint, or articulation, is the location where two or more bones meet.

4-8. TYPES OF JOINTS

Joints are classified according to the kind of material holding the bones together and the relative freedom and kind of motion at the particular joint.

a. **Fibrous Joints**. Varying degrees of motion, from none to some, are possible in fibrous joints.

(1) Syndesmosis. When the bones are held together by FCT (fibrous connective tissue), the joint is referred to as a syndesmosis.

SYN = together
DESMOS = fiber (a tying material)

Example: The inferior tibio-fibular joint.

(2) Suture. When the bones are quite close together with a minimum of FCT, the joint is known as a suture. Example: the joints between the cranial bones.

b. **Bony Joints**. Should the bones be united by bony material, the joint is referred to as a synosteosis.

SYN = together
OSTEO = bone

Example: The frontal bone. (The frontal bone of the skull is actually a bony fusion of two bones. Approximately 10 percent of the time, this fusion fails to take place; the original suture between the bones remains and is called a metopic suture.)

    c. **Cartilagenous Joints**. These are also nonmovable joints.

      (1) Synchondrosis. A cartilagenous joint in which the bones are held together by hyaline cartilage.

        SYN = together
        CHONDRO = cartilage

Example: Epiphyseal plate.

      (2) Symphysis. A cartilagenous joint in which the bones are held together by a disc of fibrocartilage.

Example: Pubic symphysis.

    d. **Synovial Joints**. In the synovial type of joints, the bones move on one another so as to allow various motions of the body parts. The "ovial" part of the name refers to the fact that the fluid substance seen in this type of joint appeared to the old anatomists to be like raw egg white (ovum = egg).

4-9. A "TYPICAL" SYNOVIAL JOINT

    A "typical" synovial joint is one which has parts common to all of the synovial joints. In a sense, it is imaginary. It is not actually a specific synovial joint. It is a composite. It is illustrated in figure 4-2. The "typical" synovial joint has the following parts:

    a. **Bones**. Bones are the levers of motion. They are the site of attachment for skeletal muscles.

    b. **Articular Cartilages**. The "contact" points of the bones are usually covered with a layer of lubricated cartilage. Where these cartilages end, the synovial membranes begin. Cartilages provide a smooth surface to reduce friction.

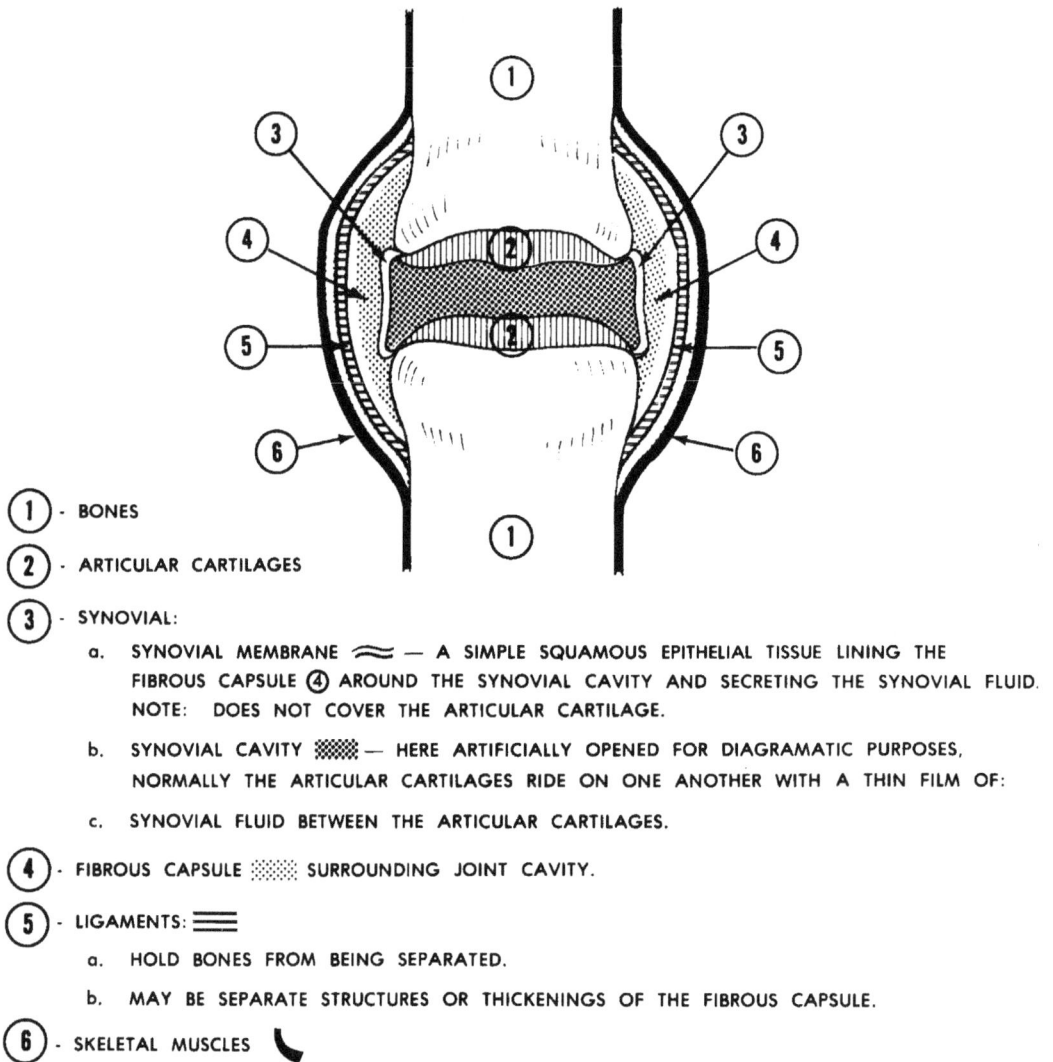

① - BONES

② - ARTICULAR CARTILAGES

③ - SYNOVIAL:

a. SYNOVIAL MEMBRANE ⁓ — A SIMPLE SQUAMOUS EPITHELIAL TISSUE LINING THE FIBROUS CAPSULE **④** AROUND THE SYNOVIAL CAVITY AND SECRETING THE SYNOVIAL FLUID. NOTE: DOES NOT COVER THE ARTICULAR CARTILAGE.

b. SYNOVIAL CAVITY ▓▓ — HERE ARTIFICIALLY OPENED FOR DIAGRAMATIC PURPOSES, NORMALLY THE ARTICULAR CARTILAGES RIDE ON ONE ANOTHER WITH A THIN FILM OF:

c. SYNOVIAL FLUID BETWEEN THE ARTICULAR CARTILAGES.

④ - FIBROUS CAPSULE ▒▒ SURROUNDING JOINT CAVITY.

⑤ - LIGAMENTS: ≡

a. HOLD BONES FROM BEING SEPARATED.

b. MAY BE SEPARATE STRUCTURES OR THICKENINGS OF THE FIBROUS CAPSULE.

⑥ - SKELETAL MUSCLES ❟

Figure 4-2. A "typical synovial joint:--diagrammatic.

c. **Synovial Membrane, Space, and Fluid**.

(1) Synovial membrane. The synovial membrane lines the inner surface of the capsule. It secretes synovial fluid into the synovial space.

(2) Synovial space. Figure 4-2 exaggerates the amount of space between the bones. The space within the capsule allows movement.

(3) Synovial fluid. Synovial fluid is a colorless, viscous fluid similar in consistency to raw egg white. It lubricates the articulation.

d. **Capsule**. The "typical" synovial articulation is surrounded by a sleeve of dense FCT known as the capsule. The capsule encloses the articulation.

e. **Ligaments**. Primarily, ligaments hold bones together. Ligaments also may help restrain motion in certain directions and stabilize the articulation.

f. **Muscles**. Skeletal muscles apply the forces to produce a given motion.

NOTE: See table 4-1 for a summary of the structures in a "typical" synovial articulation, the tissues composing each structure, and the actions attributed to each structure.

4-10. CLASSIFICATION OF SYNOVIAL JOINTS

Synovial joints are further classified according to the kind of motion and the number of axes of motions used.

a. **Uni-Axial Synovial Joints**.

(1) In uni-axial synovial joints, motion occurs in only one plane. The joints of the fingers (interphalangeal) flex and extend in the sagittal plane. These are commonly referred to as hinge joints.

(2) If a single rotatory (rotational) motion occurs around a post-like structure, the joint is a pivot joint. The atlas vertebra rotating around the dens (tooth like projection) of the axis vertebra at the top of the neck (base of the skull) is a pivot joint.

b. **Bi-Axial Synovial Joints**. In bi-axial synovial joints, motion between the bones occurs in two planes. Here the surface in contact is curved or rounded in two directions.

(1) The proximal phalanx of a finger can flex and extend and move from side to side on the rounded head of the metacarpal bone. This is the MP or metacarpophalangeal joint.

(2) When the two surfaces are curved in directions at right angles to each other, a shape similar to that of a cowboy's saddle is formed. This type of synovial joint is called a saddle joint. In the human body, the saddle joint is located at the base of the thumb.

STRUCTURE	TISSUE(S)	FUNCTION(S)
1. BONE	BONY	(a) Serves as site of attachment for the skeletal muscles. (b) Serves as lever of motion.
2. ARTICULAR CARTILAGE	HYALINE CARTILAGE	Serves as smooth surface, over which motion takes place.
3. FIBROUS CAPSULE	DENSE FCT	Encloses articulation.
4. SYNOVIAL MEMBRANE	SIMPLE SQUAMOUS EPITHELIUM	(a) Lines capsule. (b) Secretes synovial fluid into synovial space.
5. SYNOVIAL SPACE	-	Frees articulation for motion.
6. SYNOVIAL FLUID	SEROUS FLUID	Lubricates articulation.
7. LIGAMENT	(VERY) DENSE FCT	Holds the bones together.
8. SKELETAL MUSCLE	STRIATED MUSCLE FIBERS	Applies force to produce motion.

Table 4-1. The tissues and functions of structures of a "typical" synovial articulation.

c. **Multi-Axial Synovial Joints**. In multi-axial joints, motion is possible in all three planes of space.

(1) The ball-and-socket-type synovial joint has the freest motion in all directions. A spherically rounded head (ball-like) fits into a receiving concavity (socket). The hip joint is an example of the ball-and-socket type, with the spherical head of the femur fitting into the cup or socket (acetabulum) of the pelvic bone.

(2) In the plane joint, the contact surfaces of the bones are essentially flat. These flat surfaces slide on one another (also called translatory motion). The acromioclavicular joint of the shoulder region is an example of a plane joint.

4-11. THE ARTICULAR DISC

In three of the synovial joints of the human body, a special addition is seen. This addition is known as an articular disc. The joints with articular discs are the temporo-mandibular joint of the lower jaw, the sternoclavicular joint (at the sternum (breastbone)), and the ulnocarpal joint of the distal end of the forearm.

a. An articular disc is a fibrocartilage plate. It is inserted between the articular surfaces of the bones of a synovial joint. In this way, it divides the synovial space into two spaces.

b. Joints having an articular disc are capable of having several different motions occurring at the same time. Mechanically, there are really two joints together here.

Section IV. THE HUMAN SKELETON

4-12. GENERAL

a. The human skeleton (figures 4-3A and 4-3B) is a collection of individual bones articulated (joined) together.

b. The major subdivisions of the skeleton are the axial skeleton and the appendicular skeleton.

4-13. THE AXIAL SKELETON

The axial skeleton is the central framework of the human body. It includes the skull, the vertebral column (spine), and the thoracic cage (chest or rib cage).

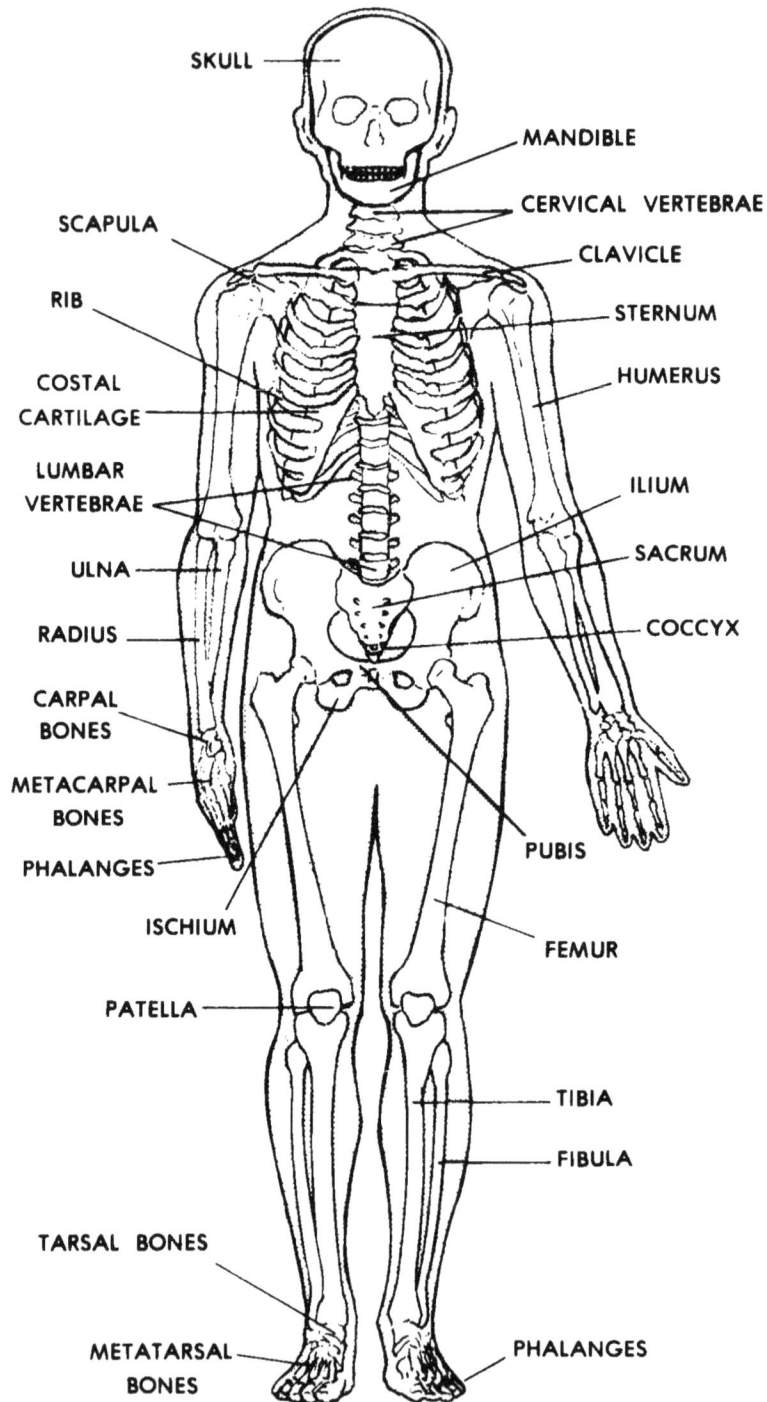

Figure 4-3A. Anterior view of the human skeleton.

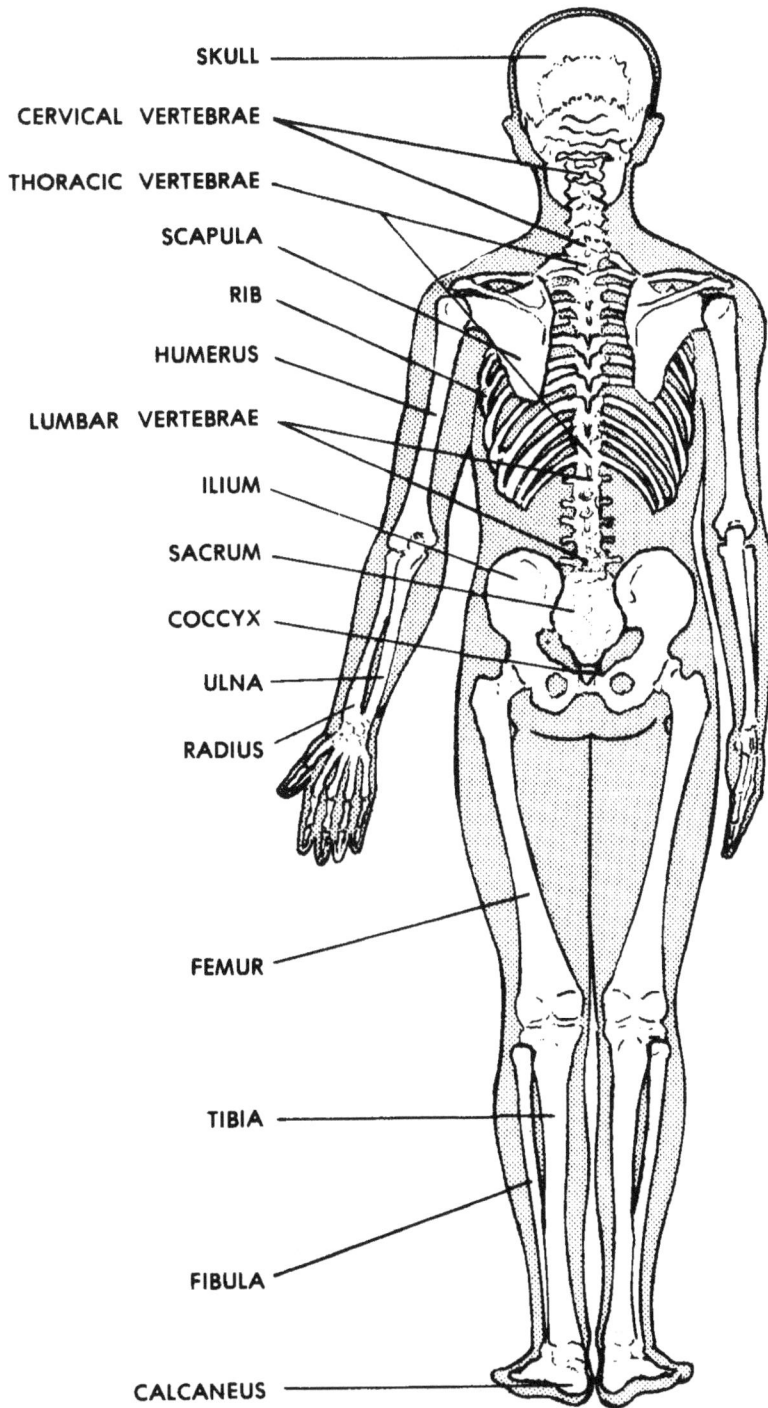

Figure 4-3B. Posterior view of the human skeleton.

a. **Vertebral Column (Spine)**. The vertebral column, or spine, is made up of a vertical series of bony blocks called vertebrae. These vertebrae are joined together in such a way as to form a semiflexible rod. The spine is the central support for the trunk, yet allows trunk movements.

(1) Anatomically and functionally, a typical vertebra (figure 4-4) is constructed of two major parts:

(a) The vertebral body is a drum-shaped cylindrical mass. Its superior and inferior surfaces are flat. Its function is primarily weight-bearing.

(b) The neural arch extends posteriorly, arching over and protecting the spinal cord of the central nervous system. From the neural arch are several processes. These processes serve as attachment areas for the trunk muscles. They also act as levers during various trunk motions.

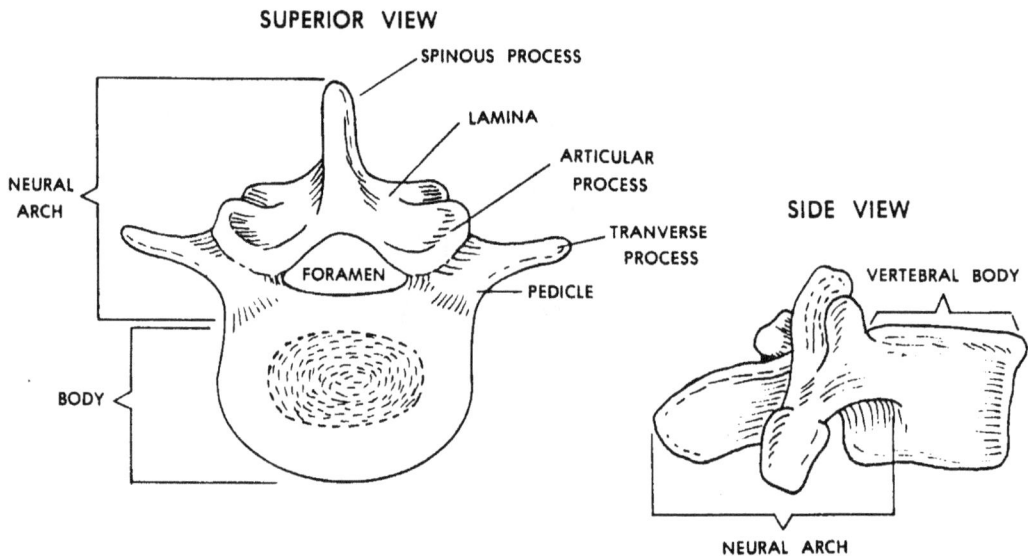

Figure 4-4. A typical vertebra (superior and side views.

(2) The vertebral column has 32-33 vertebrae, one on top of the other. These vertebrae are arranged in regions. The vertebrae of each region have a characteristic shape. The regions are as follows:

(a) Cervical (neck) region, with seven cervical vertebrae.

(b) Thoracic (chest) region, with 12 thoracic vertebrae.

(c) Lumbar (low back) region with five lumbar vertebrae.

(d) The sacrum, which is a bony fusion of five sacral vertebrae.

(e) The coccyx (pronounced COCK-sicks, "tail"), with 3-4 coccygeal vertebrae together.

(3) The vertebrae are held together in two ways:

(a) The intervertebral disc holds the bodies of adjacent vertebrae together. The intervertebral disc is a fibrous ring with a soft center. This disc allows the vertebral bodies to move on one another. This joint between the vertebral bodies is a plane-type joint.

(b) The various parts of adjacent vertebrae are held together by ligaments. A ligament is a dense FCT structure which extends from bone to bone. These ligaments extend along the vertebral column from the base of the skull all the way down to the coccyx.

(4) The spine has four curvatures in the adult human. In the cervical (neck) region and the lumbar (low back) region, the spine curves forward. In the thoracic (chest) region and the sacro-coccygeal (pelvic- sacrum and coccyx) region, the spine curves backwards.

(5) When one examines the back of a person by sight and feel (palpation), certain landmarks are observed.

(a) At the upper shoulder region in the midline, a knob can be seen and felt. This is the tip of the spinous process of the seventh cervical vertebra. Since this is the first vertebra from the top that can be easily palpated, this bony landmark is called the vertebra prominens (the "prominent vertebra").

(b) From the vertebra prominens down to the beginning of the sacrum, one can feel the tip of the spinous process of each vertebra.

b. **The Thoracic (Rib) Cage**. The rib cage (figure 4-5) forms a protective enclosure for the vital organs contained within the thorax (chest) such as the heart and lungs. It also allows the movements of breathing to take place.

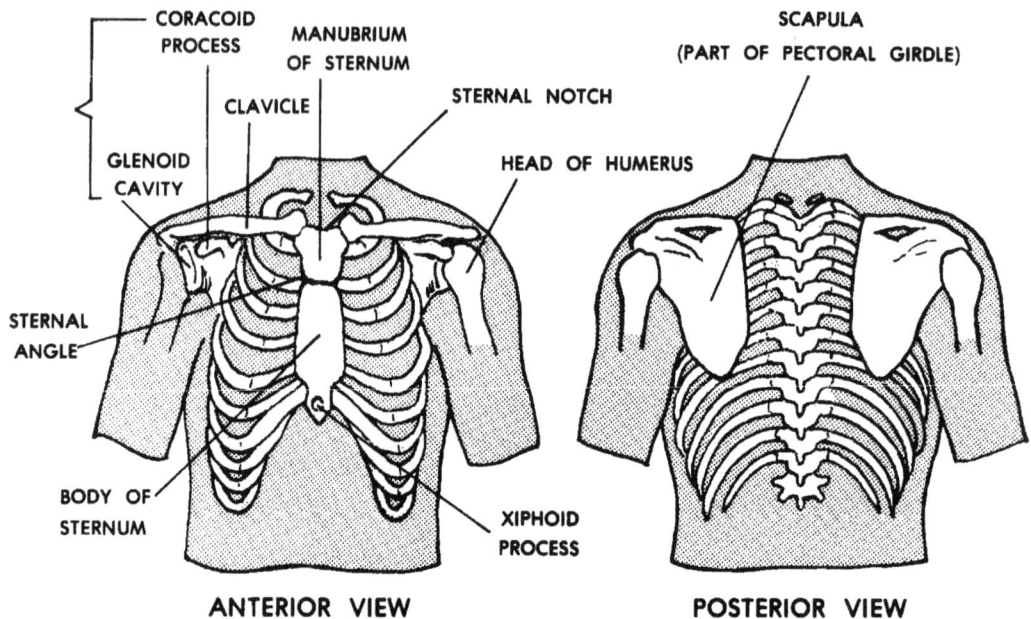

Figure 4-5. The human thorax with bones of the shoulder region.

(1) The <u>sternum</u> lies in the midline of the thorax anteriorly. It is made up of three parts: the <u>manubrium</u> at the top, the <u>body</u> as the main part, and the <u>xiphoid process</u> below. On the top of the manubrium is the <u>jugular (sternal) notch</u>, a common landmark. The junction between the manubrium and the body is a joint called the <u>sternal angle</u>. This sternal angle is an important landmark clinically because the second rib attaches to the sternum at this junction. It is just a matter of simple counting after identifying the second rib to know where you are on the thoracic wall.

(2) The <u>rib cage</u> consists of the 12 thoracic vertebrae, 12 pairs of ribs, and the sternum. Each rib is curved laterally from back to front. All 12 pairs of ribs are attached posteriorly to the thoracic vertebrae. The upper six pairs of ribs are attached directly to the sternum by their costal cartilages. The seventh through tenth pairs of ribs are attached indirectly to the sternum through their costal cartilages (by attaching to the costal cartilage of the rib above). Rib pairs 11 and 12 do not attach to the sternum. Instead, they are embedded in the trunk wall muscles.

c. **The Skull.** The skull (figure 4-6) is the bony framework (skeleton) of the head region. It has two major subdivisions: the <u>cranium</u> which encases and protects the brain and the <u>facial skeleton</u> which is involved with the beginnings of the digestive and respiratory systems. The special sense organs (eyes, ears, etc.) are included and protected within the skull.

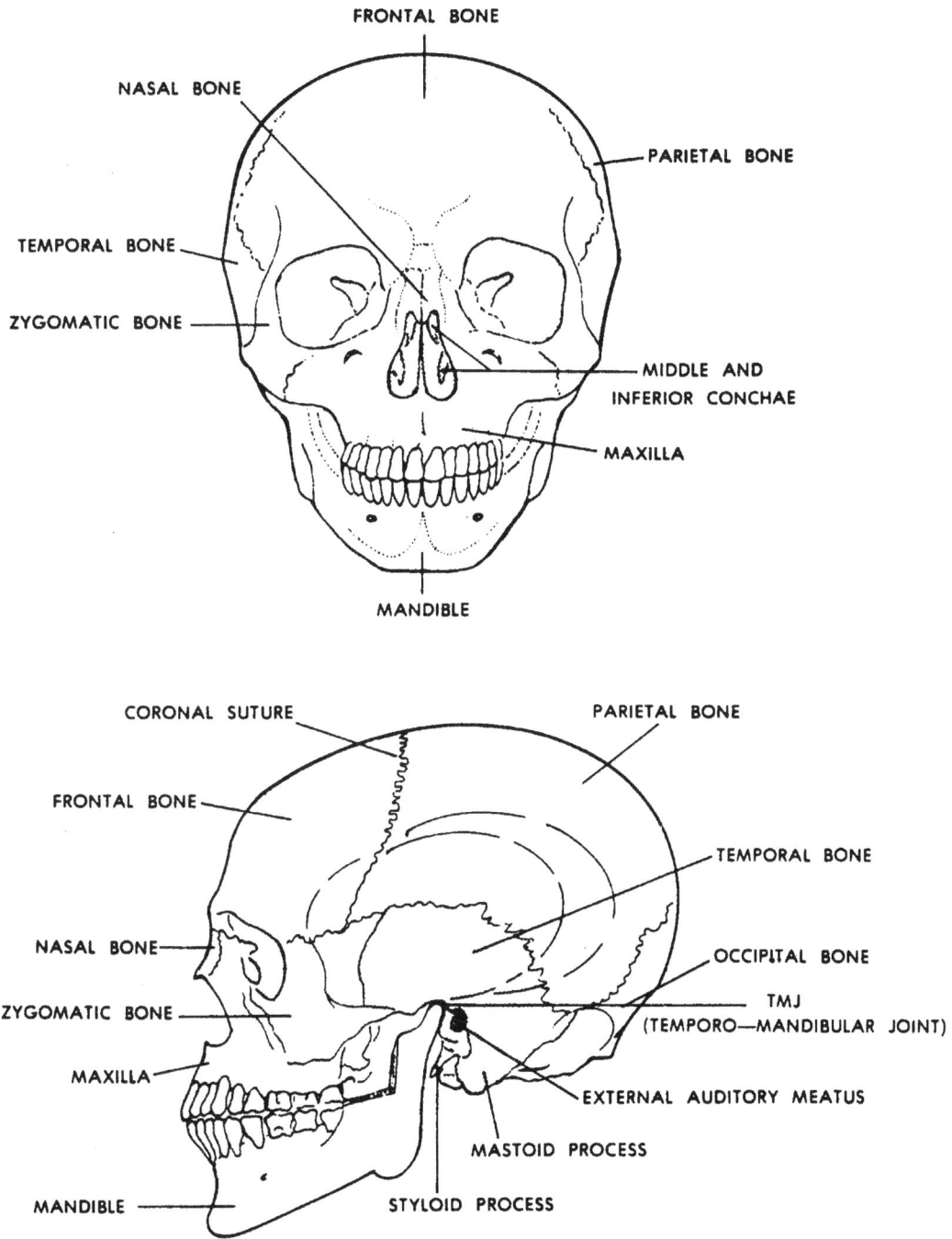

Figure 4-6. The human skull (front and side views).

(1) The bones of the <u>cranium</u> form a spherical case around the brain. With age, the sutures between the cranial bones become more solid. The cranium has a <u>base</u> with several openings for the passage of blood vessels and nerves. The <u>vault</u> (or calvaria) is made up of flat bones arching over and covering the brain.

(2) The facial skeleton consists of bones which surround the nose and the mouth. These are mainly flat and irregular bones. Bones of the facial skeleton also form part of the orbit of each eye.

(3) Certain bones of the skull have air-filled spaces called the <u>paranasal sinuses</u>.

(4) The <u>upper jaw</u> (maxilla) and the <u>lower jaw</u> (mandible) are parts of the facial skeleton which surround the mouth.

(5) The <u>hyoid bone</u> is located at the junction between the head and the neck. It is not articulated directly with the other bones. It is held in place--and moved around--by groups of muscles above and below. The root of the <u>tongue</u> is attached to its upper anterior surface. The <u>larynx</u> is suspended from its inferior surface. These three structures, together, form the <u>hyoid complex</u>. This complex is a functional unit for swallowing.

4-14. THE APPENDICULAR SKELETON

a. The <u>appendicular skeleton</u> is made up of the skeletal elements of the upper and lower members (often incorrectly referred to as the "extremities"). These members are appended (attached) to the axial skeleton.

b. The general pattern of construction of the upper and lower members is the same as follows:

(1) <u>Girdle</u>. The girdle is the actual attaching part. It attaches (appends) the limb (the member less the girdle) to the axial skeleton.

(2) <u>Proximal limb segment</u>. The proximal segment of the limb has a single long bone.

(3) <u>Middle limb segment</u>. The middle segment of the limb has two long bones parallel with each other.

(4) <u>Distal limb segment</u>. The distal segment of the limb is made up of many long and short bones. These bones are arranged into a five-rayed pattern--the <u>digits</u>.

c. See table 4-2 for the main bones of the upper and lower members. Figures 4-7 through 4-13 give the main characteristics and details of the bones of the appendicular skeleton.

PART	UPPER MEMBER	LOWER MEMBER
GIRDLE	PECTORAL GIRDLE (CLAVICLE AND SCAPULA)	PELVIC GIRDLE(PELVIC BONE--A FUSION OF ILIUM, PUBIS, AND ISCHIUM)
PROXIMAL SEGMENT	HUMERUS	FEMUR
MIDDLE SEGMENT	RADIUS ULNA	TIBIA FIBULA
DISTAL SEGMENT	CARPUS (8 WRIST BONES) METACARPALS (5) PHALANGES (5 DIGITS)	TARSUS (7 ANKLE BONES) METATARSALS (5) PHALANGES (5 DIGITS)

Table 4-2. Bones of the upper and lower members.

Continue with Exercises

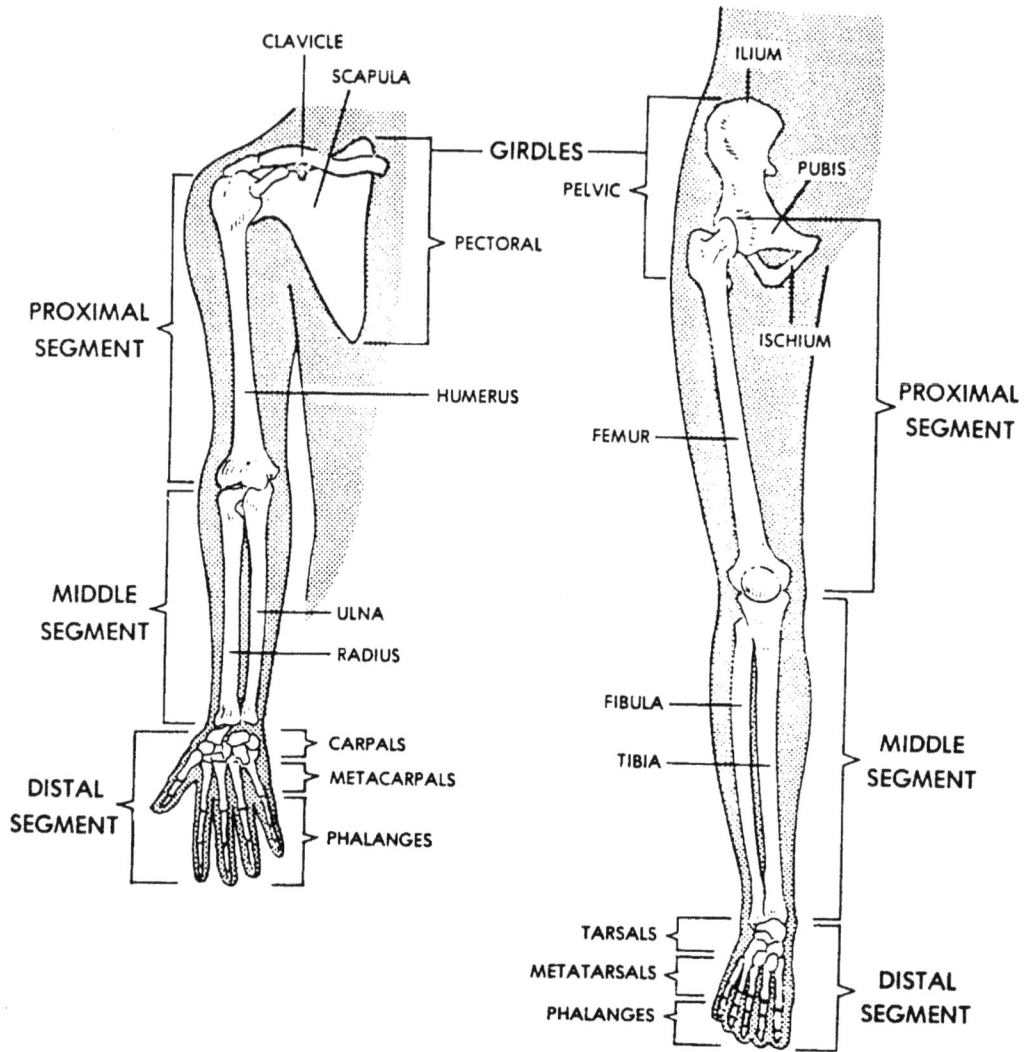

Figure 4-7. A general pattern of the upper and lower members.

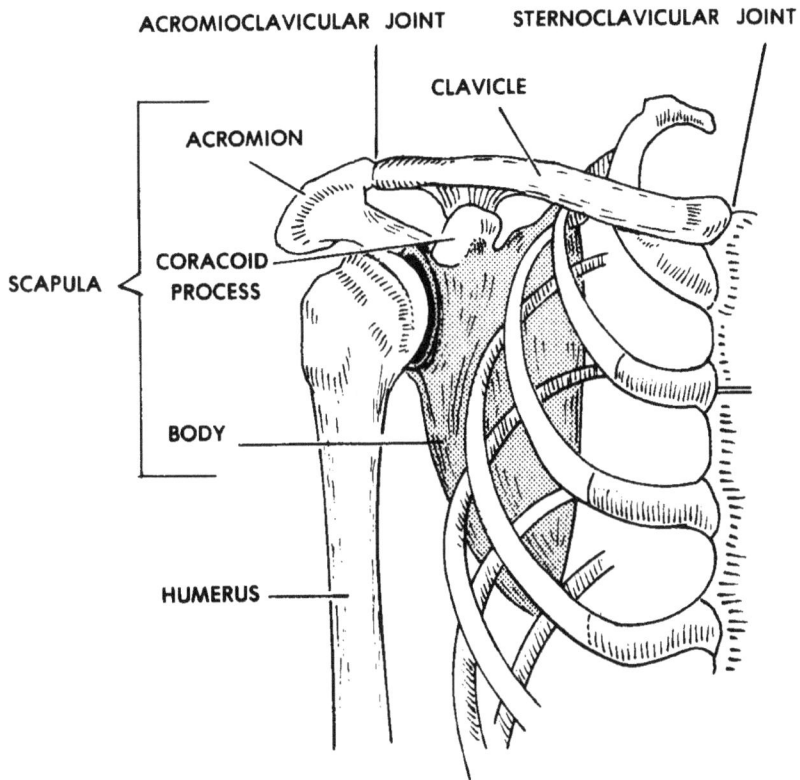

Figure 4-8. The human scapula and clavicle (pectoral girdle).

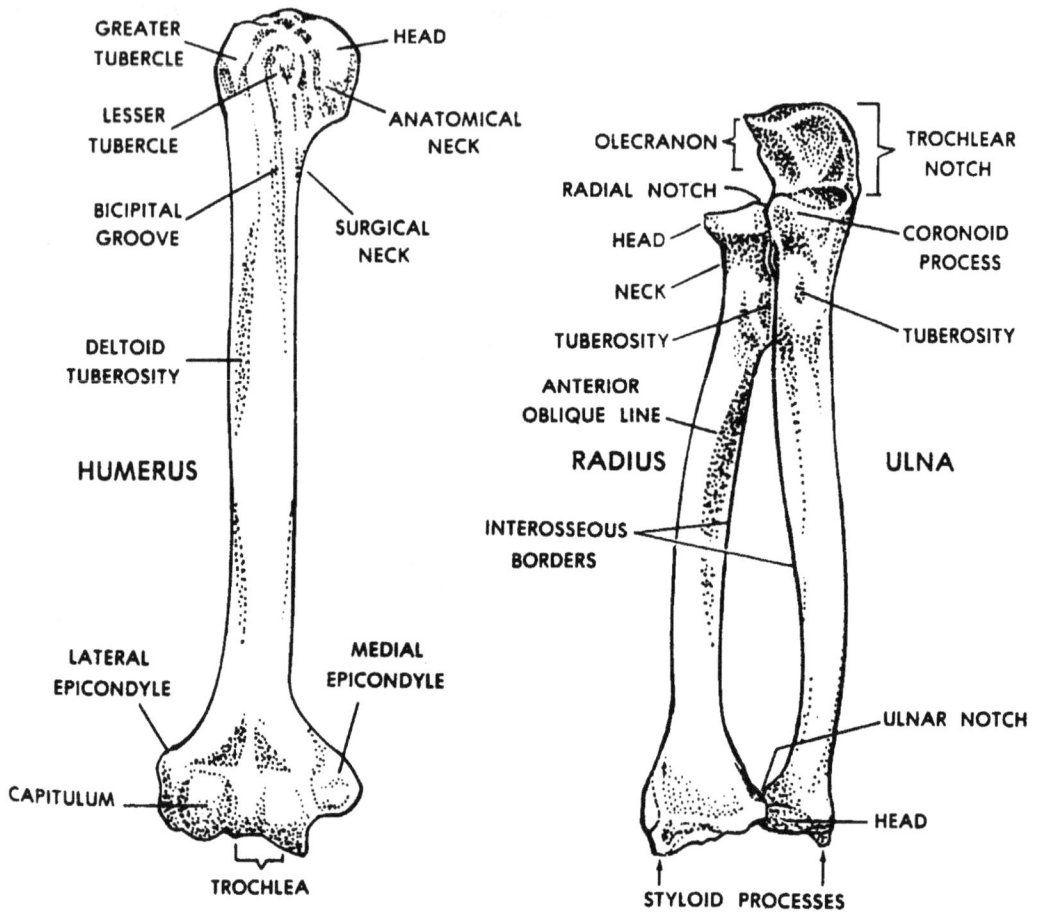

Figure 4-9. The humerus, radius, and ulna.

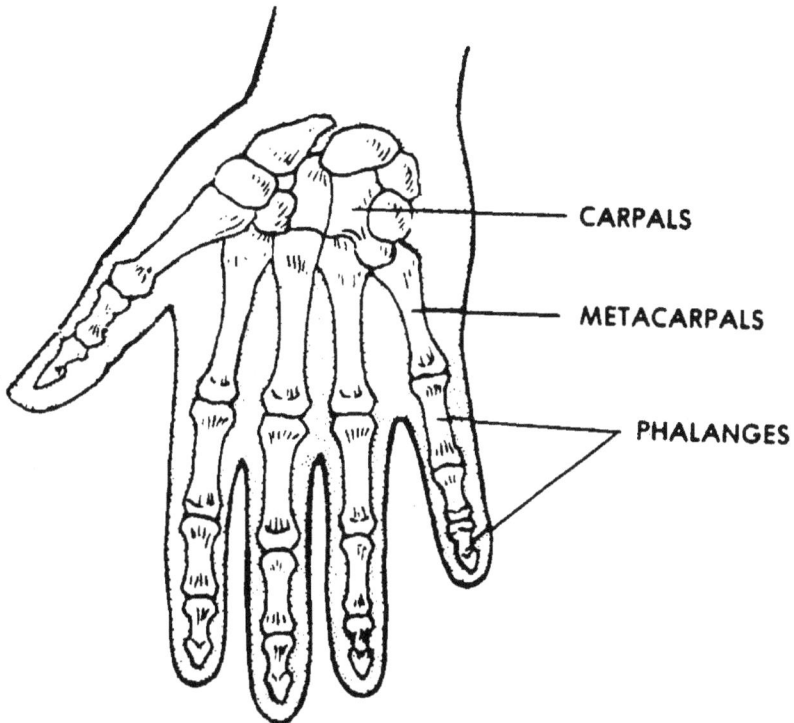

Figure 4-10. The human hand.

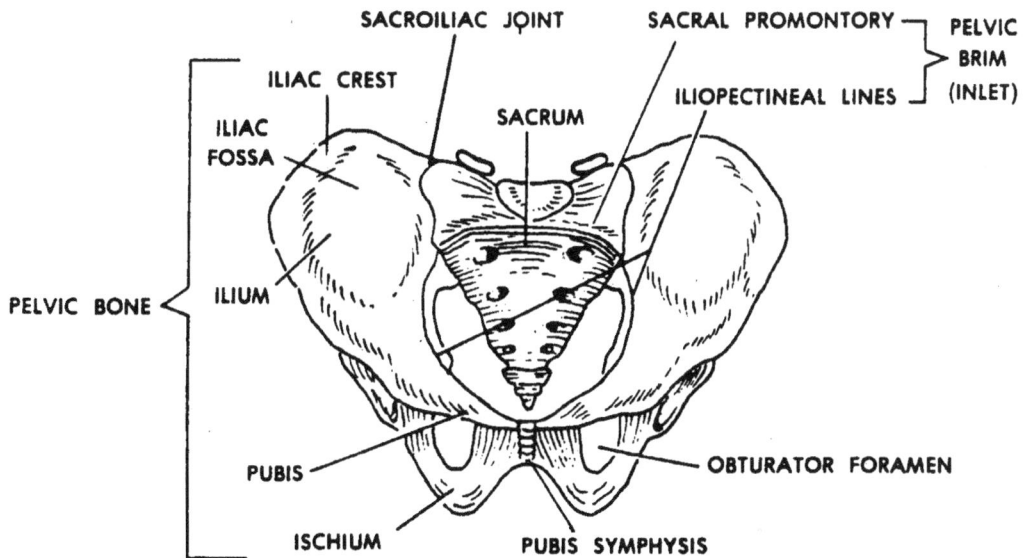

Figure 4-11. The bony pelvis (two pelvic bones and sacrum).

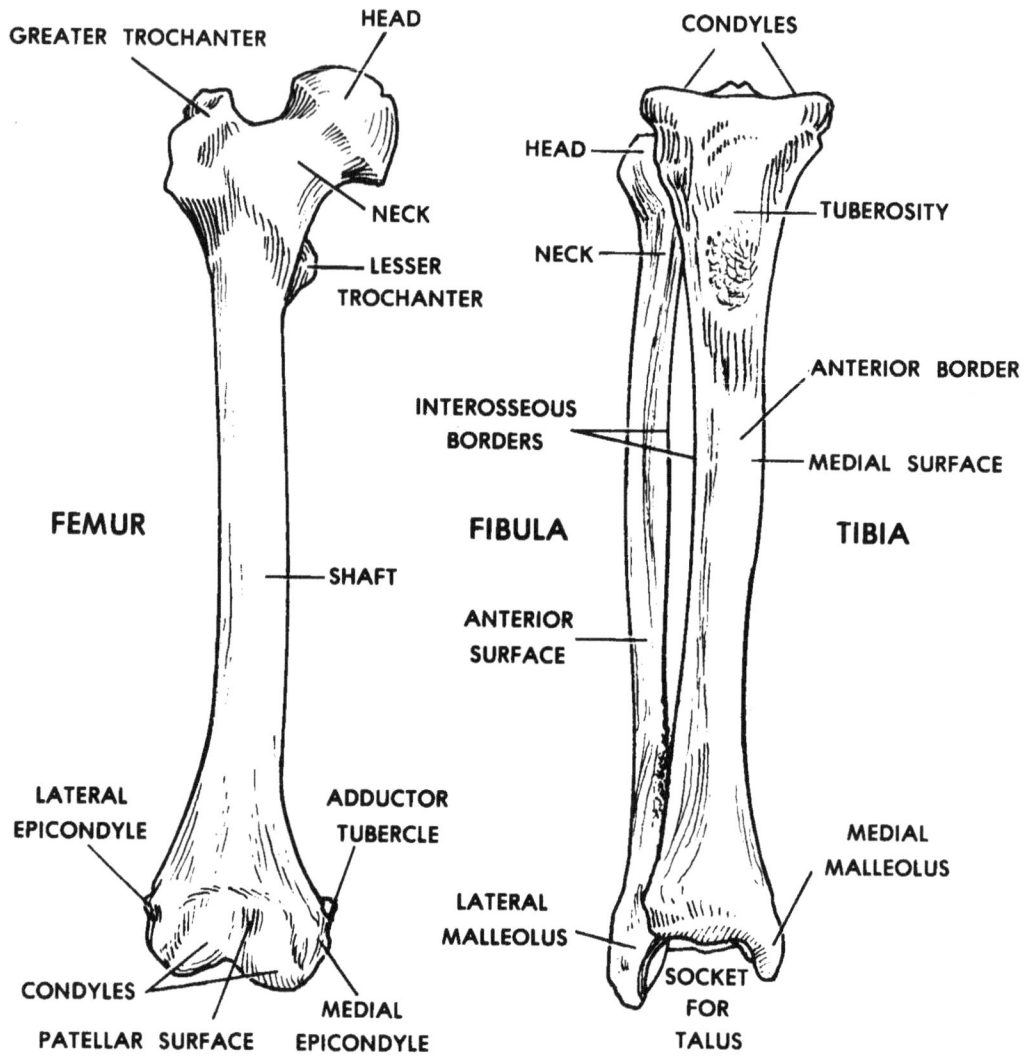

Figure 4-12. The femur, tibia, and fibula (anterior views).

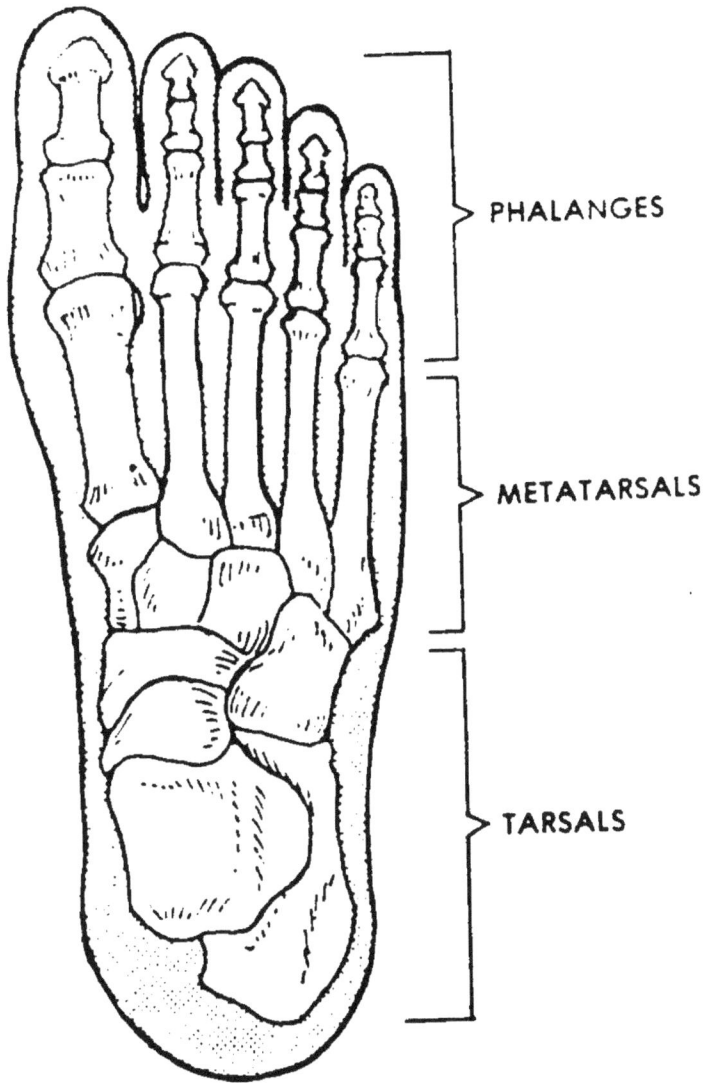

Figure 4-13. The human foot.

EXERCISES, LESSON 4

REQUIREMENT. The following exercises are to be answered by completing the incomplete statement or by writing the answer in the space provided at the end of the question.

After you have completed all the exercises, turn to "Solutions to Exercises," at the end of the lesson and check your answers.

1.   What is a skeleton?

2.   What are four functions of the human skeleton?

a.   _____.

b.   _____.

c.   _____.

d.   _____.

3.   An individual bone consists of the outer _____ and the inner _____.

4.   The two types of bone marrow are _____ and _____ bone marrow. Yellow bone marrow is mostly yellow _____ tissue. Red bone marrow is the only site in adults for the formation of _____.

5.   The parts and portions of an individual long bone are the s____(d_____s) and the _____ (e_____s). The shaft is the _____ portion of the long bone. The ends are made up mainly of c_____(s_____) bone tissue. An articular cartilage covers each area where a bone _____s another bone.

6.   The periosteum is a covering of bone surface area not covered by _____. The innermost layer is the o_____(b_____-f_____) layer. The outermost layer is an _____layer.

7. In the early fetus, bones are preformed as _____s bones and _____e bones which have the shape and location of the _____t bones. Developing long bones have growing masses of actual bone called _____ centers. These centers are located in the_____and in each _____. Preparing material surrounding these centers is destroyed and replaced with _____ tissue. A bone grows in width through the activity of the _____ layer of the _____.

8. What are four types of bones according to shape?

    a. _____.

    b. _____.

    c. _____.

    d. _____.

9. What is a syndesmosis?

10. What is a suture?

11. What is a synosteosis?

12. What is a synchondrosis?

13. What is a symphysis?

14. What is a synovial joint?

15. What are the major parts of a "typical" synovial joint?

    a.   B_____.

    b.   Articular c_____.

    c.   (1)   Synovial m_____.

                (2)   Synovial s_____.

                (3)   Synovial f_____.

    d.   C_____.

    e.   L_____.

    f.   M_____.

16. Name and describe three classifications of synovial joints. Along with each, name common subclassifications.

    a.   U_____.

             (1) Hi_____.

             (2) Pi_____.

    b.   B_____.

             Sa_____.

    c.   M_____.

             (1) Ba_____.

             (2) Pl_____.

17. Name and define the two major subdivisions of the skeleton.

a. _____ skeleton--the _____ _____of the human body--including the _____, _____ column, and _____ _____.

b. _____ skeleton--skeletal elements of the upper and _____ _____.

18. Name and describe the two major parts of a typical vertebra.

a. Vertebral _____--_____-shape cylinder. Its function is to _____ _____.

b. _____ arch--arch over posterior of the _____. The arch has several _____. The _____ are sites of attachment of _____ _____ and act as _____for trunk motions.

19. Name the regions of the vertebral column and give the number of vertebrae in each region.

a. _____ (neck) region, _____.

b. _____ (chest) region, _____.

c. _____ (low back) region, _____.

d. _____, fusion of _____.

e. _____ ("tail"), _____-_____together.

20. Describe the two ways that vertebrae are held together.

a. Intervertebral discs:

b. Ligaments:

21. The thoracic cage consists of the s_____(m_____, b_____, and x_____ p_____), 12 pairs of _____, and 12 t_____v_____. The thoracic cage provides p_____ for v_____ o_____ within the t_____. It also allows the m_____ of breathing.

22. What are the two major subdivisions of the skull and with which organs or systems is each subdivision involved?

     a.   _____: Encases and protects_____.

     b.   _____: Involved with beginning of _____; encases and protects the_____.

23. In the first column below, name a general segment or part of a member. In the second column, name bones or bone groups which are found in each segment of the upper member. In the third column, name bones or bone groups which are found in each segment of the lower member.

	PART	UPPER MEMBER	LOWER MEMBER
a.	G_____	_____GIRDLE	_____GIRDLE
b.	P_____ SEGMENT	_____S	_____R
c.	M_____ SEGMENT	_____S,	_____A,
		_____A	_____A
d.	D_____ SEGMENT	C_____,	T_____,
		M_____,	M_____,
		P_____	P_____

Check Your Answers on Next Page

SOLUTIONS TO EXERCISES, LESSON 4

1.   The skeleton is <u>a combination of bones joined together that serves as a support or framework of the human body</u>. (para 4-1)

2.   The four functions of the human skeleton are:

    a.   <u>Bodily support</u>.
    b.   <u>Protection</u>.
    c.   <u>Motion</u>.
    d.   <u>Formation of blood cells</u>. (para 4-2)

3.   An individual bone consists of the outer <u>cortex</u> and the inner <u>medulla</u>. (para 4-4a)

4.   The two types of bone marrow are <u>red</u> bone marrow and <u>yellow</u> bone marrow. Yellow bone marrow is mostly yellow <u>fat</u> tissue. Red bone marrow is the only site in adults for the formation of <u>red blood cells</u>. (para 4-4b)

5.   The parts or portions of an individual long bone are the <u>shaft</u> (<u>diaphysis</u>) and the <u>ends</u> (<u>epiphyses</u>). The shaft is the <u>central</u> portion of the long bone. The ends are made up mainly of <u>cancellous</u> (<u>spongy</u>) bone tissue. An articular or cartilage covers each area where a bone <u>contact</u>s another bone. (para 4-4c)

6.   The periosteum is a covering of bone surface area not covered by <u>articular cartilage</u>. The innermost layer is the <u>osteogenic</u> (<u>bone-forming</u>) layer. The outermost layer is an <u>FCT</u> layer. (para 4-4d)

7.   In the early fetus, bones are "preformed" as <u>membranous</u> bones and <u>cartilage</u> bones which have the shape and location of the <u>adult</u> bones. Developing long bones have growing masses of actual bone called <u>ossification</u> centers. These centers are located in the <u>shaft</u> and in each <u>end</u>. Preforming material surrounding these centers is destroyed and replaced with <u>bony</u> tissue. A bone grows in width through the activity of the <u>osteogenic</u> layer of the <u>periosteum</u>. (paras 4-5a, c, d)

8.   Four types of bones according to shape are:

    a.   <u>Long bones</u>.
    b.   <u>Short bones</u>.
    c.   <u>Flat bones</u>.
    d.   <u>Irregular bones</u>. (para 4-6)

9.   A syndesmosis is <u>a joint in which the bones are held together by FCT (fibrous connective tissue)</u>. (para 4-8a(1))

10. A suture is <u>a joint in which the bones are very close together with a minimum of FCT</u>. (para 4-8a(2))

11. A synosteosis is <u>a joint in which the bones are united by bony material</u>. (para 4-8b)

12. A synchondrosis is <u>a joint in which the bones are held together by hyaline cartilage</u>. (para 4-8c(1))

13. A symphysis is <u>a joint in which the bones are held together by a disc of fibrocartilage</u>. (para 4-8c(2))

14. A synovial joint is <u>a joint in which the bones are able to move freely upon one another</u>. (para 4-8d)

15. The major parts of a synovial joint are:

    a.   B<u>ones</u>.
    b.   Articular <u>cartilages</u>.
    c.   (1) Synovial <u>membrane</u>.
           (2) Synovial s<u>pace</u>.
           (3) Synovial f<u>luid</u>.
    d.   C<u>apsule</u>.
    e.   L<u>igaments</u>.
    f.   M<u>uscles</u>. (para 4-9)

16. Synovial joints may be classified as follows:

    a.   <u>Uni-axial--motion in one plane</u>.
           (1) H<u>Inge joint</u>.
           (2) Pi<u>vot joint</u>.
    b.   <u>Bi-axial--motion in two planes</u>.
           Sa<u>ddle joint</u>.
    c.   <u>Multi-axial--motion in all three planes</u>.
           (1) Ba<u>ll-and-socket joint</u>.
           (2) Pl<u>ane joint</u>. (para 4-10)

17. The major subdivisions of the skeleton are the:

    a.   <u>Axial</u> skeleton--the <u>central framework</u> of the human body--including the <u>skull</u>, <u>vertebral</u> column, and <u>thoracic cage</u>.
    b.   <u>Appendicular</u> skeleton--skeletal elements of the upper and <u>lower members</u>. (paras 4-12, 4-13, 4-14)

18. The two major parts of a typical vertebra are the:

    a.   Vertebral <u>body--drum</u>-shape cylinder. Its function is to <u>bear weight</u>.
    b.   <u>Neural</u> arch--arch over posterior of the <u>spinal cord.</u> The <u>neural</u> arch has several <u>processes</u>. The <u>processes</u> are sites for attachment of <u>trunk muscles</u> and act as <u>levers</u> for trunk motions. (para 4-13a(1))

19. The regions of the vertebral column and the number of vertebrae in each are as follows:

    a.   Cervical (neck) region, 7.
    b.   Thoracic (chest) region, 12.
    c.   Lumbar (low back) region, 5.
    d.   Sacrum, fusion of 5.
    e.   Coccyx ("tail"), 3-4 together. (para 4-13a(2))

20. a.   Intervertebral discs hold the bodies of adjacent vertebrae together, are fibrous rings with soft centers, allow adjacent vertebral bodies to move on one another, and are part of plane-type joints between vertebrae.

    b.   Ligaments are dense FCT structures extending from bone to bone (along the vertebral column from the base of the skull to the coccyx). (para 4-13a(3))

21. The thoracic (rib) cage consists of the sternum (manubrium, body, and xiphoid process), 12 pairs of ribs, and 12 thoracic vertebrae. The thoracic cage provides protection for vital organs within the thorax. It also allows the movements of breathing. (para 4-13b)

22. The two major subdivisions of the skull are as follows:

    a.   Cranium: Encases and protects brain.
    b.   Facial skeleton: Involved with beginning of digestive and respiratory tracts; encases and protects the special sense organs (eyes, ears, etc.). (para 4-13c)

23.

	PART	UPPER MEMBER	LOWER MEMBER
a.	GIRDLE	PECTORAL GIRDLE	PELVIC GIRDLE
b.	PROXIMAL SEGMENT	HUMERUS	FEMUR
c.	MIDDLE SEGMENT	RADIUS,	TIBIA,
		ULNA	FIBULA
d.	DISTAL SEGMENT	CARPUS,	TARSUS,
		METACARPALS,	METATARSALS,
		PHALANGES	PHALANGES

(table 4-2)

End of Lesson 4

LESSON ASSIGNMENT

LESSON 5   The Human Muscular System.

TEXT ASSIGNMENT   Paragraphs 5-1 through 5-8.

LESSON OBJECTIVES   After completing this lesson, you should be able to:

5-1.   Describe the general features of the skeletal muscles.

5-2.   Describe the general arrangement of the trunk and limb musculature.

5-3.   Given a sample drawing, identify the class of lever.

5-4.   Name the components of a skeleto-muscular unit. Given a description of a muscle's role in a motion, name that role.

SUGGESTION   After completing the assignment, complete the exercises at the end of this lesson. These exercises will help you to achieve the lesson objectives.

LESSON 5

THE HUMAN MUSCULAR SYSTEM

Section I. THE SKELETAL MUSCLE

5-1. MUSCLE TISSUES

The cellular elements of muscle tissues are specialized to produce motion by contraction. They also produce body heat. (See paragraphs 2-14 and 2-15 of lesson 2 for a discussion of muscle tissues.)

a. <u>Smooth</u> muscle tissue is utilized to make up the muscular portion of the various visceral organs (stomach, blood vessels, etc.).

b. <u>Cardiac</u> muscle tissue makes up the muscular wall of the heart--the myocardium.

c. <u>Striated</u> muscle tissue is used in the makeup of several types of muscles. The main type of muscle is the <u>skeletal muscle</u>. Other types of muscles made with striated muscle tissue are the facial or integumentary muscles and muscles of the jaw apparatus.

5-2. THE SKELETAL MUSCLE

Each skeletal muscle is an individual organ of the human body. Each is made up of several types of tissues--mainly, striated muscle fibers and FCT (fibrous connective tissue). Each is attached to and moves bones. Bones are parts of the skeleton serving as levers.

a. **General Construction of a Skeletal Muscle**. The large portion of a muscle is known as its <u>belly</u> or fleshy belly. This muscle is <u>attached</u> to bones by tendons or aponeuroses. Tendons and aponeuroses are similar to each other. However, tendons are cord-like and aponeuroses are broad and flat. The fleshy portion may be directly connected to the bone. If so, it is called a "fleshy attachment."

b. **Muscular NAVL (Nerves, Arteries, Veins, Lymphatics)**.

(1) From the main NAVL (nerve, artery, vein, lymphatic), there are branches going to each muscle. These muscular branches are bound together by an FCT sheath to form a <u>neurovascular bundle</u>.

(2) The <u>motor point</u> is that specific location on the surface of the muscle where the neurovascular bundle enters.

(3) A <u>motor unit</u> is the single motor neuron and the number of striated muscle fibers activated by it (innervation). The importance of the motor unit is that its fibers work in unison. Either all fibers within a unit contract or none contract. When a certain amount of force is needed, one unit after another is recruited until just enough units are available to produce the desired action.

5-3. NAMING SKELETAL MUSCLES

The name of a muscle may appear with the abbreviation M., meaning <u>Musculus</u> or muscle. We abbreviate muscles (plural) with the symbol Mm. Skeletal muscles are named according to their physical attributes (shape, size, length, etc.), their location, or their function. For example:

SHAPE: deltoid M.
              DELTA = Δ , Greek letter D

              biceps M.
              BICEPS = two-head
              BI = two CEPS = head

SIZE: adductor magnus M.
              MAGNUS = great, large

LENGTH: adductor longus M.
              LONGUS = long

LOCATION: biceps brachii M.
              BRACHII = of the arm

              biceps femoris M.
              FEMORIS = of the thigh

FUNCTION: rotatores Mm.
              ROTATORES = rotators
              (They turn/rotate the vertebral column.)

5-4. ARRANGEMENT OF HUMAN SKELETAL MUSCLES

See figures 5-1 and 5-2 for some of the skeletal muscles.

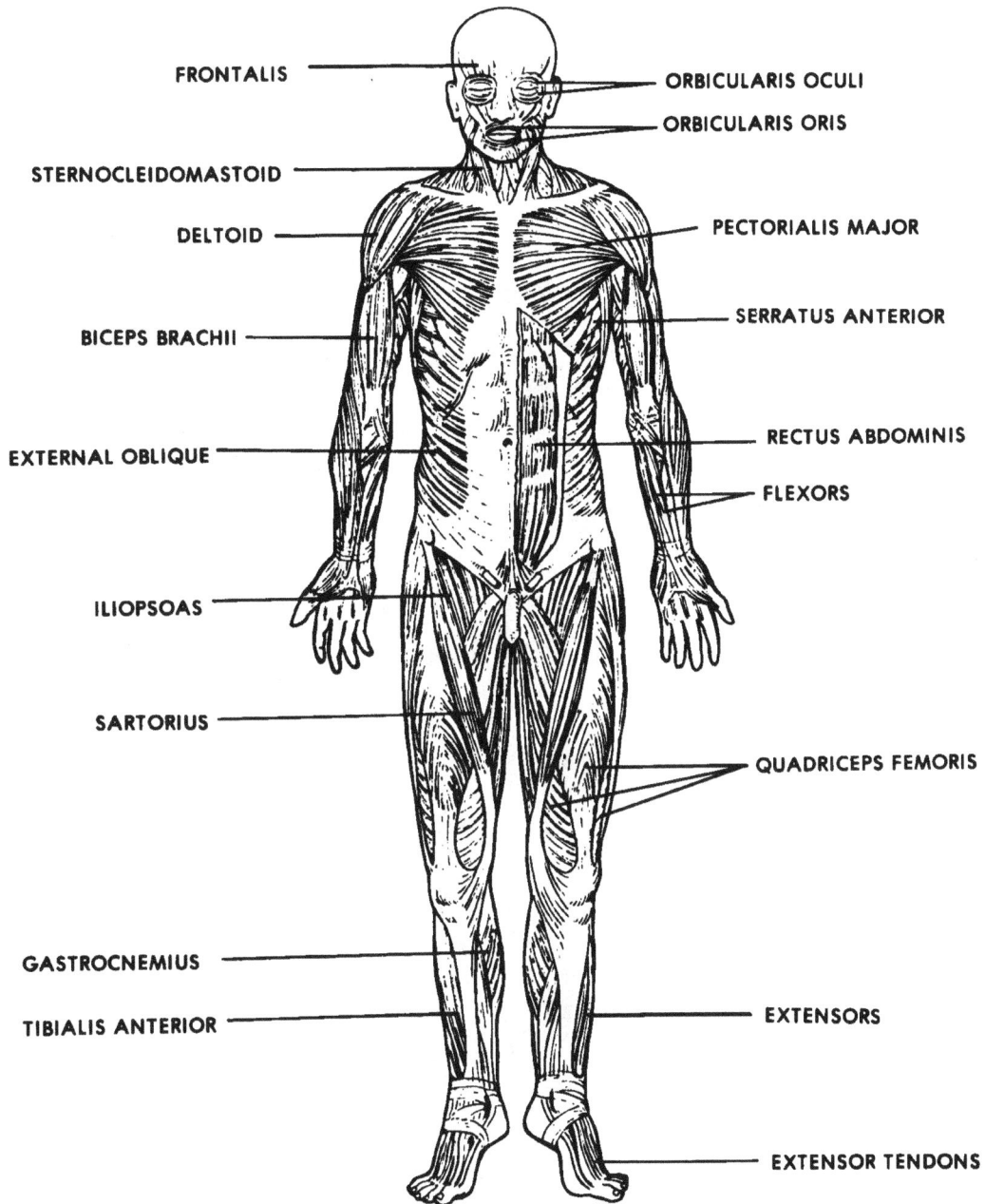

Figure 5-1. Skeletal and facial muscles, anterior view.

FRONTALIS

ORBICULARIS OCULI

ORBICULARIS ORIS

STERNOCLEIDOMASTOID

DELTOID

PECTORIALIS MAJOR

SERRATUS ANTERIOR

BICEPS BRACHII

EXTERNAL OBLIQUE

RECTUS ABDOMINIS

FLEXORS

ILIOPSOAS

SARTORIUS

QUADRICEPS FEMORIS

GASTROCNEMIUS

TIBIALIS ANTERIOR

EXTENSORS

EXTENSOR TENDONS

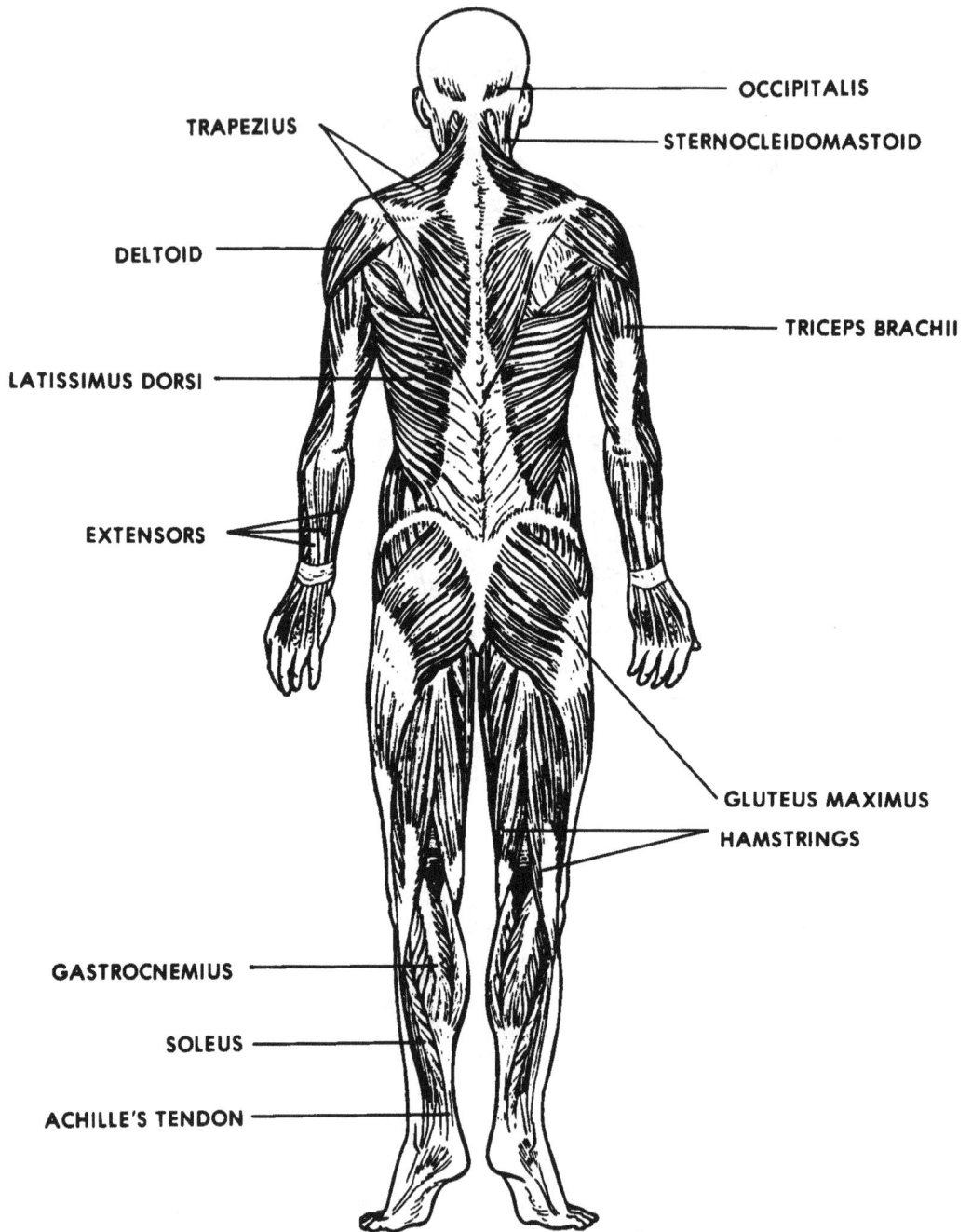

OCCIPITALIS

TRAPEZIUS

STERNOCLEIDOMASTOID

DELTOID

TRICEPS BRACHII

LATISSIMUS DORSI

EXTENSORS

GLUTEUS MAXIMUS

HAMSTRINGS

GASTROCNEMIUS

SOLEUS

ACHILLE'S TENDON

Figure 5-2. Skeletal and facial muscles, posterior view.

a. **Trunk Musculature**. The trunk musculature is arranged in two ways--<u>longitudinal</u> muscles and <u>oblique</u> muscles. Together, they:

(1) Maintain trunk posture.

(2) Move the parts of the trunk.

(3) Adjust the internal pressures of the trunk to perform certain functions such as breathing.

b. **Limb Musculature**. The limb musculature is arranged around the joints to produce the appropriate motions of the limbs. Elementary mechanics are described in the next section to help you to understand typical arrangements of limb musculature.

Section II. SOME ELEMENTARY SKELETO-MUSCULAR MECHANICS

5-5. GENERAL

Muscles and bones together work like machines within the laws of physics and chemistry. Lever and pulley systems are examples of simple machines found commonly in the human body.

5-6. LEVER SYSTEMS

See figure 5-3 for an illustration of the three classes of levers.

a. **First Class**. In a first class lever, the weight to be moved is at one end of the lever, the applied force is at the other end, and the fulcrum (the pivot or turning point) is between the two.

b. **Second Class**. In a second class lever, the weight to be moved is between the applied force and the fulcrum. This type of lever enables a weight to be moved with less force than would be required without a lever. (Many feel that there are no second class levers in the human body.)

c. **Third Class**. In a third class lever, the weight to be moved is at one end of the lever, the fulcrum is at the other end, and the applied force is between the weight and the fulcrum. This type of lever provides speed, but a greater amount of force is required for a given weight. This is the <u>most common type</u> of lever in the human body.

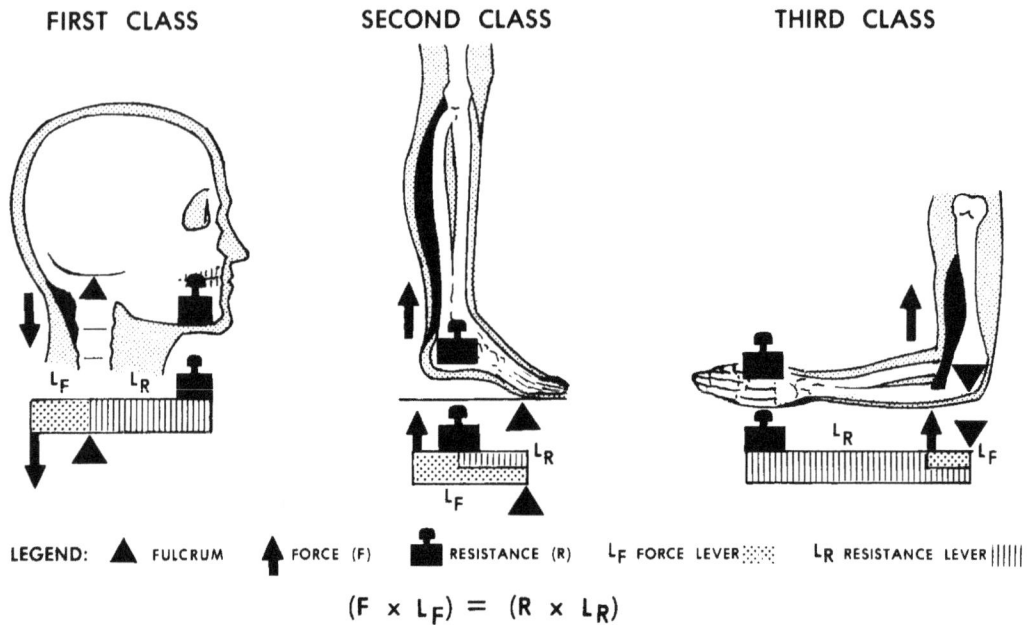

FIRST CLASS   SECOND CLASS   THIRD CLASS

LEGEND: ▲ FULCRUM   ↑ FORCE (F)   ▪ RESISTANCE (R) L_F FORCE LEVER L_R RESISTANCE LEVER

$$(F \times L_F) = (R \times L_R)$$

Figure 5-3. Types of lever systems.

5-7. SIMPLE PULLEY SYSTEM

a. In the human body when the tendon of a skeletal muscle slides over a round bony surface, the "system" acts like a simple pulley (figure 5-4). A simple pulley provides a change in the direction of the force or muscle pull. There is no change in the amount of force produced by the muscle. For example, the knee acts as a simple pulley by which the quadriceps femoris M. extends the leg.

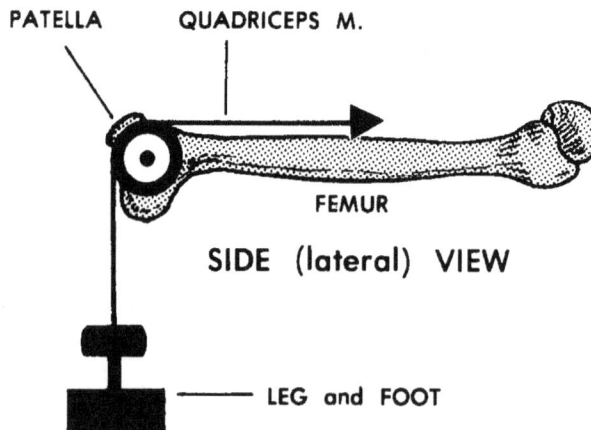

PATELLA   QUADRICEPS M.

FEMUR

SIDE (lateral) VIEW

LEG and FOOT

Figure 5-4. A simple pulley (the human knee mechanism).

b. Sesamoid bones, such as the patella (kneecap), develop in tendons where pressure is applied to the tendon.

5-8. THE SKELETO-MUSCULAR UNIT

The skeleto-muscular unit (figure 5-5) is a working concept of muscle and skeleton producing motion. The components of an S-M unit are bones, a joint, and skeletal muscle(s).

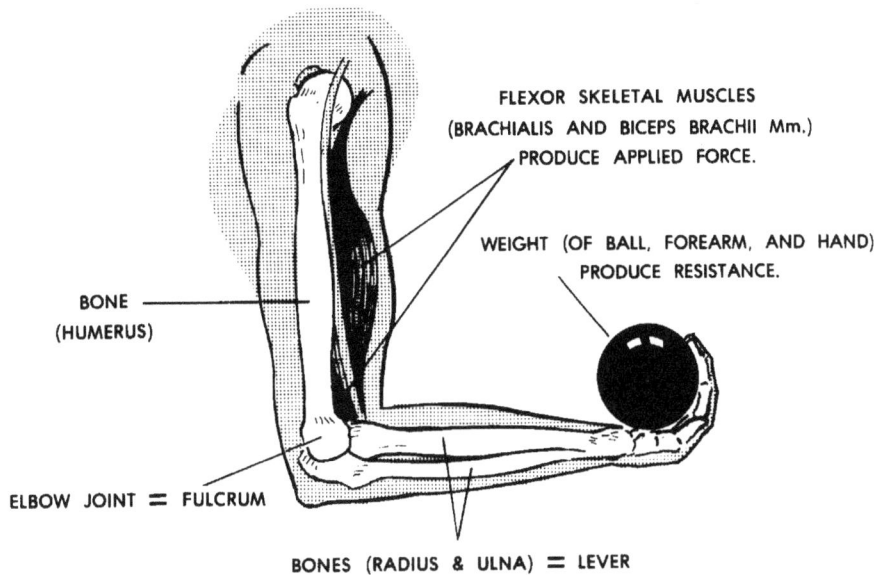

FLEXOR SKELETAL MUSCLES (BRACHIALIS AND BICEPS BRACHII Mm.) PRODUCE APPLIED FORCE.

WEIGHT (OF BALL, FOREARM, AND HAND) PRODUCE RESISTANCE.

BONE (HUMERUS)

ELBOW JOINT = FULCRUM

BONES (RADIUS & ULNA) = LEVER

Figure 5-5. The skeleto-muscular unit (arm-forearm flexion (3rd class lever system)).

a. **Bones**. Bones act as levers and as attachment sites for skeletal muscles.

b. **Joint (Articulation)**. The joint is the center, fulcrum, point, or axis of motion.

c. **Skeletal Muscle(s)**. Skeletal muscles apply the forces for motion. Any given motion utilizes a group of muscles working together. A skeletal muscle may serve only one of the three following major roles during a particular motion:

(1) Prime mover. The muscle which makes the main effort for a given motion is called the prime mover, or agonist.

(2) Synergist. A synergist is a muscle which assists the prime mover.

SYN = together
ERG = unit of effort

(3) <u>Antagonist</u>. An <u>antagonist</u> applies a force opposite to that of the prime mover.

(a) By opposing the prime mover, the antagonist helps control the motion.

(b) The antagonist also brings the limb or other part back to its original position.

Continue with Exercises

EXERCISES, LESSON 5

REQUIREMENT. The following exercises are to be answered by completing the incomplete statements or by writing the answer in the space provided at the end of the question.

After you have completed all the exercises, turn to "Solutions to Exercises," at the end of the lesson and check your answers.

1. The main types of tissues in skeletal muscles are _____ and _____.

2. The large portion of a skeletal muscle is known as its _____ or its _____ _____. Generally, a skeletal muscle is attached to bone by a _____ or _____. If the fleshy portion is directly connected to the bone, it is called a _____ _____.

3. What is a <u>neurovascular bundle</u>?

    What is a <u>motor point</u>?

    What is a <u>motor unit</u>?

4. The trunk musculature is arranged in two ways--_____muscles and _____ muscles. The limb musculature is arranged around the _____ to provide the appropriate motions of the _____.

5. Label the drawings below according to class of lever.

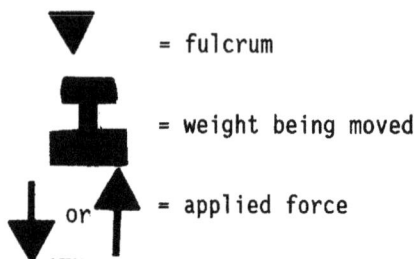

     ▼ = fulcrum

      = weight being moved

      or = applied force

a. _____   _____ class

b. _____   _____ class

c. _____   _____ class

6. The components of a skeleto-muscular unit are:

    a. _____.

    b. _____.

    c. _____.

7. The muscle which makes the main effort for a given motion is called the _____. A muscle which assists the first is called a _____. A muscle which applies a force opposite to that of the first is called an _____.

Check Your Answers on Next Page

SOLUTIONS TO EXERCISES, LESSON 5

1. The main types of tissues in skeletal muscles are <u>striated muscle fibers</u> and <u>fibrous connective tissue</u>. (para 5-2)

2. The large portion of skeletal muscle is known as its <u>belly</u> or <u>fleshy belly</u>. Generally, a skeletal muscle is attached to bone by a <u>tendon</u> or <u>aponeurosis</u>. If the fleshy portion is directly connected to the bone, it is called a <u>fleshy attachment</u>. (para 5-2a)

3. A neurovascular bundle <u>is a branch from the main NAVL, sheathed in fibrous connective tissue</u>. The motor point is <u>the specific location on the surface of the muscle where the neurovascular bundle enters</u>. A motor unit is <u>a single motor neuron and the striated muscle fibers activated by the neuron. All fibers of a motor unit contract or none contract</u>. (para 5-2b)

4. The trunk musculature is arranged in two ways--<u>longitudinal</u> muscles and <u>oblique</u> muscles. The limb musculature is arranged around the <u>joints</u> to produce the appropriate motions of the <u>limbs</u>. (para 5-4)

5. a. <u>Third</u> class.
    b. <u>First</u> class.
    c. <u>Second</u> class. (para 5-6; figure 5-3)

6. The components of a skeleto-muscular unit are:

    a. <u>Bones</u>.
    b. <u>Joint (articulation)</u>.
    c. <u>Skeletal muscles</u>. (para 5-8)

7. The muscle which makes the main effort for a given motion is called the <u>prime mover (agonist)</u>. A muscle which assists the first is called a <u>synergist</u>. A muscle which applies a force opposite to that of the first is called an <u>antagonist</u>. (para 5-8c)

End of Lesson 5

LESSON ASSIGNMENT

LESSON 6   The Human Digestive System.

TEXT ASSIGNMENT   Paragraphs 6-1 through 6-16.

LESSON OBJECTIVES   After completing this lesson, you should be able to:

                             6-1. Define the human <u>digestive system</u>.

                             6-2. Name six major organs of the human digestive system.

                             6-3. Name and describe six structures of the oral complex.

                             6-4. Describe the pharynx, the esophagus, the stomach, the small intestines, the liver and gallbladder, the pancreas, and the large intestines.

SUGGESTION   After completing the assignment, complete the exercises at the end of this lesson. These exercises will help you to achieve the lesson objectives.

LESSON 6

THE HUMAN DIGESTIVE SYSTEM

Section I. INTRODUCTION

6-1. GENERAL

a. **Definition**. The <u>human digestive system</u> is a group of organs designed to take in foods, initially process foods, digest the foods, and eliminate unused materials of food items. It is a <u>hollow tubular</u> system from one end of the body to the other end. See figure 6-1.

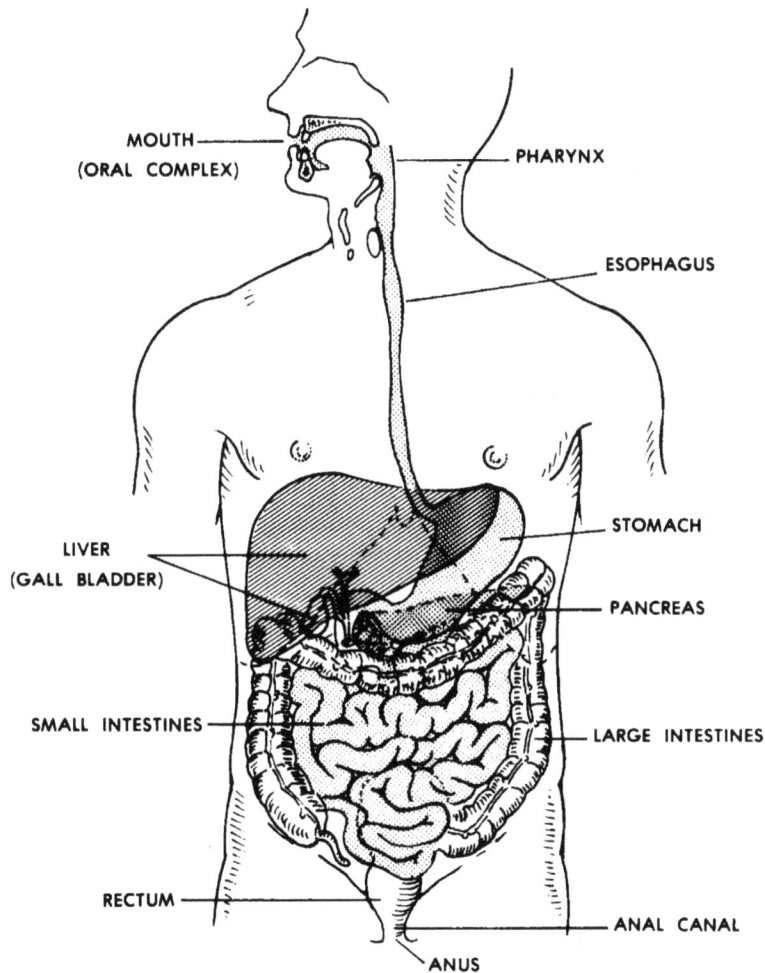

Figure 6-1. The human digestive system.

b. **Major Organs**. The major organs involved in the human digestive system are listed below. They are each discussed later in this lesson.

(1) Mouth or oral complex.

(2) Pharynx.

(3) Esophagus.

(4) Stomach.

(5) Small intestines and associated glands.

(6) Large intestines.

(7) Rectum.

(8) Anal canal and anus.

c. **Digestive Enzymes**. A catalyst is a substance that accelerates (speeds up) a chemical reaction without being permanently changed or consumed itself. A digestive enzyme serves as a catalyst, aiding in digestion. Digestion is a chemical process by which food is converted into simpler substances that can be absorbed or assimilated by the body. Enzymes are manufactured in the salivary glands of the mouth, in the lining of the stomach, in the pancreas, and in the walls of the small intestine.

6-2. FOODS AND FOODSTUFFS

Examples of food items are a piece of bread, a pork chop, and a tomato. Food items contain varying proportions of foodstuffs. Foodstuffs are the classes of chemical compounds which make up food items. The three major types of foodstuffs are carbohydrates, lipids (fats and oils), and proteins. Food items also contain water, minerals, and vitamins.

Section II. THE SUPRAGASTRIC STRUCTURES

6-3. ORAL COMPLEX

The oral complex consists of the structures commonly known together as the mouth. It takes in and initially processes food items. See figure 6-2.

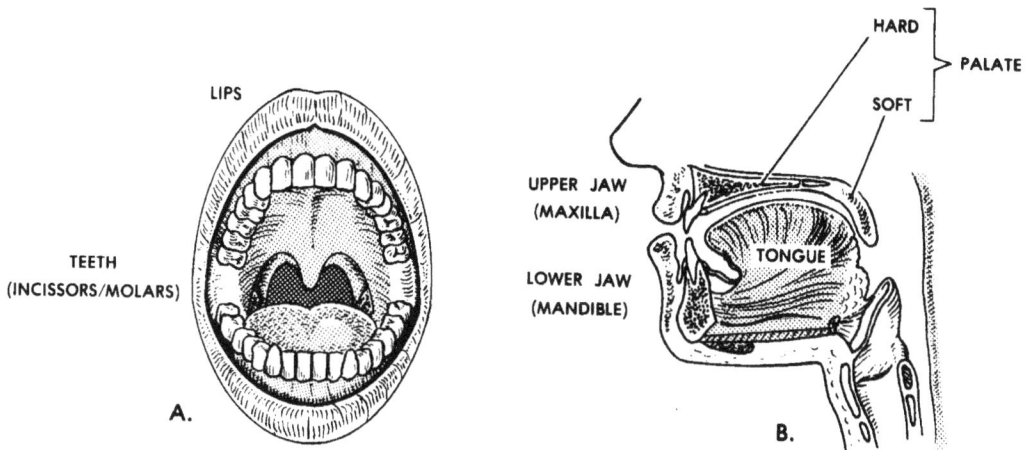

Figure 6-2. Anatomy of the oral complex.

a. **Teeth**.

(1) A tooth (figure 6-3) has two main parts--the <u>crown</u> and the <u>root</u>. A <u>root canal</u> passes up through the central part of the tooth. The root is suspended within a socket (called the <u>alveolus</u>) of one of the jaws of the mouth. The crown extends up above the surface of the jaw. The root and inner part of the crown are made of a substance called <u>dentin</u>. The outer portion of the crown is covered with a substance known as <u>enamel</u>. Enamel is the hardest substance of the human body. The nerves and blood vessels of the tooth pass up into the root canal from the jaw substance.

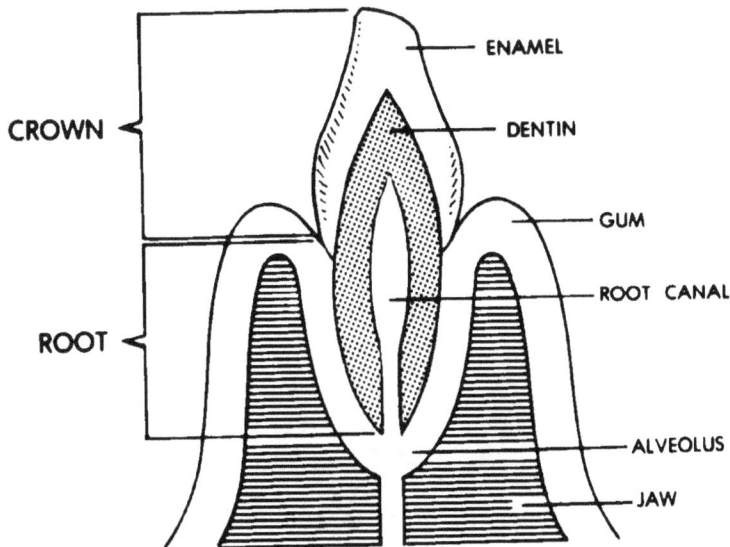

Figure 6-3. Section of a tooth and jaw.

(2) There are two kinds of teeth-- anterior and posterior. The anterior teeth are also known as incisors and canine teeth. The anterior teeth serve as choppers. They chop off mouth-size bites of food items. The posterior teeth are called molars. They are grinders. They increase the surface area of food materials by breaking them into smaller and smaller particles.

(3) Humans have two sets of teeth--deciduous and permanent. Initially, the deciduous set includes 20 baby teeth.

DECIDUOUS = to be shed

These are eventually replaced by a permanent set of 32.

b. **Jaws**. There are two jaws--the upper and the lower. The upper is called the maxilla. The lower is called the mandible.

(1) In each jaw, there are sockets for the teeth. These sockets are known as alveoli. The bony parts of the jaws holding the teeth are known as alveolar ridges.

(2) The upper jaw is fixed to the base of the cranium.
The lower jaw is movable. There is a special articulation (T-MJ--temporo-mandibular joint) with muscles to bring the upper and lower teeth together to perform their functions.

c. **Palate**. The palate serves as the roof of the mouth and the floor of the nasal chamber above. Since the anterior two-thirds is bony, it is called the hard palate. The posterior one-third is musculo-membranous and is called the soft palate. The soft palate serves as a trap door to close off the upper respiratory passageway during swallowing.

d. **Lips and Cheeks**. The oral cavity is closed by a fleshy structure around the opening. Forming the opening are the lips. On the sides are the cheeks.

e. **Tongue**. The tongue is a muscular organ. The tongue is capable of internal movement to shape its body. It is moved as a whole by muscles outside the tongue. Interaction between the tongue and cheeks keeps the food between the molar teeth during the chewing process. When the food is properly processed, the tongue also initiates the swallowing process.

f. **Salivary Glands**. Digestion is a chemical process which takes place at the wet surfaces of food materials. The chewing process has greatly increased the surface area available. The surfaces are wetted by saliva produced by glands in the oral cavity. Of these glands, three pairs are known as the salivary glands proper.

g. **Taste Buds**. Associated with the tongue and the back of the mouth are special clumps of cells known as taste buds. These taste buds literally taste the food. That is, they check its quality and acceptability.

6-4. PHARYNX

The pharynx (pronounced "FAIR -inks") is a continuation of the rear of the mouth region, just anterior to the vertebral column (spine). It is a common passageway for both the respiratory and digestive systems.

6-5. ESOPHAGUS

The esophagus is a muscular, tubular structure extending from the pharynx, down through the neck and the thorax (chest), and to the stomach. During swallowing, the esophagus serves as a passageway for the food from the pharynx to the stomach.

Section III. THE STOMACH

6-6. STORAGE FUNCTION

The stomach is a sac-like enlargement of the digestive tract specialized for the storage of food. Since food is stored, a person does not have to eat continuously all day. One is freed to do other things. The presence of valves at each end prevents the stored food from leaving the stomach before it is ready. The pyloric valve prevents the food from going further. The inner lining of the stomach is in folds to allow expansion.

6-7. DIGESTIVE FUNCTION

a. While the food is in the stomach, the digestive processes are initiated by juices from the wall of the stomach. The musculature of the walls thoroughly mixes the food and juices while the food is being held in the stomach. In fact, the stomach has an extra layer of muscle fibers for this purpose.

b. When the pyloric valve of the stomach opens, a portion of the stomach contents moves into the small intestine.

Section IV. THE SMALL INTESTINES AND ASSOCIATED GLANDS

6-8. GENERAL

a. Digestion is a chemical process. This process is facilitated by special chemicals called digestive enzymes. The end products of digestion are absorbed through the wall of the gut into the blood vessels. These end products are then distributed to body parts that need them for growth, repair, or energy.

b. There are associated glands--the liver and the pancreas--which produce additional enzymes to further the process.

c. Most digestion and absorption takes place in the small intestines.

6-9. ANATOMY OF THE SMALL INTESTINES

a. The small intestines are classically divided into three areas-- the duodenum, the jejunum, and the ileum. The duodenum is C-shaped, about 10 inches long in the adult. The duodenum is looped around the pancreas.

DUODENUM = 12 fingers (length equal to width of 12 fingers)

The jejunum is approximately eight feet long and connects the duodenum and ileum. The ileum is about 12 feet long. The jejunum and ileum are attached to the rear wall of the abdomen with a membrane called a mesentery. This membrane allows mobility and serves as a passageway for nerves and vessels (NAVL) to the small intestines.

JEJUNUM = empty

ILEUM = lying next to the ilium (bone of the pelvic girdle; PELVIS = basin)

b. The small intestine is tubular. It has muscular walls which produce a wave-like motion called peristalsis moving the contents along. The small intestine is just the right length to allow the processes of digestion and absorption to take place completely.

c. The inner surface of the small intestine is NOT smooth like the inside of new plumbing pipes. Rather, the inner surface has folds (plicae). On the surface of these plicae are finger-like projections called villi (villus, singular). This folding and the presence of villi increase the surface area available for absorption.

6-10. LIVER AND GALLBLADDER

a. **Liver Anatomy**. The liver is a large and complex organ. Most of its mass is on the right side of the body and within the lower portion of the rib cage. Its upper surface is in contact with the diaphragm.

b. **Liver Functions**. The liver is a complex chemical factory with many functions. These include aspects of carbohydrate, protein, lipid, and vitamin metabolism and processes related to blood clotting and red blood cell destruction. Its digestive function is to produce a fluid called bile or gall.

c. **Gallbladder**. Until needed, the bile is stored and concentrated in the gallbladder, a sac on the inferior surface of the liver. Fluid from the gallbladder flows through the cystic duct, which joins the common hepatic duct from the liver to form the common bile duct. The common bile duct then usually joins with the duct of the pancreas as the fluid enters the duodenum.

6-11. PANCREAS

The pancreas is a soft, pliable organ stretched across the posterior wall of the abdomen. When called upon, it secretes its powerful digestive fluid, known as pancreatic juice, into the duodenum. Its duct joins the common bile duct.

Section V. THE LARGE INTESTINES

6-12. GENERAL FUNCTION

The primary function of the large intestines is the salvaging of water and electrolytes (salts). Most of the end products of digestion have already been absorbed in the small intestines. Within the large intestines, the contents are first a watery fluid. Thus, the large intestines are important in the conservation of water for use by the body. The large intestines remove water until a nearly solid mass is formed before defecation, the evacuation of feces.

6-13. MAJOR SUBDIVISIONS

The major subdivisions of the large intestines are the cecum (with vermiform or "worm-shaped" appendix), the ascending colon, the transverse colon, the descending colon, and the sigmoid colon. The fecal mass is stored in the sigmoid colon until passed into the rectum.

6-14. RECTUM, ANAL CANAL, AND ANUS

Rectum means "straight." However, this six-inch tubular structure would actually look a bit wave-like from the front. From the side, one would see that it was curved to conform the sacrum (at the lower end of the spinal column). The final storage of feces is in the rectum. The rectum terminates in the narrow anal canal, which is about one and one-half inches long in the adult. At the end of the anal canal is the opening called the anus. Muscles called the anal sphincters aid in the retention of feces until defecation.

Section VI. ASSOCIATED PROTECTIVE STRUCTURES

6-15. GENERAL

Within the body, there are many structures that aid in protection from bacteria, viruses, and other foreign substances. These structures include cells that can phagocytize (engulf) foreign particles or manufacture antibodies (which help to inactivate foreign substances). Collectively, such cells make up the reticuloendothelial system (RES). Such cells are found in bone marrow, the spleen, the liver, and lymph nodes.

6-16. STRUCTURES WITHIN THE DIGESTIVE SYSTEM

Lymphoid structures make up the largest part of the RES. Lymphoid structures are collections of cells associated with circulatory systems (to be discussed in lesson 9).

a. Tonsils are associated with the posterior portions of the respiratory and digestive areas in the head, primarily in the region of the pharynx. The tonsils are masses of lymphoid tissue.

b. Other lymphoid aggregations are found in the walls of the small intestines.

c. The vermiform appendix, attached to the cecum of the large intestine, is also a mass of lymphoid tissue. It is the "tonsil" of the intestines.

Continue with Exercises

EXERCISES, LESSON 6

REQUIREMENT. The following exercises are to be answered by completing the incomplete statement or by writing the answer in the space provided at the end of the question.

After you have completed all the exercises, turn to "Solutions to Exercises," at the end of the lesson and check your answers.

1. What is the human digestive system?

2. What are six major organs of the human digestive system?

    a. _____.

    b. _____.

    c. _____.

    d. _____.

    e. _____.

    f. _____.

3. What are seven important structures associated with the oral cavity?

    a. T_____.

    b. J_____ (m_____ and m_____).

    c. P_____.

    d. L_____ and c_____.

    e. T_____.

    f. S_____ g_____.

    g. T_____ b_____.

4.   The anterior teeth, called incisors and canine teeth, serve as _____.
The posterior teeth, called molars, serve as _____.

5.   The palate serves as the roof of the_____ and the floor of the
_____. The soft palate serves as a _____ to close off
the upper respiratory passageway during swallowing.

6.   The tongue aids in _____ and _____.

7.   The pharynx is a common passageway for both the _____ and
_____ systems.

8.   The esophagus serves as a passageway for food from the _____ to the
_____.

9.   What is the <u>stomach</u>?

10.   The process of digestion is facilitated by special chemicals called
_____ _____. Most digestion and absorption take place in
the _____.

11.   In order after the stomach, the three areas of the small intestines are the
_____, the _____, and the _____. The jejunum and ileum are
attached to the rear wall of the abdomen with a membrane called the _____.

12.   Folds on the inner surfaces of the small intestines are known as
_____. Finger-like projections from these folds are known as
_____.

13.   The digestive function of the liver is to produce a fluid called _____.
The common bile duct joins with the duct of the pancreas as the fluid enters the
_____.

14.   The texture of the pancreas is _____ and _____.
Pertaining to location, the pancreas is stretched across the _____ of the
abdomen.

15.   The primary function of the large intestine is to _____water and
electrolytes. The large intestines remove water until a nearly solid mass is formed
before _____.

16.   In order, the major subdivisions of the large intestines are the
_____, the _____ colon, the _____ colon,
the _____ colon, and the _____ colon.

17.   The rectum terminates in the narrow _____, at the end
of which is an opening called the _____. Muscles called
_____ aid in the retention of feces until defecation.

18.   Attached to the cecum is a mass of lymphoid tissue called the
_____.

Check Your Answers on Next Page

SOLUTIONS TO EXERCISES, LESSON 6

1. The human digestive system is a group of organs designed to take in foods, initially process foods, digest the foods, and eliminate unused materials of food items. It is a hollow tubular system from one end of the body to the other end. (para 6-1a)

2. Six major organs of the human digestive system are the:

   a. Mouth (oral complex).
   b. Pharynx.
   c. Esophagus.
   d. Stomach.
   e. Small intestines.
   f. Large intestines. (para 6-1b)

3. Seven important structures associated with the oral cavity are the:

   a. Teeth.
   b. Jaws (maxilla and mandible).
   c. Palate.
   d. Lips and cheeks.
   e. Tongue.
   f. Salivary glands.
   g. Taste buds. (para 6-3)

4. The anterior teeth, called incisors and canine teeth, serve as choppers. The posterior teeth, called molars, serve as grinders. (para 6-3a(2))

5. The palate serves as the roof of the mouth and the floor of the nasal chamber. The soft palate serves as a trap door to close off the respiratory passageway during swallowing. (para 6-3c)

6. The tongue aids in chewing and swallowing. (para 6-3e)

7. The pharynx is a common passageway for both the respiratory and digestive systems. (para 6-4)

8. The esophagus serves as a passageway for food from the pharynx to the stomach. (para 6-5)

9. The stomach is a sac-like enlargement of the digestive tract specialized for the storage of food. (para 6-6)

10. The process of digestion is facilitated by special chemicals called <u>digestive enzymes</u>. Most digestion and absorption take place in the <u>small intestines</u>. (paras 6-8a, c)

11. In order after the stomach, the three areas of the small intestines are the <u>duodenum</u>, the <u>jejunum</u>, and the <u>ileum</u>. The jejunum and the ileum are attached to the rear wall of the abdomen with a membrane called the <u>mesentery</u>. (para 6-9a)

12. Folds on the inner surfaces of the small intestines are known as <u>plicae</u>. Finger-like projections from these folds are known as <u>villi</u>. (para 6-9c)

13. The digestive function of the liver is to produce a fluid called <u>bile (gall)</u>. The common bile duct joins with the duct of the pancreas as the fluid enters the <u>duodenum</u>. (para 6-10)

14. The texture of the pancreas is <u>soft</u> and <u>pliable</u>. Pertaining to location, the pancreas is stretched across the <u>posterior wall</u> of the abdomen. (para 6-11)

15. The primary function of the large intestine is to <u>salvage</u> water and electrolytes. The large intestines remove water until a nearly solid mass is formed before <u>defecation</u>. (para 6-12)

16. In order, the major subdivisions of the large intestines are the <u>cecum</u>, the <u>ascending</u> colon, the <u>transverse</u> colon, the <u>descending</u> colon, and the <u>sigmoid</u> colon. (para 6-13)

17. The rectum terminates in the narrow <u>anal canal</u>, at the end of which is an opening called the <u>anus</u>. Muscles called <u>anal sphincters</u> aid in the retention of feces until defecation. (para 6-14)

18. Attached to the cecum is a mass of lymphoid tissue called the <u>vermiform appendix</u>. (para 6-16c)

End of Lesson 6

LESSON ASSIGNMENT

LESSON 7   The Human Respiratory System and Breathing.

TEXT ASSIGNMENT   Paragraphs 7-1 through 7-8.

LESSON OBJECTIVES   After completing this lesson, you should be able to:

         7-1. Define <u>respiration</u>, <u>external respiration</u>, <u>internal respiration</u>, and <u>breathing</u>.

         7-2. Identify the main subdivisions of the respiratory system and their functions.

         7-3. Describe the external nose, nasal chambers, pharynx, larynx, trachea, bronchi, alveoli, lungs, and pleural cavities.

         7-4. Describe breathing and breathing mechanisms.

SUGGESTION   After completing the assignment, complete the exercises at the end of this lesson. These exercises will help you to achieve the lesson objectives.

LESSON 7

THE HUMAN RESPIRATORY SYSTEM AND BREATHING

Section I. THE RESPIRATORY SYSTEM

7-1. INTRODUCTION

a. **Respiration**. Respiration is the exchange of gases between the atmosphere and the cells of the body. It is a physiological process. There are two types of respiration--external and internal. External respiration is the exchange of gases between the air in the lungs and blood. Internal respiration is the exchange of gases between the blood and the individual cells of the body.

b. **Breathing**. Breathing is the process that moves air into and out of the lungs. It is a mechanical process. There are two types of breathing in humans--costal (thoracic) and diaphragmatic (abdominal). In costal breathing, the major structure causing the movement of the air is the rib cage. In diaphragmatic breathing, interaction between the diaphragm and the abdominal wall causes the air to move into and out of the lungs.

7-2. COMPONENTS AND SUBDIVISIONS OF THE HUMAN RESPIRATORY SYSTEM

See figure 7-1 for an illustration of the human respiratory system.

a. **Components**. The components of the human respiratory system consist of air passageways and two lungs. Air moves from the outside of the body into tiny sacs in the lungs called alveoli (pronounced al-VE-oh-lie).

b. **Main Subdivisions**. The main subdivisions of the respiratory system may be identified by their relationship to the voice box or larynx. Thus, the main subdivisions are as listed in table 7-1.

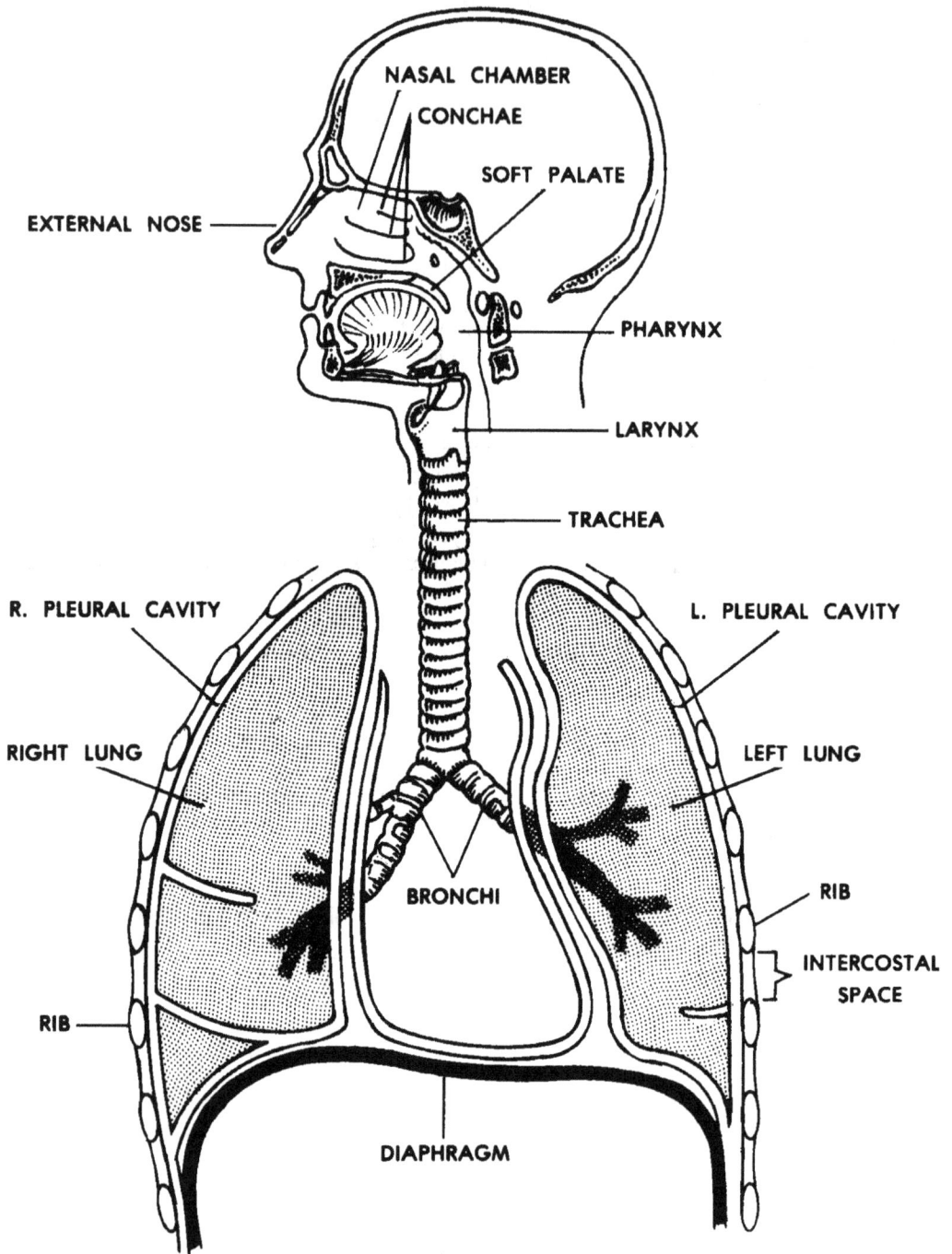

Figure 7-1. The human respiratory system.

SUBDIVISION	FUNCTION
(1) SUPRALARYNGEAL STRUCTURES (su-prah-lah-RIN-je-al)	Cleanse, warm, moisten, and test inflowing air
(2) LARYNX (voice box) (LARE-inks)	Controls the volume of inflowing air; produces selected pitch(vibration frequency) in the moving column of air
(3) INFRALARYNGEAL STRUCTURES (in-frah-lah-RIN-je-al)	Distribute air to the alveoli of the lung where the actual external respiration takes place

Table 7-1. The main subdivisions of the respiratory system.

7-3. SUPRALARYNGEAL STRUCTURES

See figure 7-2.

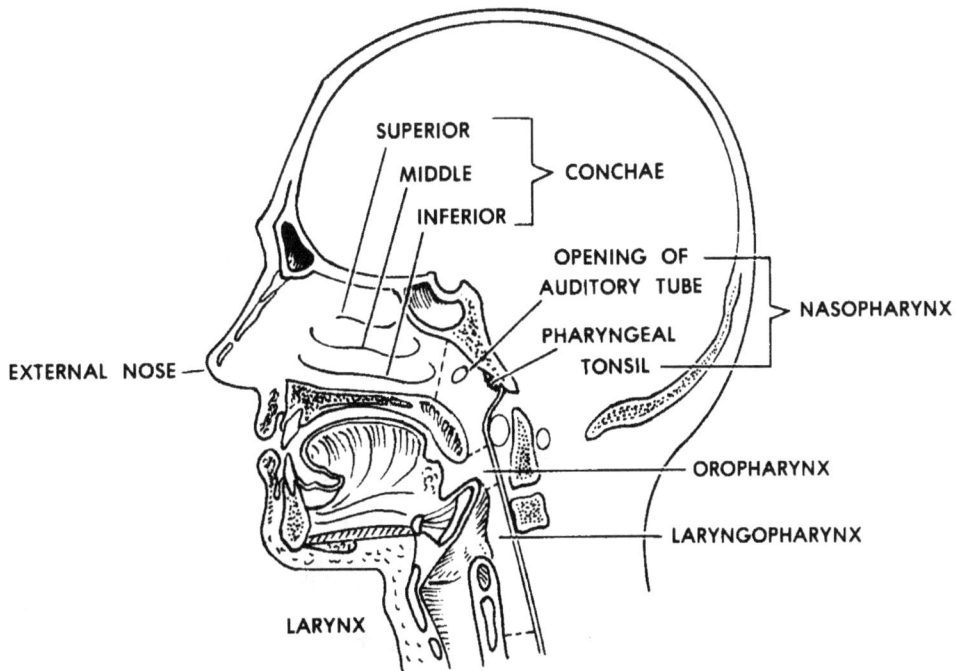

Figure 7-2. Supralaryngeal structures.

a. **External Nose**. The external nose is the portion projecting from the face. It is supported primarily by cartilages. It has a midline divider called the nasal septum, which extends from the internal nose. Paired openings (nostrils) lead to paired spaces (vestibules). Guard hairs in the nostrils filter inflowing air.

b. **Nasal Chambers (Internal Nose)**. Behind each vestibule of the external nose is a nasal chamber. The two nasal chambers together form the internal nose. These chambers too are separated by the nasal septum.

(1) Mucoperiosteum. The walls of the nasal chambers are lined with a thick mucous-type membrane known as the mucoperiosteum. It has a ciliated epithelial surface and a rich blood supply, which provides warmth and moisture. At times, it may become quite swollen.

CILIATED = provided with cilia (hairlike projections which move fluids to the rear)

(2) Conchae. The lateral wall of each chamber has three scroll- like extensions into the nasal chamber which help to increase the surface area exposed to the inflowing air. These scroll-like extensions are known as conchae.

CONCHA (pronounced KON-kah) = sea shell

CONCHA (singular), CONCHAE (plural)

(3) Olfactory epithelium. The sense of smell is due to special nerve endings located in the upper areas of the nasal chambers. The epithelium containing the sensory endings is known as the olfactory epithelium.

(4) Paranasal sinuses. There are air "cells" or cavities in the skull known as paranasal sinuses. The paranasal sinuses are connected with the nasal chambers and are lined with the same ciliated mucoperiosteum. Thus, these sinuses are extensions of the nasal chambers into the skull bones. For this reason, they are known as paranasal sinuses.

c. **Pharynx**. The pharynx (FAIR-inks) is the common posterior space for the respiratory and digestive systems.

(1) Nasopharynx. That portion of the pharynx specifically related to the respiratory system is the nasopharynx. It is the portion of the pharynx above the soft palate. The two posterior openings (nares) of the nasal chambers lead into the single space of the nasopharynx. The auditory (eustachian) tubes also open into the nasopharynx. The auditory tubes connect the nasopharynx with the middle ears (to equalize the pressure between the outside and inside of the eardrum). Lying in the upper posterior wall of the nasopharynx are the pharyngeal tonsils (adenoids). The soft palate floor of the nasopharynx is a trapdoor which closes off the upper respiratory passageways during swallowing.

(2) Oropharynx. The portion of the pharynx closely related to the digestive system is the oropharynx. It is the portion of the pharynx below the soft palate and above the upper edge of the epiglottis. (The epiglottis is the flap that prevents food from entering the larynx (discussed below) during swallowing.)

(3) Laryngopharynx. That portion of the pharynx which is common to the respiratory and digestive systems is the laryngopharynx. It is the portion of the pharynx below the upper edge of the epiglottis. Thus, the digestive and respiratory systems lead into it from above and lead off from it below.

7-4. LARYNX

The larynx, also called the Adam's apple or voice box, connects the pharynx with the trachea. The larynx, located in the anterior neck region, has a box-like shape. See figure 7-3 for an illustration. Since the voice box of the male becomes larger and heavier during puberty, the voice deepens. The adult male's voice box tends to be located lower in the neck; in the female, the larynx remains higher and smaller and the voice is of a higher pitch.

a. **Parts and Spaces**. The larynx has a vestibule ("entrance hallway") which can be covered over by the epiglottis. The glottis itself is the hole between the vocal cords. Through the glottis, air passes from the vestibule into the main chamber of the larynx (below the cords) and then into the trachea. The skeleton of the larynx is made up of a series of cartilages.

b. **Muscles**. The larynx serves two functions and there are two sets of muscles--one for each function.

(1) One set controls the size of the glottis. Thus, it regulates the volume of air passing through the trachea.

(2) The other set controls the tension of the vocal cords. Thus, it produces vibrations of selected frequencies (variations in pitch) of the moving air to be used in the process of speaking.

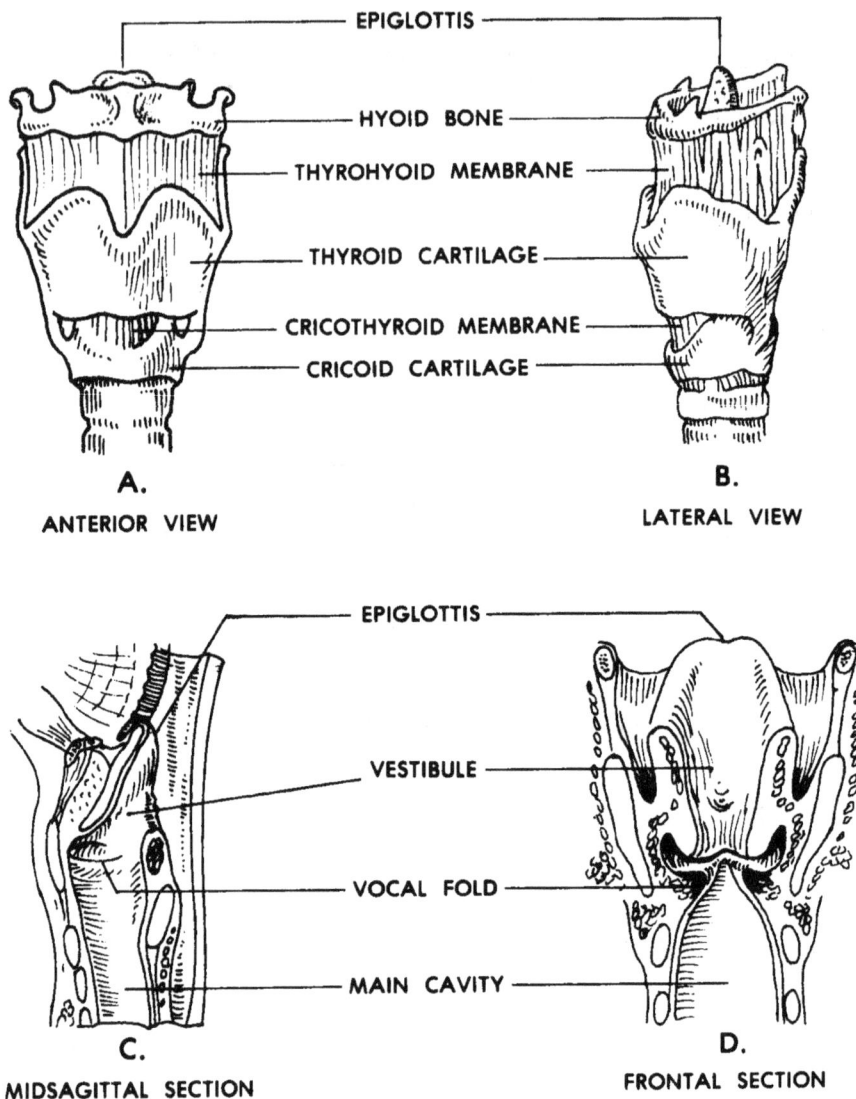

EPIGLOTTIS

HYOID BONE

THYROHYOID MEMBRANE

THYROID CARTILAGE

CRICOTHYROID MEMBRANE

CRICOID CARTILAGE

A.
ANTERIOR VIEW

B.
LATERAL VIEW

EPIGLOTTIS

VESTIBULE

VOCAL FOLD

MAIN CAVITY

C.
MIDSAGITTAL SECTION

D.
FRONTAL SECTION

Figure 7-3. The larynx.

7-5. INFRALARYNGEAL STRUCTURES

a. **Trachea and Bronchi**. The respiratory tree (figure 7-4) is the set of tubular structures which carry the air from the larynx to the alveoli of the lungs. Looking at a person UPSIDE DOWN, the trachea is the trunk of the tree and the bronchi are the branches. These tubular parts are held open (made <u>patent</u>) by rings of cartilage. Their lining is ciliated to remove mucus and other materials that get into the passageway.

A. "RESPIRATORY TREE"

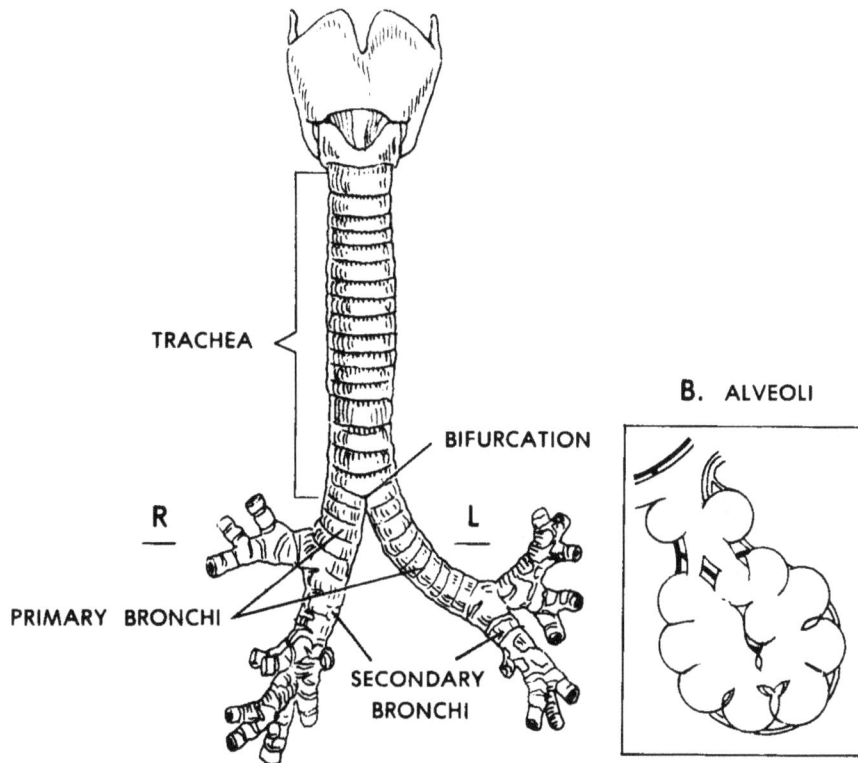

TRACHEA

BIFURCATION

B. ALVEOLI

R

L

PRIMARY BRONCHI

SECONDARY BRONCHI

Figure 7-4. Infralaryngeal structures ("respiratory tree").

b. **Alveoli**. The alveoli (alveolus, singular) are tiny spherical (balloon-like) sacs which are connected to the larger tubes of the lungs by tiny tubes known as alveolar ducts and bronchioles. The alveoli are so small that there are billions in the adult lungs. This very small size produces a maximum surface area through which external respiration takes place. External respiration is the actual exchange of gases between the air in the alveolar spaces and the adjacent blood capillaries through their walls.

c. **Lungs**. A lung is an individual organ composed of tubular structures and alveoli bound together by fibrous connective tissue (FCT). In the human, there are two lungs--right and left. Each lung is supplied by a primary or mainstem bronchus leading off of the trachea. The right lung is larger in volume than the left lung. The left lung must leave room for the heart. The right lung is divided into three pulmonary lobes (upper, middle, and lower) and 10 bronchopulmonary segments (2 + 3 + 5). The left lung is divided into two pulmonary lobes (upper and lower) and eight bronchopulmonary segments (4 + 4). A pulmonary lobe is a major subdivision of a lung marked by fissures (deep folds). Each lobe is further partitioned into bronchopulmonary segments. Each lobe is supplied by a secondary or <u>lobar bronchus</u>. Each segment is supplied by a tertiary or <u>segmental bronchus</u>, a branch of the lobar bronchus.

d. **Pleural Cavities**. See paragraph 3-14 to review a description of pleural cavities. That paragraph indicates that each serous cavity has inner and outer membranes. In the case of the lungs, the inner membrane is known as the <u>visceral pleura</u> which very closely covers the surface of the lungs. The outer membrane is known as the <u>parietal pleura</u>, forming the outer wall of the cavity. The <u>pleural cavities</u> are the potential spaces between the inner and outer membranes. The pleural cavities allow the lungs to move freely with a minimum of friction during the expansion and contraction of breathing.

Section II. BREATHING AND BREATHING MECHANISMS IN HUMANS

7-6. INTRODUCTION

a. Boyle's law tells us that as the volume (V) of a gas-filled container increases, the pressure (P) inside decreases; as the volume (V) of a closed container decreases, the pressure (P) inside increases. When two connected spaces of air have different pressures, the air moves from the space with greater pressure to the one with lesser pressure. In regard to breathing, we can consider the air pressure around the human body to be constant. The pressure inside the lungs may be greater or less than the pressure outside the body. Thus, a greater internal pressure causes air to flow out; a greater external pressure causes air to flow in.

b. We can compare the human trunk to a hollow cylinder. This cylinder is divided into upper and lower cavities by the diaphragm. The upper is the <u>thoracic cavity</u> and is essentially gas-filled. The lower is the <u>abdominopelvic cavity</u> and is essentially water-filled.

7-7. COSTAL (THORACIC) BREATHING

a. **Inhalation**. Muscles attached to the thoracic cage raise the rib cage. A typical rib might be compared to a bucket handle, attached at one end to the sternum (breastbone) and at the other end to the vertebral column. The "bucket handle" is lifted by the overall movement upward and outward of the rib cage. These movements increase the thoracic diameters from right to left (transverse) and from front to back (A-P). Thus, the intrathoracic volume increases. Recalling Boyle's law, the increase in volume leads to a decrease in pressure. The air pressure outside the body then forces air into the lungs and inflates them.

b. **Exhalation**. The rib cage movements and pressure relationships are reversed for <u>exhalation</u>. Thus, intrathoracic volume decreases. The intrathoracic pressure increases and forces air outside the body.

7-8. DIAPHRAGMATIC (ABDOMINAL) BREATHING

The diaphragm is a thin, but strong, dome-shaped muscular membrane that separates the abdominal and thoracic cavities. The abdominal wall is elastic in nature. The abdominal cavity is filled with soft, watery tissues.

a. **Inhalation**. As the diaphragm contracts, the dome flattens and the diaphragm descends. This increases the depth (vertical diameter) of the thoracic cavity and thus increases its volume. This decreases air pressure within the thoracic cavity. The greater air pressure outside the body then forces air into the lungs.

b. **Exhalation**. As the diaphragm relaxes, the elastic abdominal wall forces the diaphragm back up by pushing the watery tissues of the abdomen against the underside of the relaxed diaphragm. The dome extends upward. The process of inhalation is thus reversed.

Continue with Exercises

EXERCISES, LESSON 7

REQUIREMENT. The following exercises are to be answered by completing the incomplete statement or by writing the answer in the space provided at the end of the question.

After you have completed all the exercises, turn to "Solutions to Exercises," at the end of the lesson and check your answers.

1. What is respiration?

2. What is external respiration?

3. What is internal respiration?

4. What is breathing?

5. In costal breathing, the major structure causing movement of the air is the
_____.

6. In diaphragmatic breathing, air movement is caused by interaction between the _____ and the _____.

7. The components of the human respiratory system consist of air _____ and two _____. Air moves from the outside of the body into tiny sacs in the lungs called _____.

8. The main subdivisions of the respiratory system may be identified by their relationship to the _____ (v_____ b_____). The subdivisions are as follows: _____ structures, the _____, and _____ structures.

9. The functions of the supralaryngeal structures are to c_____, w_____, m_____, and t_____ inflowing air.

10. The functions of the larynx are to control the _____ of the inflowing air and to produce selected _____ (_____).

11. The function of the infralaryngeal structures is to distribute air to the _____ of the _____. Here, actual external respiration takes place.

12. The external nose is supported primarily by _____.

13. The two nasal chambers are separated by the _____. The walls of the nasal chambers are lined with a membrane known as the _____. Scroll-like extensions, which increase the surface area of the lateral walls, are known as _____. Sensory endings for the sense of smell are found in the _____ epithelium. Air "cells" or cavities in the skull are known as _____.

14. That portion of the pharynx specifically related to the respiratory system is the _____. It is the portion of the pharynx above the _____.

15. During swallowing, food is prevented from entering the larynx by the _____.

16. In the larynx, one set of muscles regulates the volume of air passing through the trachea by controlling the _____. Another set of muscles produces selected frequencies (variations in pitch) by controlling the _____.

17. The trunk of the respiratory tree is called the _____. The branches are called the _____.

18. What are alveoli?

19. A lung is an individual organ composed of _____ structures and _____ bound together by _____ tissue.

20. The pleural cavities allow the lungs to move freely with a minimum of _____ during the expansion and contraction of breathing.

21. In both costal and diaphragmatic breathing, inhalation depends upon an increase in lung volume. The diameters increased in costal breathing are from _____ and from _____. The diameter increased in diaphragmatic breathing is _____.

Check Your Answers on Next Page

SOLUTIONS TO EXERCISES, LESSON 7

1. Respiration is <u>the exchange of gases between the atmosphere and the cells of the body</u>. (para 7-1a)

2. External respiration is <u>the exchange of gases between the air in the lungs and blood</u>. (para 7-1a)

3. Internal respiration is <u>the exchange of gases between the blood and the individual cells of the body</u>. (para 7-1a)

4. Breathing is <u>the process that moves air into and out of the lungs. It is a mechanical process</u>. (para 7-1b)

5. In costal breathing, the major structure causing movement of the air is the <u>rib cage</u>. (para 7-1b)

6. In diaphragmatic breathing, air movement is caused by interaction between the <u>diaphragm</u> and the <u>abdominal wall</u>. (para 7-1b)

7. The components of the human respiratory system consist of air <u>passageways</u> and two <u>lungs</u>. Air moves from the outside of the body into tiny sacs in the lungs called <u>alveoli</u>. (para 7-2a)

8. The main subdivisions of the respiratory system may be identified by their relationship to the <u>larynx</u> (<u>voice box</u>). The subdivisions are as follows: <u>supralaryngeal</u> structures, the <u>larynx</u>, and <u>infralaryngeal</u> structures. (para 7-2b)

9. The functions of the supralaryngeal structures are to c<u>leanse</u>, <u>warm</u>, m<u>oisten</u>, and <u>test</u> inflowing air. (para 7-2b)

10. The functions of the larynx are to control the <u>volume</u> of the inflowing air and to produce selected <u>pitch</u> (<u>vibration frequency</u>). (para 7-2b)

11. The function of the infralaryngeal structures is to distribute air to the <u>alveoli</u> of the <u>lung</u>. Here, actual external respiration takes place. (para 7-2b)

12. The external nose is supported primarily by <u>cartilages</u>. (para 7-3a)

13. The two nasal chambers are separated by the <u>nasal septum</u>. The walls of the nasal chambers are lined with a membrane known as the <u>mucoperiosteum</u>. Scroll-like extensions, which increase the surface area of the lateral walls, are known as <u>conchae</u>. Sensory endings for the sense of smell are found in the <u>olfactory</u> epithelium. Air "cells" or cavities in the skull are known as <u>paranasal sinuses</u>. (para 7-3b)

14. That portion of the pharynx specifically related to the respiratory system is the nasopharynx. It is the portion of the pharynx above the soft palate. (para 7-3c(1))

15. During swallowing, food is prevented from entering the larynx by the epiglottis. (para 7-3c(2))

16. In the larynx, one set of muscles regulates the volume of air passing through the trachea by controlling the size of the glottis. Another set of muscles produces selected frequencies (variations in pitch) by controlling the tension of the vocal cords. (para 7-4b)

17. The trunk of the respiratory tree is called the trachea. The branches are called the bronchi. (para 7-5a)

18. Alveoli are tiny spherical sacs in the lungs. They are the site of external respiration. (para 7-5b)

19. A lung is an individual organ composed of tubular structures and alveoli bound together by fibrous connective tissue. (para 7-5c)

20. The pleural cavities allow the lungs to move freely with a minimum of friction during the expansion and contraction of breathing. (para 7-5d)

21. In both costal and diaphragmatic breathing, inhalation depends upon an increase in lung volume. The diameters increased in costal breathing are from right to left (transverse) and from front to back (A-P). The diameter increased in diaphragmatic breathing is vertical (depth). (paras 7-7a, 7-8a)

End of Lesson 7

LESSON ASSIGNMENT

LESSON 8   The Human Urogenital Systems.

TEXT ASSIGNMENT   Paragraphs 8-1 through 8-16.

LESSON OBJECTIVES   After completing this lesson, you should be able to:

  8-1. Define <u>urogenital systems</u>.

  8-2. Identify the function and major parts of the human urinary system.

  8-3. Describe the kidney, including its gross internal structure and the structure of the nephron.

  8-4. Describe the ureters, the urinary bladder, and the urethra.

  8-5. Identify general characteristics of both the male and female genital systems.

  8-6. Describe the ovaries, the uterine tubes, the uterus, the vagina, the external genitalia, and secondary sexual characteristics of human females.

  8-7. Describe the testes, the epididymis, the ductus deferens, the seminal vesicles, the ejaculatory duct, the prostate gland, the penis, and the secondary sexual characteristics of human males.

SUGGESTION   After completing the assignment, complete the exercises at the end of this lesson. These exercises will help you to achieve the lesson objectives.

LESSON 8

THE HUMAN UROGENITAL SYSTEMS

Section I. THE HUMAN URINARY SYSTEM

8-1. DEFINITION

The human urogenital systems are made up of the urinary organs, which produce the fluid called urine, and the genital, or reproductive, organs of male and female
humans, which together can produce a new human being.

8-2. INTRODUCTION TO THE HUMAN URINARY SYSTEM

a. Proteins are one of the basic foodstuffs that humans consume. When
proteins are used by the body, there are residue or waste products which can be
poisonous (toxic) if allowed to accumulate in large amounts. The urinary system of the
human body is specialized to remove these nitrogenous waste products from the circulating blood.

b. **Major Parts**. See figure 8-1 for the major parts of the human urinary system.
This system includes two kidneys, two ureters (one connecting each kidney to the
urinary bladder), the urinary bladder, and the urethra.

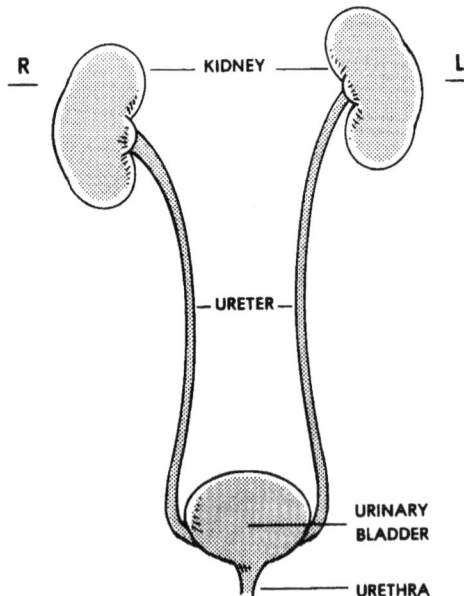

Figure 8-1. The human urinary system.

8-3. THE KIDNEY

   a. **General**.

   (1) The kidneys have the same shape and color as kidney beans, but are about 8-10 centimeters (3-3 1/2 inches) in length.

   (2) Each kidney has a fibrous capsule. On the concave, medial side of each kidney, there is a notch called the hilus. Through this hilus pass the ureter and the NAVL (nerve, artery, vein, and lymphatic) which service the kidney.

   (3) Each kidney is attached to the posterior wall of the abdominal cavity, just above the waistline level. Each is held in place by special fascia and fat.

   b. **Gross Internal Structure**. If we compare the structure of the kidney with that of a cantaloupe (muskmelon), the renal cortex would correspond to the hard rind, the renal medulla would correspond with the edible flesh of the melon, while the renal sinus would correspond to the hollow center (after the seeds have been removed). The medulla consists of pyramids with their bases at the cortex and forming peaks, papillae, which empty into the sinus.

   PAPILLA = pimple, nipple

See figure 8-2 for a section of the kidney showing the inner structure.

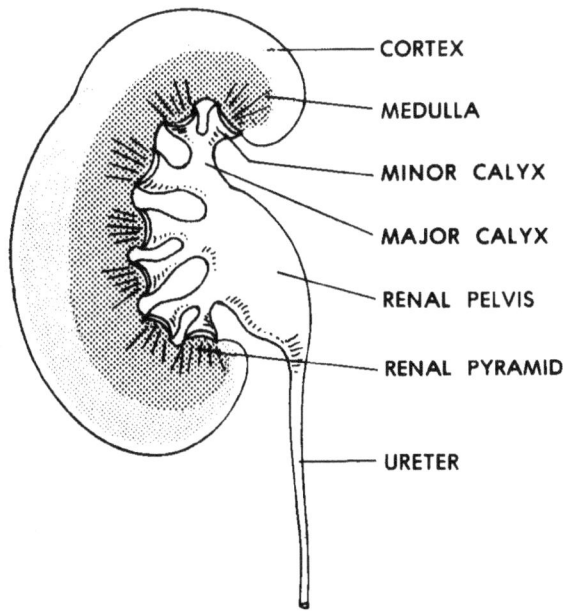

Figure 8-2. A section of a human kidney.

c. **The Nephron**. See figure 8-3 for an illustration of a nephron. Nephrons are the functional units of the human kidney. Their primary function is to remove the wastes of protein usage from the blood. In addition, they serve to conserve water and other materials for continued use by the body. The end result of nephron function is a more or less concentrated fluid called urine. The kidneys contain great numbers of nephrons, about a million for each kidney. The main subdivisions of a nephron are the renal corpuscle and a tubular system.

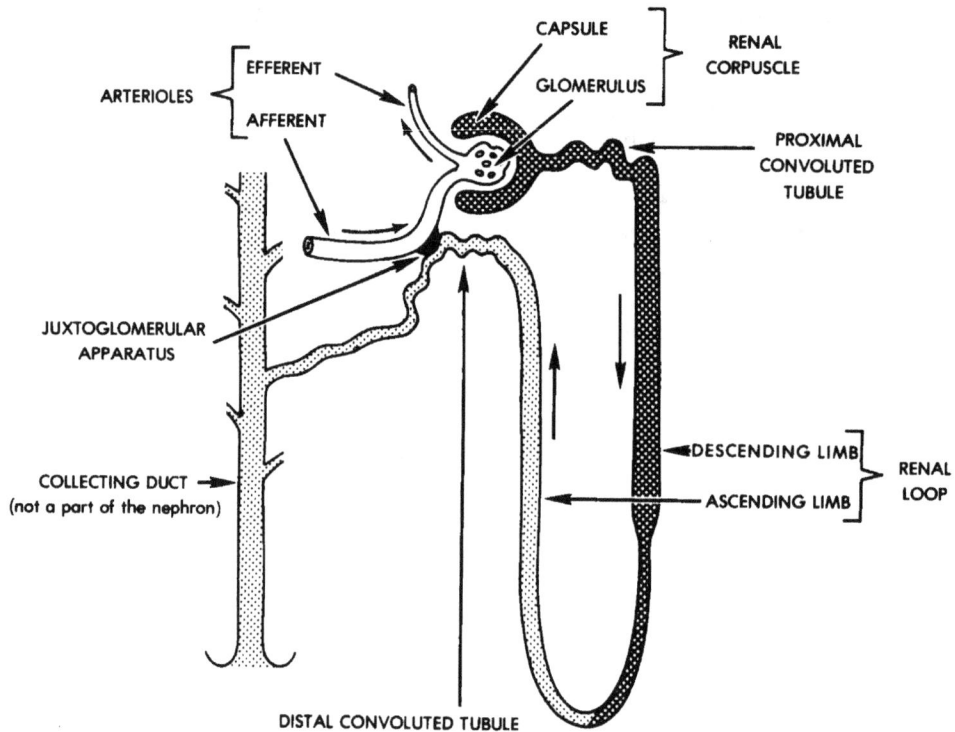

Figure 8-3. A "typical" nephron.

(1) Renal corpuscle. The renal corpuscle has a hollow double- walled sac called the renal capsule ("Bowman's capsule"). Leading into the capsule is a very small artery called the afferent arteriole. Within the capsule, this artery becomes a mass of capillaries known as the glomerulus. An efferent arteriole drains the blood away from the capsule. The capsule and the glomerulus together are known as the renal corpuscle.

(2) Tubules. Each renal capsule is drained by a renal tubule. The first part of this tubule runs quite a distance in a coiled formation and is called the proximal convoluted tubule. A long loop, the renal loop (of Henle), extends down into the medulla with two straight parts and a sharp bend at the bottom. As the tube returns to

the cortex layer, it once again becomes coiled and here is known as the <u>distal convoluted tubule</u>.

(3) <u>Filtration/reabsorption</u>. Except for the blood cells and the larger proteins, the fluid portion of the blood passes through the walls of the glomerulus into the cavity between the two layers of the renal capsule. This fluid is called the <u>glomerular filtrate</u>. By a process of taking back (resorption), the majority of the fluid is removed from the tubules and the concentrated fluid is called the urine.

d. **The Collecting Tubule**. The distal convoluted tubules of several nephrons empty into a collecting tubule. The urine is then passed from the collecting tubule at the papilla of the medullary pyramid. Several collecting tubules are present in each pyramid.

e. **Renal Pelvis**. The <u>renal pelvis</u> is a hollow sac within the sinus of the kidney. Urine from the pyramids collects into the funnel-shaped renal pelvis. The ureter then drains the urine from the renal pelvis.

8-4. URETERS

The <u>ureters</u> are tubes which connect the kidneys to the urinary bladder. The smooth muscle walls of the ureters produce a peristalsis (wave-like movement) that moves the urine along drop by drop.

8-5. URINARY BLADDER

a. The <u>urinary bladder</u> is a muscular organ for storing the urine. Near the inferior posterior corners of the urinary bladder are openings where the ureters empty into the bladder. Also at the inferior aspect of the urinary bladder is the exit, the beginning of the urethra. The triangular area, between the openings of the ureters and the urethra, is called the <u>trigone</u>, or base of the urinary bladder.

b. The urinary bladder wall is stretchable to accommodate varying volumes of urine.

c. Nerve endings called <u>stretch receptors</u> are found in the wall of the urinary bladder. Usually, the <u>pressure</u> within the urinary bladder is low. However, as the volume of the enclosed urine approaches the bladder's capacity, stretching of the wall stimulates the stretch receptors. The cycle of events controlling urination (voiding or emptying of the urinary bladder) is known as the <u>voiding reflex</u>.

8-6. URETHRA

The <u>urethra</u> is a tube which conducts the urine from the urinary bladder to the outside of the body. It begins at the anterior base of the urinary bladder.

a. **Urethral Sphincters**. The urethral sphincters are circular muscle masses which control the passage of the urine through the urethra. There are two urethral sphincters--an internal urethral sphincter and an external urethral sphincter.

(1) The internal urethral sphincter is located in the floor of the urinary bladder. It is made of smooth muscle tissue. It is controlled by nerves of the autonomic nervous system (lesson 11).

(2) The external urethral sphincter is more inferior around the urethra in the area of the pelvic floor. It is made up of striated muscle tissue. It is controlled by the peripheral nervous system (lesson 11).

b. **Male-Female Differences**. The female urethra is short and direct. The male urethra is much longer and has two curvatures. Whereas the female urethra serves only a urinary function, the male urethra serves both the urinary and reproductive functions.

Section II. INTRODUCTION TO HUMAN GENITAL (REPRODUCTIVE) SYSTEMS

8-7. SEXUAL DIMORPHISM

The human male and human female each has a system of organs specifically designed for the production of new humans. These systems are known as reproductive or genital systems. Since there are different systems for males and females, the genital systems are an example of sexual dimorphism.

MORPH = form, shape
DI = two
SEXUAL = according to sex (gender)
SEXUAL DIMORPHISM = having two different forms according to sex

8-8. ADVANTAGES OF DOUBLE PARENTING

The existence of two parents for each child means that genetic materials are recombined to produce a new type. This new type may be an improvement over previous generations.

8-9. MAJOR COMPONENT CATEGORIES OF THE GENITAL SYSTEMS

Components of the genital systems may be considered in the following categories:

a. **Primary Sex Organs (Gonads)**. Primary sex organs produce sex cells (gametes). A male gamete and a female gamete may be united to form the one-cell beginning of an embryo (the process of fertilization). Primary sex organs also produce sex hormones.

b. **Secondary Sex Organs**. Secondary sex organs care for the product of the primary sex organ.

c. **Secondary Sexual Characteristics**. Secondary sexual characteristics are those traits that tend to make males and females more attractive to each other. Secondary sexual characteristics help to ensure mating. These characteristics first appear during puberty (10-15 years of age).

Section III. THE HUMAN FEMALE GENITAL (REPRODUCTIVE) SYSTEM

8-10. PRIMARY SEX ORGANS (OVARIES)

The primary sex organ in the human female is the ovary. See figure 8-4 for an illustration of the female genital system. The ovaries are located to the sides of the upper end of the uterus. They are anchored to the posterior surface of the broad ligaments. (The broad ligaments are sheets or folds of peritoneum enclosing the uterus and uterine tubes and extending to the sides of the pelvis.)

a. The ovary produces the egg cell or ovum (ova, plural).

b. The ovary produces female sex hormones (estrogens and progesterone).

c. The production of ova is cyclic. One ovum is released in each menstrual period, about 28 days.

8-11. SECONDARY SEX ORGANS

a. **Uterine Tubes (Fallopian Tubes, Oviducts)**. Extending to either side of the uterus are two muscular tubes which open at the outer ends like fringed trumpets. The fringe-like appendages encircle the ovaries. At their medial ends, the uterine tubes open into the uterus. The function of the uterine tubes is to pick up the ovum when released from the ovary and hold it UNTIL one of the following happens:

(1) It is fertilized. After fertilization, the initial stages of embryo development take place. The developing embryo is eventually moved into the uterus.

(2) The nutrient stored within the ovum is used up and the ovum dies. This may take three to five days.

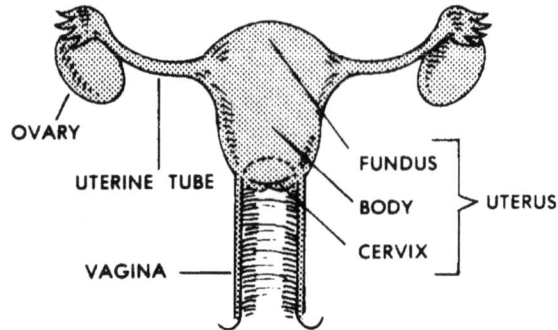

A. ANTERIOR VIEW

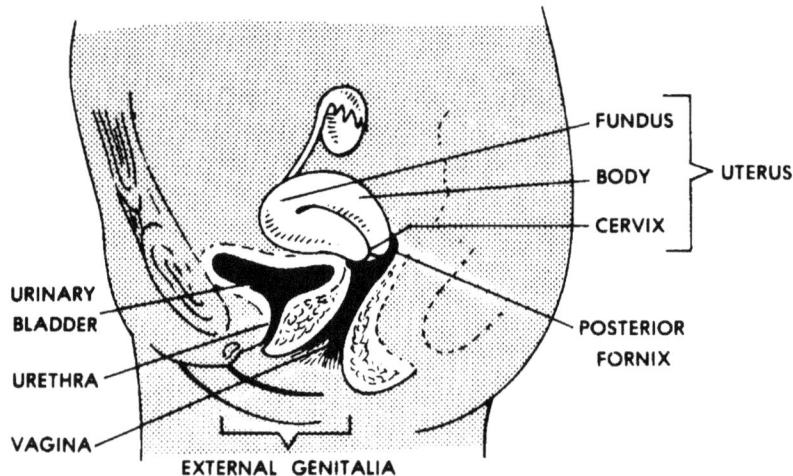

B. MIDSAGITTAL SECTION

Figure 8-4. The human female genital system.

b. **Uterus**. The uterus is the site where all but the first few days of embryo development takes place. After eight weeks of embryonic development, it is known as the fetus.

(1) Main subdivisions. The uterus is shaped like a pear, with the stem (cervix) facing downward and toward the rear. The fundus is the portion of the uterus above the openings of the uterine tubes. The main part, or body, is the portion between the cervix and the fundus. The uterus usually leans forward with the body slightly curved as it passes over the top of the urinary bladder. The cervix opens into the upper end of the vagina.

(2) Wall structure. The inner lining of the uterus is called the endometrium. Made up of epithelium, it is well supplied with blood vessels and glands. The muscular wall of the uterus is called the myometrium. In the body of the uterus, the muscular tissue is in a double spiral arrangement. In the cervix, it is in a circular arrangement.

(3) Age differences. The uterus of an infant female is undeveloped. During puberty, the uterus develops. The uterus of an adult is fully developed. The uterus of an old woman is reduced in size and nonfunctional.

c. **Vagina**. The vagina is a tubular canal connecting the cervix of the uterus with the outside. It serves as a birth canal and as an organ of copulation. It is capable of stretching during childbirth. The lower opening of the vagina may be partially closed by a thin membrane known as the hymen.

d. **External Genitalia**. Other terms for the external genitals of the human female are vulva and pudendum. Included are the:

(1) Mons pubis. The mons pubis is a mound of fat tissue covered with skin and hair in front of the symphysis pubis (the joint of the pubic bones).

(2) Labia majora. Extending back from the mons pubis and encircling the vestibule (discussed below) are two folds known as the labia majora. Their construction is similar to the mons pubis, including fatty tissue and skin. The outer surfaces are covered with hair. The inner surfaces are moist and smooth. The corresponding structure in the male is the scrotum.

LABIA = lips   (LABIUM, singular)

(3) Labia minora. The labia minora are two folds of skin lying within the labia majora and also enclosing the vestibule. In front, each labium minus (minus = singular of minora) divides into two folds. The fold above the clitoris (discussed below) is called the prepuce of the clitoris. The fold below is the frenulum.

(4) Clitoris. The clitoris is a small projection of sensitive erectile tissue which corresponds to the male penis. However, the female urethra does not pass through the clitoris.

(5) Vestibule. The cleft between the labia minora and behind the clitoris is called the vestibule. It includes the urethral opening in front and the vaginal opening slightly to the rear.

e. **Pregnancy and Delivery**. When an embryo forms an attachment to the endometrium, a pregnancy exists. The attachment eventually forms a placenta, an organ joining mother and offspring for such purposes as nutrition of the offspring. The fetal membranes surround the developing individual (fetus) and are filled with amniotic fluid.

(1) During the first eight weeks, the developing organism is known as an embryo. During this time, the major systems and parts of the body develop.

(2) During the remainder of the pregnancy, the developing organism is known as the fetus. During this time, growth and refinement of the body parts occur.

(3) Parturition is the actual delivery of the fetus into a free- living state. The delivery of the fetus is followed by a second delivery-- that of the placenta and fetal membranes.

f. **Menstruation and Menopause**. About two weeks after an ovum is released, if it is not fertilized, menstruation occurs. Menstruation involves the loss of all but the basal layer of the endometrium. This process includes bleeding. It first occurs at puberty and lasts until menopause (45 to 55 years of age). After menopause, pregnancy is no longer possible.

8-12. SECONDARY SEXUAL CHARACTERISTICS

The secondary sexual characteristics of females include growth of pubic hair, development of mammary glands, development of the pelvic girdle, and deposition of fat in the mons pubis and labia majora.

8-13. MAMMARY GLANDS

The mammary glands were previously mentioned in paragraph 3-6c. Secretion of milk begins after parturition. Stimulation from suckling helps to maintain the normal rate of milk secretion. At the time of menopause, breast tissue becomes less prominent.

Section IV. THE HUMAN MALE GENITAL (REPRODUCTIVE) SYSTEM

8-14. PRIMARY SEX ORGANS (TESTES)

The primary sex organ of the human male is the testis. See figure 8-5 for an illustration of the male genital system. The testes are egg-shaped.

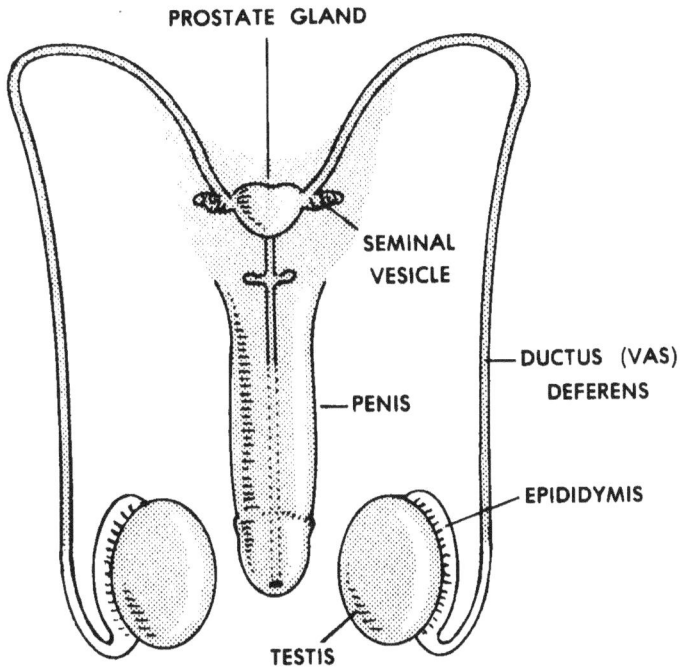

A. SCHEME OF ANTERIOR VIEW

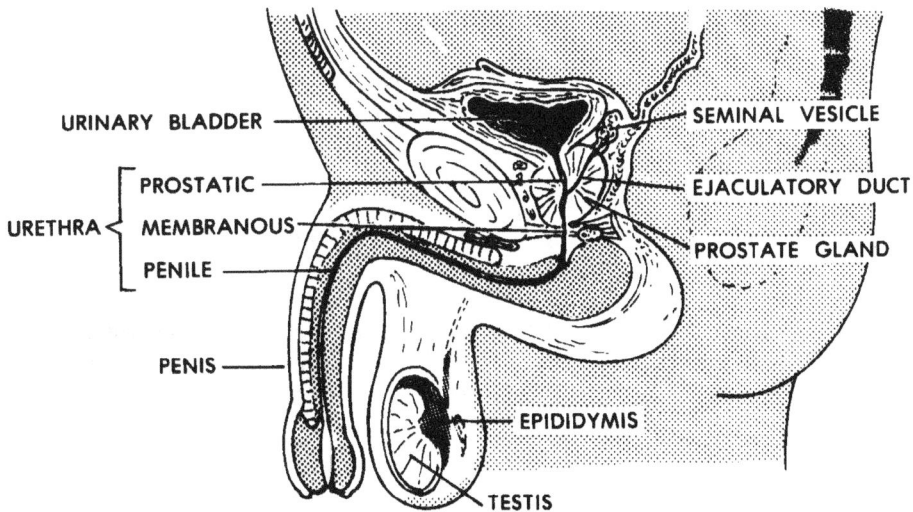

B. MIDSAGITTAL SECTION

Figure 8-5. The human male genital system.

a. **Location**. The paired testes lie within the scrotum. The scrotum is a sac of loose skin attached in the pubic area of the lower abdomen. The scrotum provides a site cooler than body temperature to maintain the viability of the spermatozoa. However, when the air is too cold, muscles and muscular fibers draw the testes and scrotum closer to the body to maintain warmth. Otherwise, the scrotum hangs loosely. The tunica vaginalis is a serous cavity surrounding each testis.

b. **Functions**. The testis produces the male sex cells called spermatozoa (spermatozoon, singular). The spermatozoa are continuously produced by the millions. One such cell may eventually fertilize an ovum of a human female. The testes also produce male sex hormones called androgens.

8-15. SECONDARY SEX ORGANS

a. **Epididymis**. The epididymis is a coiled tube whose function is to aid in the maturation of spermatozoa. Its coiled length is only about one and one-half inches. Its uncoiled length is about 16 feet. When coiled, it extends downward along the posterior side of each testis. Its lining secretes a nutritive medium for spermatozoa. It receives spermatozoa from the testes in an immature state. As the spermatozoa pass through the nutrient, they mature.

b. **Ductus (Vas) Deferens**. The ductus deferens is a transporting tube which carries the mature sperm from the epididymis to the prostate. Each tube enters the abdomen through the inguinal canal. Each passes over a ureter to reach the back of the urinary bladder and then down to the prostate gland.

c. **Seminal Vesicles**. Lying alongside each ductus deferens as it crosses the back of the bladder is a tubular structure called the seminal vesicle. The seminal vesicle produces a fluid which becomes part of the ejaculate.

d. **Ejaculatory Duct**. Each ductus deferens and its corresponding seminal vesicle converge to form a short tube called the ejaculatory duct. The ejaculatory duct opens into the urethra within the prostate gland. The ejaculatory duct carries both sperma-tozoa and seminal vesicle fluid.

e. **Prostate Gland**. As the urethra leaves the urinary bladder, its first inch is surrounded by a chestnut-size gland called the prostate gland. The prostate gland provides an additional fluid to be added to the spermatozoa and seminal vesicle fluid.

f. **Penis**. As the urethra leaves the abdomen, it passes through the penis, the male organ of copulation.

(1) Surrounding the urethra is a central cylinder of erectile tissue called the corpus spongiosum. This cylinder is bulb-shaped at each end. The posterior end is attached to the base of the pelvis. The sensitive anterior end is known as the glans.

CORPUS SPONGIOSUM = spongy body

(2) Overlying the corpus spongiosum is a pair of cylinders of erectile tissue called the corpora cavernosa. These two cylinders are separate in their proximal fourth and joined in their distal three-fourths. They are attached to the pubic bones. Together, the corpus spongiosum and the corpora cavernosa combine to form the shaft of the penis.

CORPUS CAVERNOSUM = cavernous body

(3) The prepuce, or foreskin, is a covering of skin for the glans. It may be removed in a surgical procedure called circumcision.

8-16. SECONDARY SEXUAL CHARACTERISTICS

The secondary sexual characteristics of male include growth of facial, pubic, and chest hair; growth of the larynx to deepen the voice; and deposition of protein to increase muscularity and general body size.

Continue with Exercises

EXERCISES, LESSON 8

REQUIREMENT. The following exercises are to be answered by completing the incomplete statement or by writing the answer in the space provided at the end of the question.

After you have completed all the exercises, turn to "Solutions to Exercises," at the end of the lesson and check your answers.

1. The human urogenital systems are made up of the u_____ organs, which produce the fluid called _____, and the _____, or _____, organs of male and female humans, which together can produce a new human.

2. The urinary system is specialized to remove certain _____ from the circulating blood. These result from the body's use of _____.

3. The major parts of the human urinary system are two _____, two _____, one _____, and one _____.

4. On the concave, medial side of each kidney, there is a notch called the _____. Through this notch pass the _____ and the _____ which service the kidney.

5. If we compare the structure of the kidney with that of a cantaloupe, the structure corresponding to the hard rind would be the _____ _____. The structure corresponding to the edible flesh of the melon would be the _____. Corresponding to the hollow center (after removal of the seeds) would be the _____. The pyramids of the renal medulla form peaks called _____, which empty into the _____ _____.

6. The functional unit of the human kidney is the _____. Its main subdivisions are the _____ and a _____ system.

7. The renal corpuscle is composed of the _____ and the _____ _____. Blood enters by way of the _____ arteriole, passes through the tangled mass of capillaries called the _____, and leaves by way of the _____ arteriole. Leaving the blood, fluid is first collected in the double-walled sac called the _____ _____.

8.   The first coiled portion of the renal tubule is known as the
_____. The hairpin-shaped portion of the renal
tubule is known as the _____. The second coiled portion is
known as the _____.

9.   The distal convoluted tubules of several nephrons empty into a _____
tubule. The urine is then passed from the collecting tubule at the _____ of the
medullary pyramid. Several collecting tubules are present in each _____. There
is a hollow sac within the sinus of the kidney called the _____. The ureter then
drains the urine from the _____.

10.   What are ureters?

      What mechanism is used by ureters to move urine?

11.   The urinary bladder is a muscular organ for _____ing the urine.
The triangular base of the urinary bladder is known as the _____. The two
posterior corners of the trigone are the points where the _____ empty into the
bladder. The anterior corner of the trigone is the opening of the _____. Nerve
endings stimulated by the stretching of the bladder walls are known as _____.

12.   What is the urethra?

      At what part of the urinary bladder does the urethra begin?

      There is an _____ urethral sphincter and an _____ urethral sphincter. The
internal urethral sphincter is located in the _____ of the urinary bladder. It is
controlled by nerves of the _____ nervous system. The external urethral
sphincter is more inferior, in the area of the _____. It is controlled by nerves
of the _____ nervous system.

13.   The female urethra is _____ and _____.
The male urethra is much longer and has two _____. The female urethra serves
only a _____ function. The male urethra serves both the _____ and
_____ functions.

14. Since there are different genital systems for males and females, genital systems are an example of _____.

15. Primary sex organs produce _____ cells (_____). Primary sex organs also produce _____.

What do secondary sex organs do?

Secondary sexual characteristics help to ensure mating by
_____.

16. The primary sex organ of the human female is the _____. The ovaries are located to the sides of the upper end of the _____. They are anchored to the posterior surface of the _____. The broad ligaments are sheets or folds of _____ enclosing the _____ and uterine _____ and extending to the sides of the _____. The ovary produces the egg cell or _____. The ovary produces chemicals called female sex _____ (_____ and _____). One ovum is released in each _____ period.

17. Uterine tubes are two muscular tubes which extend to either side of the _____ and open at the outer ends. Fringe-like appendages encircle the _____. At their medial ends, the uterine tubes open into the _____. The function of a uterine tube is to _____ and hold it until (a) it is _____ OR (b) the nutrient is _____ and the ovum _____.

18. The uterus is the site for all but the first few days of the development of the _____. The uterus is shaped like a _____. The stem, or _____, faces _____. It opens into the _____. The uterus leans anteriorly with the body slightly curved as the body passes over the top of the _____.

19. The inner lining of the uterus is called the _____. The muscular wall of the uterus is called the _____.

20. The vagina is a tubular canal connecting the _____ of the _____ with the outside. The vagina serves as a _____ and as an organ of _____.

21. The external genitalia of the human female include the _____, the _____, the _____, the _____, and the _____.

22. The mons pubis is a mound of _____ tissue, covered with ____ and _____, in front of the s_____ p_____.

23. The labia majora are two folds of _____ tissue and _____ which extend back from the _____ and encircle the _____. The outer surfaces are covered with _____. The inner surfaces are _____ and _____.

24. The labia minora are two folds of skin lying within the _____ and also enclosing the _____.

25. What is the clitoris?

26. During the first eight weeks of pregnancy, the developing organism is known as a(n) _____. Thereafter, the developing organism is known as a(n) _____. At the time of birth, the second delivery is that of the _____ and f_____ m_____.

27. The secondary sexual characteristics of females include growth of _____ hair, development of _____ glands, development of the _____ girdle, and deposition of fat in the _____ and _____.

28. The primary sex organ of the human male is the _____. The testes are shaped like _____. Their location is within the _____. The scrotum is a sac of loose _____ attached in the _____ area of the lower abdomen.

How does the scrotum affect the temperature of the spermatozoa?

The testis produces the male sex cells called _____. The testis also produces chemicals, or _____, called _____.

29.   The epididymis is a coiled _____ whose function is to aid in the
_____ of _____. Its lining secretes a _____ medium for _____.
As the spermatozoa pass through the nutrient, they _____.

30.   The ductus deferens is a _____ing tube which carries the
_____ from the _____ to the _____. Each tube enters the abdomen
through the _____. Each tube passes over a _____ to reach the back
of the _____ and then down to the _____.

31.   Lying alongside each ductus deferens as it crosses the bladder is a tubular
structure called the _____.

32.   The prostate gland is a _____-size gland that surrounds the first inch of
the _____ as it leaves the _____. It provides an additional fluid to be
added to the _____ and _____ fluid.

33.   The penis is the male organ of _____. Passing through the penis is
the _____. The penis has a central cylinder of erectile tissue called the
_____. Each end of this cylinder is _____-shaped. The sensitive
anterior end is known as the _____.

      What are the corpora cavernosa?

      When present, a covering of skin for the glans is called the _____ or
_____.

34.   The secondary characteristics of males include growth of _____,
_____, and _____ hair; growth of the _____ to deepen the voice;
and deposition of protein to increase _____y and general body size.

Check Your Answers on Next Page

SOLUTIONS TO EXERCISES, LESSON 8

1. The human urogenital systems are made up of the <u>urinary</u> organs, which produce the fluid called <u>urine</u>, and the <u>genital</u>, or <u>reproductive</u>, organs   of male and female humans, which together can produce a new human. (para 8-1)

2. The urinary system is specialized to remove certain <u>nitrogenous waste products</u> from the circulating blood. These result from the body's use of <u>proteins</u>. (para 8-2a)

3. The major parts of the human urinary system are two <u>kidneys</u>, two <u>ureters</u>, one <u>urinary bladder</u>, and one <u>urethra</u>. (para 8-2b)

4. On the concave, medial side of each kidney there is a notch called the <u>hilus</u>. Through this notch pass the <u>ureter</u> and the <u>NAVL</u> which service the kidney. (para 8-3a(2))

5. If we compare the structure of the kidney with that of a cantaloupe, the structure corresponding to the hard rind would be the <u>renal cortex</u>. The structure corresponding to the edible flesh of the melon would be the <u>renal medulla</u>. Corresponding to the hollow center (after removal of the seeds) would be the <u>renal sinus</u>. The pyramids of the renal medulla form peaks called <u>papillae</u>, which empty into the <u>renal sinus</u>. (para 8-3b)

6. The functional unit of the human kidney is the <u>nephron</u>. Its main subdivisions are the <u>renal corpuscle</u> and a <u>tubular</u> system. (para 8-3c)

7. The renal corpuscle is composed of the <u>glomerulus</u> and the <u>renal capsule</u>. Blood enters by way of the <u>afferent</u> arteriole, passes through the tangled mass of capillaries called the <u>glomerulus</u>, and leaves by way of the <u>efferent</u> arteriole. Leaving the blood, fluid is first collected in the double-walled sac called the <u>renal capsule</u>. (para 8-3c)

8. The first coiled portion of the renal tubule is known as the <u>proximal convoluted tubule</u>. The hairpin-shaped portion of the renal tubule is known as the <u>renal loop (of Henle)</u>. The second coiled portion is known as the <u>distal convoluted tubule</u>. (para 8-3c(2))

9. The distal convoluted tubules of several nephrons empty into a <u>collecting</u> tubule. The urine is then passed from the collecting tubule at the <u>papilla</u> of the medullary pyramid. Several collecting tubules are present in each <u>pyramid</u>. There is a hollow sac within the sinus of the kidney called the <u>renal pelvis</u>. The ureter then drains the urine from the <u>renal pelvis</u>. (paras 8-3d, e)

10. Ureters are <u>tubes which connect the kidneys to the urinary bladder</u>. The mechanism used by ureters to move urine is <u>peristalsis</u>. (para 8-4)

11.	The urinary bladder is a muscular organ for storing the urine. The triangular base of the urinary bladder is known as the trigone. The two posterior corners of the trigone are the points where the ureters empty into the bladder. The anterior corner of the trigone is the opening of the urethra. Nerve endings stimulated by the stretching of the bladder walls are known as stretch receptors. (para 8-5)

12.	The urethra is a tube conducting urine from the urinary bladder to the outside of the body. It begins at the anterior base of the urinary bladder. There is an internal urethral sphincter and an external urethral sphincter. The internal urethral sphincter is located in the floor of the urinary bladder. It is controlled by nerves of the autonomic nervous system. The external urethral sphincter is more inferior, in the area of the pelvic floor. It is controlled by nerves of the peripheral nervous system. (para 8-6a)

13.	The female urethra is short and direct. The male urethra is much longer and has two curvatures. The female urethra serves only a urinary function. The male urethra serves both the urinary and reproductive functions. (para 8-6b)

14.	Since there are different genital systems for males and females, genital systems are an example of sexual dimorphism. (para 8-7)

15.	Primary sex organs produce sex cells (gametes). Primary sex organs also produce sex hormones. What do secondary sex organs do? Secondary sex organs care for the product of the primary sex organ. Secondary sexual characteristics help to ensure mating by making males and females more attractive to each other. (para 8-9)

16.	The primary sex organ of the human female is the ovary. The ovaries are located to the sides of the upper end of the uterus. They are anchored to the posterior surface of the broad ligaments. The broad ligaments are sheets or folds of peritoneum enclosing the uterus and uterine tubes and extending to the sides of the pelvis. The ovary produces the egg cell or ovum. The ovary produces chemicals called female sex hormones (estrogens and progesterone). One ovum is released in each menstrual period. (para 8-10)

17.	Uterine tubes are two muscular tubes which extend to either side of the uterus and open at the outer ends. Fringe-like appendages encircle the ovaries. At their medial ends, the uterine tubes open into the uterus. The function of a uterine tube is to pick up the ovum when it is released from the ovary and hold it until (a) it is fertilized, or (b) the nutrient is used up and the ovum dies. (para 8-11a)

18.	The uterus is the site for all but the first few days of the development of the embryo and fetus. The uterus is shaped like a pear. The stem, or cervix, faces downward and to the rear. It opens into the upper end of the vagina. The uterus leans anteriorly with the body slightly curved as the body passes over the top of the urinary bladder. (para 8-11b)

19. The inner lining of the uterus is called the <u>endometrium</u>. The muscular wall of the uterus is called the <u>myometrium</u>. (para 8-11b(2))

20. The vagina is a tubular canal connecting the <u>cervix</u> of the <u>uterus</u> with the outside. The vagina serves as a <u>birth canal</u> and as an organ of <u>copulation</u>. (para 8-11c)

21. The external genitalia of the human female include the <u>mons pubis</u>, the <u>labia majora</u>, the <u>labia minora</u>, the <u>clitoris</u>, and the <u>vestibule</u>. (para 8-11d)

22. The mons pubis is a mound of <u>fat</u> tissue, covered with <u>skin</u> and <u>hair</u>, in front of the <u>symphysis pubis</u>. (para 8-11d(1))

23. The labia majora are two folds of <u>fatty</u> tissue and <u>skin</u> which extend back from the <u>mons pubis</u> and encircle the <u>vestibule</u>. The outer surfaces are covered with <u>hair</u>. The inner surfaces are <u>moist</u> and <u>smooth</u>. (para 8-11d(2))

24. The labia minora are two folds of skin lying within the <u>labia majora</u> and also enclosing the <u>vestibule</u>. (para 8-11d(3))

25. The clitoris is <u>a small projection of erectile tissue corresponding to the male penis</u>. (para 8-11d(4))

26. During the first eight weeks of pregnancy, the developing organism is known as an <u>embryo</u>. Thereafter, the developing organism is known as a <u>fetus</u>. At the time of birth, the second delivery is that of the <u>placenta</u> and <u>fetal</u> <u>membranes</u>. (para 8-11e)

27. The secondary sexual characteristics of females include growth of <u>pubic</u> hair, development of <u>mammary</u> glands, development of the <u>pelvic</u> girdle, and deposition of fat in the <u>mons pubis</u> and <u>labia majora</u>. (para 8-12)

28. The primary sex organ of the human male is the <u>testis</u>. The testes are shaped like <u>eggs</u>. Their location is within the <u>scrotum</u>. The scrotum is a sac of loose <u>skin</u> attached in the <u>pubic</u> area of the lower abdomen. <u>The scrotum provides a site cooler than body temperature to maintain the viability of the spermatozoa. When the air is too cold, muscles and muscular fibers draws the testes and scrotum closer to the body to maintain warmth. Otherwise, the scrotum hangs loosely</u>. The testis produces male sex cells called <u>spermatozoa</u>. The testis also produces chemicals, or <u>male sex hormones</u>, called androgens. (para 8-14)

29. The epididymis is a coiled <u>tube</u> whose function is to aid in the <u>maturation</u> of <u>spermatozoa</u>. Its lining secretes a <u>nutritive</u> medium for <u>spermatozoa</u>. As the spermatozoa pass through the nutrient, they <u>mature</u>. (para 8-15a)

30. The ductus deferens is a transporting tube which carries the mature sperm from the epididymis to the prostate. Each tube enters the abdomen through the inguinal canal. Each tube passes over a ureter to reach the back of the urinary bladder and then down to the prostate gland. (para 8-15b)

31. Lying alongside each ductus deferens as it crosses the back of the bladder is a tubular structure called the seminal vesicle. (para 8-15c)

32. The prostate gland is a chestnut-size gland that surrounds the first inch of the urethra as it leaves the urinary bladder. It provides an additional fluid to be added to the spermatozoa and seminal vesicle fluid. (para 8-15e)

33. The penis is the male organ of copulation. Passing through the penis is the urethra. The penis has a central cylinder of erectile tissue called the corpus spongiosum. Each end of this cylinder is bulb-shaped. The sensitive anterior end is known as the glans. The corpora cavernosa are a pair of cylinders of erectile tissue overlying the corpus spongiosum. When present, a covering of skin for the glans is called the prepuce or foreskin. (para 8-15f)

34. The secondary sexual characteristics of males include growth of facial, pubic, and chest hair; growth of the larynx to deepen the voice; and deposition of protein to increase muscularity and general body size. (para 8-16)

End of Lesson 8

LESSON ASSIGNMENT

LESSON 9

The Human Cardiovascular and Lymphatic Systems.

TEXT ASSIGNMENT

Paragraphs 9-1 through 9-10.

LESSON OBJECTIVES

After completing this lesson, you should be able to:

9-1. Name and briefly explain the four basic components of any circulatory system.

9-2. Define the human <u>cardiovascular</u> <u>system</u>, name its four major components, and match its components with the four basic components of any circulatory system.

9-3. Briefly describe plasma and the formed elements of the blood and state four general functions of blood.

9-4. Describe the general construction of a blood vessel; name three types of blood vessels; state the basic function of each type.

9-5. Describe the general construction of the human heart, including its auricles, atria, ventricles, septa, wall layers, variations of wall thickness, and the names, structures, and position of the cardiac valves.

9-6. Describe three different control systems regulating the heart beat.

9-7. Describe the coronary arteries and cardiac veins and their function.

9-8. Briefly describe the pericardium.

9-9. Describe cardiovascular circulatory patterns, including the terms <u>collateral circulation</u>, <u>end artery</u>, <u>pulmonary cycle</u>, and <u>systemic cycle</u>. Name the major arteries and veins of the human body and the areas serviced or supplies.

9-10. Briefly describe lymphatic capillaries, lymph vessels (including the thoracic duct), lymph nodes, and tonsils.

SUGGESTION

After completing the assignment, complete the exercises at the end of this lesson. These exercises will help you to achieve the lesson objectives.

LESSON 9

THE HUMAN CARDIOVASCULAR AND LYMPHATIC SYSTEMS

Section I. INTRODUCTION

9-1. NEED FOR CIRCULATORY SYSTEMS

a. The need for circulatory systems is based on two criteria:

(1) <u>Number of cells</u>. Multicellular animals are animals with a great number of cells.

(2) <u>Size</u>. In larger animals, most cells are too far away from sources of food and oxygen for simple diffusion to provide sufficient amounts. Also, distances are too great for simple removal of wastes.

b. Because of these criteria, we need a system (or systems) to carry materials to all cells. To get food and oxygen to the cells and to remove waste products, we need a <u>transport</u> system or <u>circulatory</u> system. Human circulatory systems are so effective that no cell is more than two cells away from a blood capillary.

9-2. BASIC COMPONENTS OF ANY CIRCULATORY SYSTEM

The four basic components of any circulatory system are a vehicle, conduits, a motive force, and exchange areas.

a. **Vehicle**. The <u>vehicle</u> is the substance which actually carries the materials being transported.

b. **Conduits**. A <u>conduit</u> is a channel, pipe, or tube through which a vehicle travels.

c. **Motive Force**. If we say that a force is <u>motive</u>, we mean that it produces movement. Systems providing a motive force are often known as <u>pumps</u>.

d. **Exchange Areas**. Since the materials being transported must eventually be exchanged with a part of the body, special areas are developed for this purpose. They are called <u>exchange areas</u>.

9-3. CIRCULATORY SYSTEMS IN THE HUMAN BODY

a. The <u>cardiovascular system</u> is the circulatory system involving the heart and blood vessels.

b. The lymphatic system is a drainage-type circulatory system involved with the clear fluid known as lymph.

c. There are other minor circulatory systems in the human body, such as the one involved with cerebrospinal fluid.

Section II. THE HUMAN CARDIOVASCULAR SYSTEM

9-4. GENERAL

The human cardiovascular system is a collection of interacting structures designed to supply oxygen and nutrients to living cells and to remove carbon dioxide and other wastes. Its major components are the:

a. **Blood**. Blood is the vehicle for oxygen, nutrients, and wastes.

b. **Blood Vessels**. Blood vessels are the conduits, or channels, through which the blood is moved.

c. **Heart**. The heart is the pump which provides the primary motive force.

d. **Capillaries**. The capillaries, minute (very small) vessels, provide exchange areas. For example, in the capillaries of the lungs, oxygen is added and carbon dioxide is removed from the blood.

9-5. BLOOD

Blood is the vehicle for the human cardiovascular system. Its major subdivisions are the plasma, a fluid containing proteins, and the formed elements, including red blood cells, white blood cells, and platelets.

a. **Plasma**.

(1) Plasma makes up about 55 percent of the total blood volume. It is mainly composed of water. A variety of materials are dissolved in plasma. Among the most important of these are proteins.

(2) After the blood clots, the clear fluid remaining is called serum. Serum does not contain the proteins used for clotting. Otherwise, it is very similar to plasma.

b. **Formed Elements**. The formed elements make up about 45 percent of the total blood volume. The formed elements are cellular in nature. While the red blood cells (RBCs) and white blood cells (WBCs) are cells, the platelets are only fragments of cells.

(1) <u>Red blood cells (erythrocytes)</u>. RBCs are biconcave discs. That is, they are shaped something like an inner tube from an automobile tire, but with a thin middle portion instead of a hole. There are approximately 5,000,000 RBCs in a cubic millimeter of normal adult blood. RBCs contain <u>hemoglobin</u>, a protein which carries most of the oxygen transported by the blood.

(2) <u>White blood cells (leukocytes)</u>. There are various types of WBCs, but the most common are <u>neutrophils</u> and <u>lymphocytes</u>. Neutrophils phagocytize (swallow up) foreign particles and organisms and digest them. Lymphocytes produce antibodies and serve other functions in immunity. In normal adults, there are about 5,000 to 11,000 WBCs per cubic millimeter of blood.

(3) <u>Platelets</u>. Platelets are about half the size of erythrocytes. They are fragments of cells. Since they are fragile, they last only about three to five days. Their main function is to aid in clotting by clumping together and by releasing chemical factors related to clotting. There are 150,000 - 350,000 platelets in a cubic millimeter of normal blood.

c. **Some General Functions of the Blood**.

(1) Blood serves as a <u>vehicle</u> for oxygen, nutrients, carbon dioxide and other wastes, hormones, antibodies, heat, etc.

(2) Blood aids in <u>temperature control</u>. Beneath the skin, there is a network of vessels that functions much like a radiator. To avoid accumulation of excess heat in the body, the flow of blood to these vessels can be increased greatly. Here, aided by the evaporative cooling provided by the sweat glands, large amounts of heat can be rapidly given off. The flow of blood also helps keep the outer parts of the body from becoming too cold.

(3) The blood aids in <u>protecting our bodies</u> by providing immunity. Some WBCs phagocytize (swallow up) foreign particles and microorganisms. Other WBCs produce antibodies. The blood transports antibodies throughout the body.

(4) <u>Blood clotting</u> is another function of blood. Not only does this prevent continued blood loss, it also helps prevent invasion of the body by microorganisms and viruses by sealing the wound opening.

9-6. BLOOD VESSELS

The blood is conducted or carried through the body by tubular structures known as <u>blood vessels</u>. Since at no time does the whole blood ever leave a blood vessel of some sort, we refer to this system as a <u>closed system</u>.

a. **General Construction**. The blood vessels in general are tubular and have a three-layered wall.

(1) Intima. The lumen (hollow central cavity) is lined by a layer of smooth epithelium known as the intima.

(2) Media. A middle layer of smooth muscle tissue is called the media.

(3) Adventitia. The adventitia is the outer layer of fibrous connective tissue that holds everything together.

b. **Types of Blood Vessels**. See figure 9-1 for a diagram of the human circulatory system. We recognize three types of blood vessels:

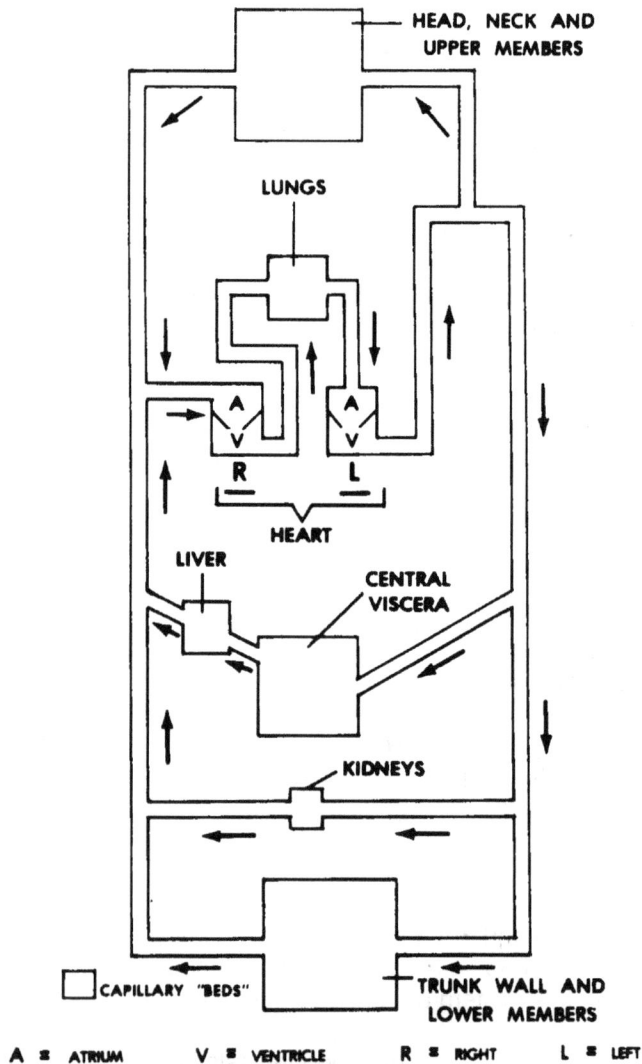

HEAD, NECK AND
UPPER MEMBERS

LUNGS

R   L

HEART

LIVER

CENTRAL
VISCERA

KIDNEYS

CAPILLARY "BEDS"

TRUNK WALL AND
LOWER MEMBERS

A = ATRIUM   V = VENTRICLE   R = RIGHT   L = LEFT

Figure 9-1. Scheme of blood vessels.

(1) The arteries carry blood away from the chambers of the heart.

(2) The veins carry blood underlined to the chambers of the heart.

(3) Capillaries are extremely thin-walled vessels having only the intimal layer through which exchanges can take place between the blood and the tissue cells.

c. **Relationships**. Arteries and veins are largest where they are closest to the heart. Away from the heart, they branch into smaller and smaller and more numerous vessels. The branching continues until the smallest arteries (underlined arterioles) empty into the capillaries. The capillaries in turn are drained by the venules of the venous system.

d. **Valves**. Within the heart and the veins are structures known as valves. Valves function to insure that the blood flows in only one direction.

9-7. THE HEART

Through the action of its very muscular walls, the heart produces the primary motive force to drive the blood through the arterial system. In humans, the heart is located just above the diaphragm, in the middle of the thorax, and extending slightly to the left. It is said that the heart of an average individual is about the size of that individual's clenched fist.

a. **General Construction of the Human Heart**. See figure 9-2 for an illustration of the human heart.

(1) Chambers. The heart is divided into four cavities known as the chambers. The upper two chambers are known as the atria, right and left. Each atrium has an ear-like projection known as an auricle. The lower two chambers are known as ventricles, right and left. Between the two atria is a common wall known as the interatrial septum. Between the two ventricles is a common wall known as the interventricular septum.

ATRIUM = hall
AURICLE = ear-like flap
VENTER = belly
SEPTUM = fence

(2) Wall layers. The walls of the chambers are in three general layers. Lining the cavity of each chamber is a smooth epithelium known as the endocardium. (Endocarditis is an inflammation of the endocardium.) The middle layer is made up of cardiac muscle tissue and is known as the myocardium. The outer layer of the heart is another epithelium known as the epicardium.

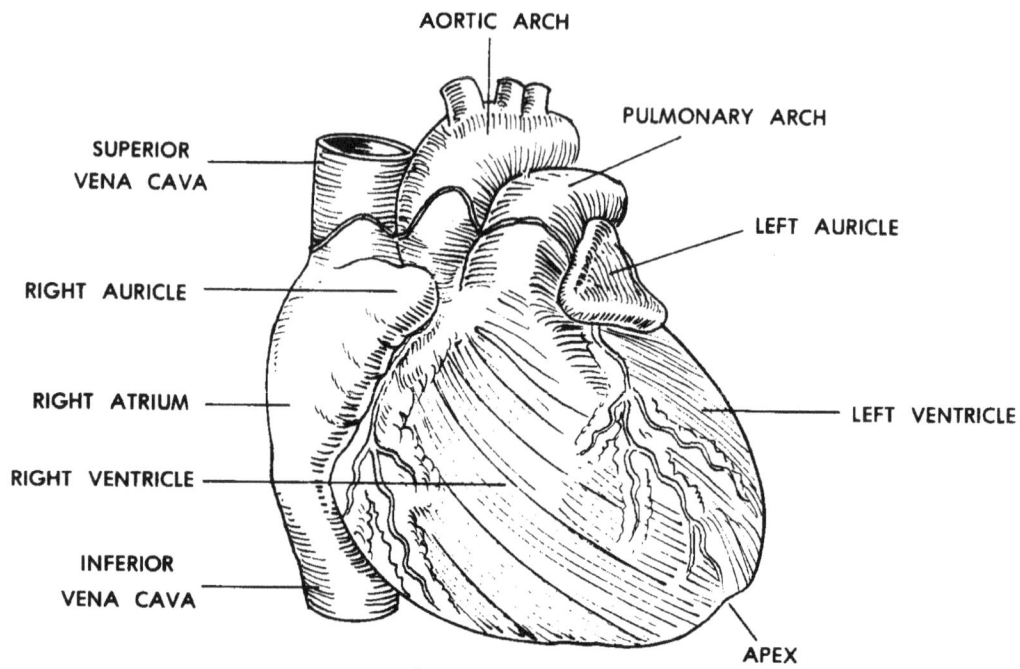

A. ANTERIOR VIEW

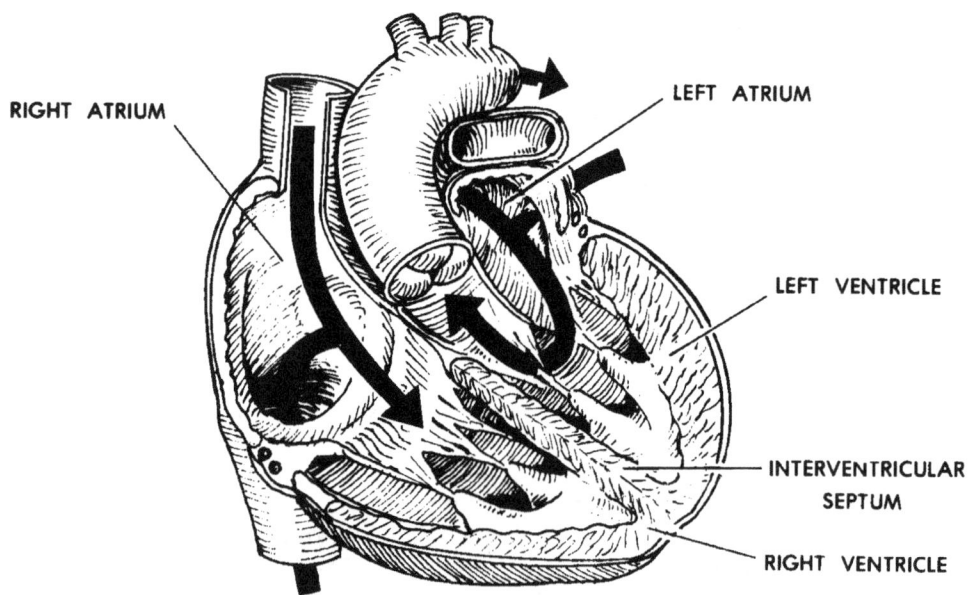

B. INTERIOR VIEW

Figure 9-2. The human heart.

(3) Relationship of wall thickness to required pressure levels. A cross-section of the chambers shows that the atrial walls are relatively thin. The right ventricular wall is much thicker. The left ventricular wall is three to five times thicker than that of the right. These differences in wall thickness reflect the amount of muscle tissue needed to produce the amount of pressure required of each chamber.

(4) Cardiac valves (figure 9-3).

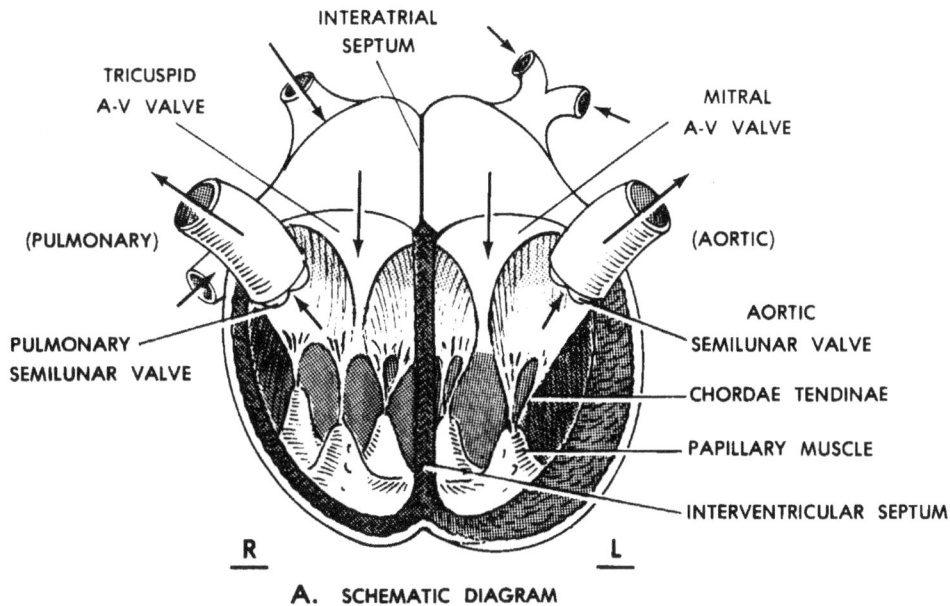

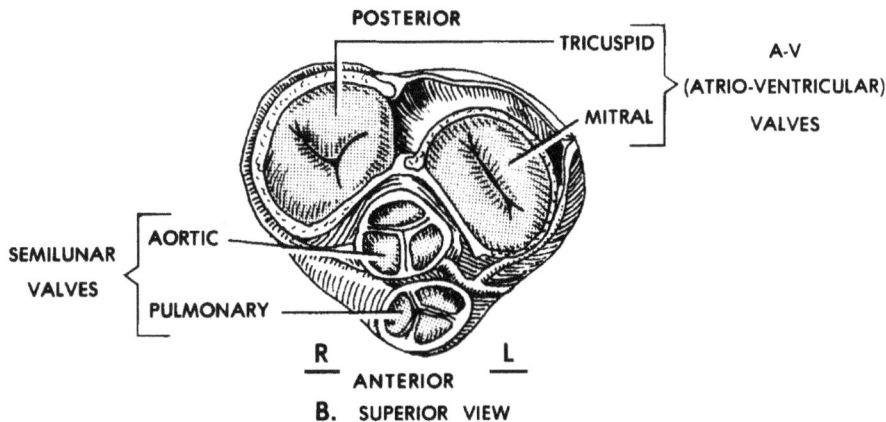

Figure 9-3. Scheme of heart valves.

(a) Between the atrium and ventricle of each side is the atrioventricular (A-V) valve. Each A-V valve prevents the blood from going back into the atrium from the ventricle of the same side. The right A-V valve is known as the tricuspid valve. The left A-V valve is known as the mitral valve. ("Might is never right.") The leaflets (flaps) of the A-V valves are prevented from being pushed back into the atria by fibrous cords. These fibrous cords are attached to the underside (the ventricular side) of the leaflets and are called chordae tendineae. At their other ends, the chordae tendineae are attached to the inner walls of the ventricles by papillary muscles.

(b) A major artery leads away from each ventricle--the pulmonary trunk from the right ventricle and the aortic arch from the left ventricle. A semilunar valve is found at the base of each of the pulmonary trunk and the aortic arch. These semilunar valves prevent blood from flowing back into the ventricles. The pulmonary (semilunar) valve and the aortic (semilunar) valve are each made up of three semilunar ("pocket-like") cusps.

b. **Control of the Heart Beat**. The heart is under several different control systems--extrinsic nervous control, intrinsic nervous control, and humoral control.

(1) Extrinsic nervous control. Extrinsic nervous control is control from outside of the heart. Extrinsic control is exerted by nerves of the autonomic nervous system. The sympathetic cardiac nerves accelerate (speed up) the heart. The vagus parasympathetic nerve decelerates (slows down) the heart.

(2) Intrinsic "nervous" control. Intrinsic "nervous" control is control built within the heart. The intrinsic "nervous" system consists of the sinoatrial (S-A) node (often referred to as the "pacemaker"), the atrioventricular (A-V) node, and the septal bundles. The septal bundles spread through the walls of the ventricles, just beneath the endocardium. This combination of nodes and bundles initiates the heart beat automatically and transmits the impulse through the atria and the ventricles.

(3) Humoral control. In addition to the "nervous" control of heart action, it appears that there are substances in the blood itself which have varying effects on the functioning of the heart. Although these substances are not as yet well understood, they appear to have some importance. The transplanted heart seems to depend to a degree on this control mechanism, since much of its "nervous controls" have been lost for the initial period in the recipient's body.

c. **Coronary Arteries and Cardiac Veins**. We may say that the heart deals with two different kinds of blood flow--"functional" blood and "nutritive" blood. "Functional" blood is the blood that the heart works on or pushes with its motive force. However, the walls of the heart require nutrition that they cannot get directly from the blood within the chambers. "Nutritive" blood is supplied to these walls by the coronary arteries, right and left. The coronary arteries arise from the base of the aortic arch and are distributed over the surface of the heart. This blood is collected by the cardiac veins and empties into the right atrium of the heart. Should a coronary artery, or one of its branches, become closed for whatever reason, that part of the heart wall formerly supplied nutrient blood by the closed vessel will very likely die.

d. **Pericardial Sac**. The average heart contracts in what is known as a heart beat, about 70-80 times a minute. To reduce the frictional forces that would be applied to its moving surfaces, the heart is enclosed in a special serous sac known as the pericardium ("around the heart").

9-8. CARDIOVASCULAR CIRCULATORY PATTERNS

See figure 9-4 for an illustration depicting cardiovascular circulatory patterns.

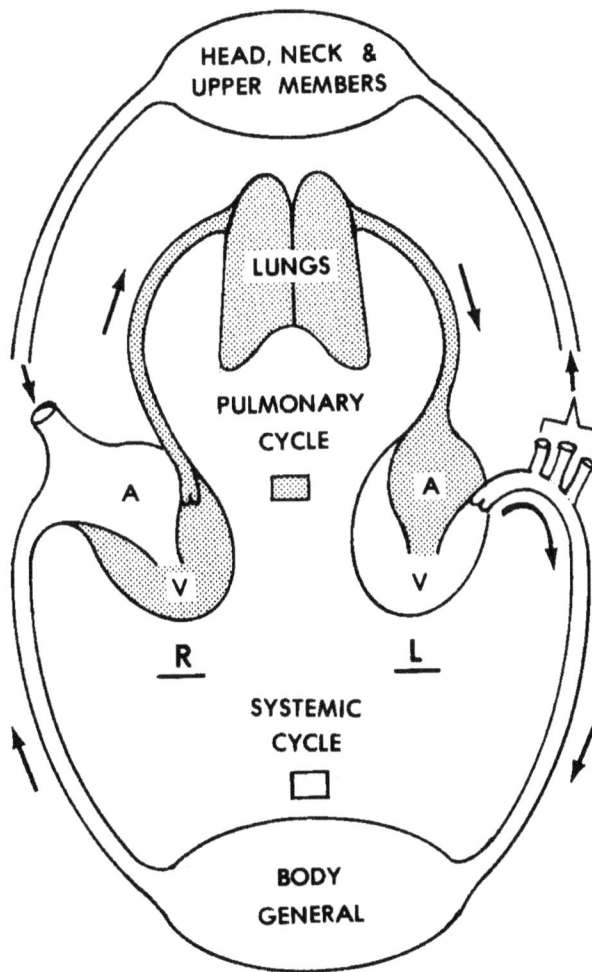

Figure 9-4. Cardiovascular circulatory patterns.

a. **General**. The human cardiovascular circulatory system is described as a closed, two-cycle system.

(1) It is <u>closed</u> because at no place is the blood as whole blood ever outside the system.

(2) It is <u>two-cycle</u> because the blood passes through the heart twice with each complete circuit of the body. In the <u>pulmonary cycle</u>, the blood passes from the right heart, through the lungs, and to the left heart. In the <u>systemic cycle</u>, the blood passes from the left heart, through the body in general, and returns to the right heart.

(3) It is common for an area of the body to be supplied by more than one blood vessel so that if one is damaged, the others will continue the supply. This is known as <u>collateral circulation</u>. However, there are situations, such as in the heart and the brain, where a single artery supplies a specific part of a structure. Such an artery is called an <u>end artery</u>. When an end artery is damaged, that area supplied by it will usually die, as in the case of the coronary artery (para 9-7c) above or in the case of a "stroke" in the brain.

b. **Pulmonary Cycle**. The pulmonary cycle begins in the right ventricle of the heart. Contraction of the right ventricular wall applies pressure to the blood. This forces the tricuspid valve closed and the closed valve prevents blood from going back into the right atrium. The pressure forces blood past the semilunar valve into the pulmonary trunk. Upon relaxation of the right ventricle, back pressure of the blood in the pulmonary trunk closes the pulmonary semilunar valve. The blood then passes into the lungs through the pulmonary arterial system. Gases are exchanged between the alveoli of the lungs and the blood in the capillaries next to the alveoli. This blood, now saturated with oxygen, is collected by the pulmonary veins and carried to the left atrium of the heart. This completes the <u>pulmonary cycle</u>.

c. **Systemic Cycle**.

(1) <u>Left ventricle of the heart</u>. The oxygen-saturated blood is moved from the left atrium into the left ventricle. When the left ventricular wall contracts, the pressure closes the mitral valve, which prevents blood from returning to the left atrium. The contraction of the left ventricular wall therefore forces the blood through the aortic semilunar valve into the aortic arch. Upon relaxation of the left ventricular wall, the back pressure of the aortic arch forces the aortic semilunar valve closed.

(2) <u>Arterial distributions</u>. The blood then passes through the various arteries to the tissues of the body. See figure 9-5 for an illustration of the main arteries of the human body.

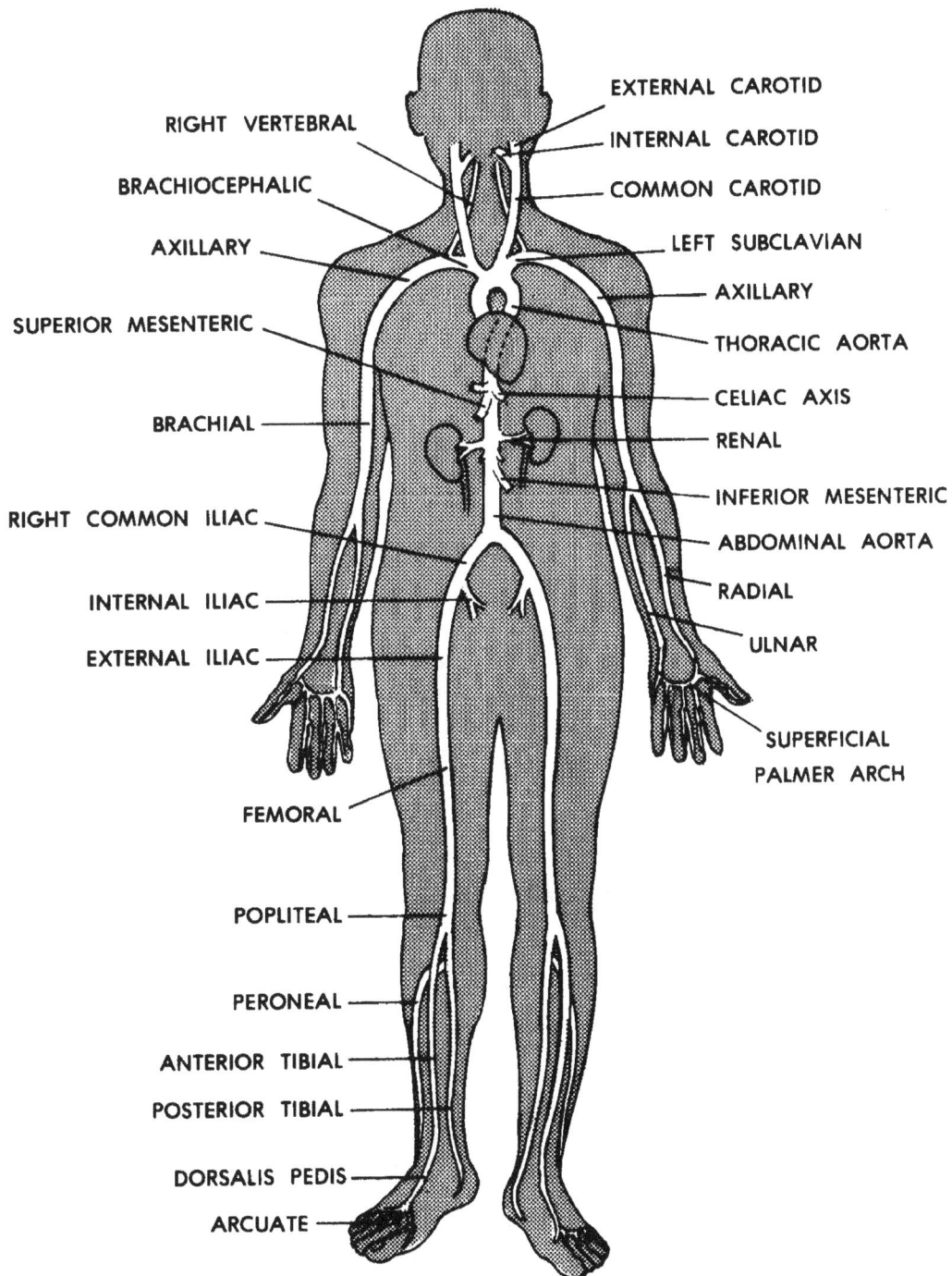

Figure 9-5. Main arteries of the human body.

(a) The carotid arteries supply the head. The neck and upper members are supplied by the subclavian arteries.

(b) The aortic arch continues as a large single vessel known as the aorta passing down through the trunk of the body in front of the vertebral column. It gives off branches to the trunk wall and to the contents of the trunk.

(c) At the lower end of the trunk, the aorta divides into right and left iliac arteries, supplying the pelvic region and lower members.

(3) Capillary beds of the body tissues. In the capillary beds of the tissues of the body, materials (such as food, oxygen, and waste products) are exchanged between the blood and the cells of the body.

(4) Venous tributaries. See figure 9-6 for an illustration of the main veins of the human body.

(a) The blood from the capillaries among the tissues is collected by a venous system parallel to the arteries. This system of deep veins returns the blood back to the right atrium of the heart.

(b) In the subcutaneous layer, immediately beneath the skin, is a network of superficial veins draining the skin areas. These superficial veins collect and then join the deep veins in the axillae (armpits) and the inguinal region (groin).

(c) The superior vena cava collects the blood from the head, neck, and upper members. The inferior vena cava collects the blood from the rest of the body. As the final major veins, the venae cavae empty the returned blood into the right atrium of heart.

(d) The veins are generally supplied with valves to assist in making the blood flow toward the heart. It is of some interest to note that the veins from the head do not contain valves.

(e) From that portion of the gut where materials are absorbed through the walls into the capillaries, the blood receives a great variety of substances. While most of these substances are useful, some may be harmful to the body. The blood carrying these substances is carried directly to the liver by the hepatic portal venous system. This blood is specially treated and conditioned in the liver before it is returned to the general circulation by way of the hepatic veins.

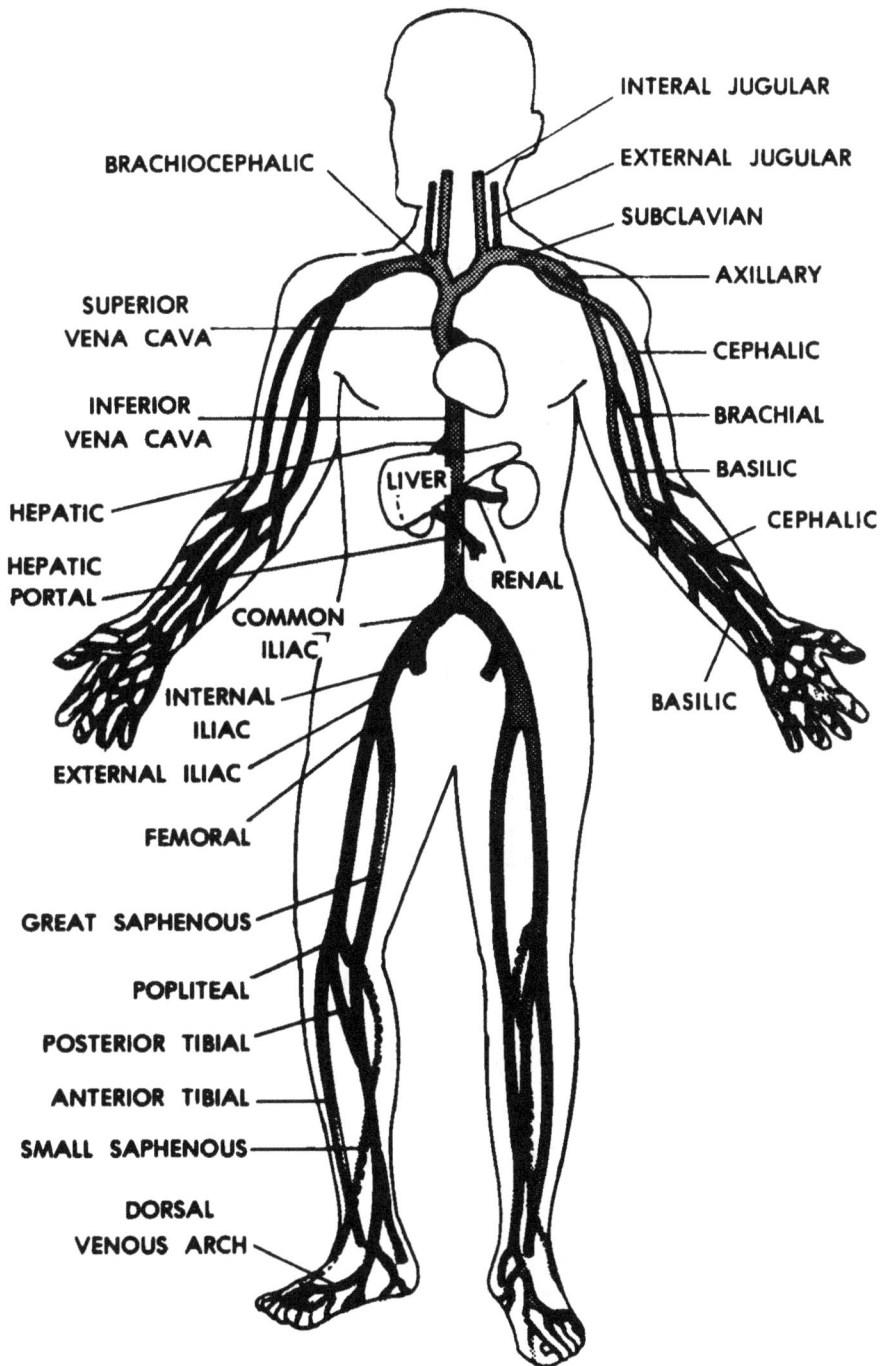

Figure 9-6. Main veins of the human body.

Section III. THE HUMAN LYMPHATIC SYSTEM

9-9. GENERAL

Between the cells of the body are spaces filled with fluid. This is the <u>interstitial</u> (or tissue) fluid, often referred to as intercellular fluid. There are continuous exchanges between the intracellular fluid, the interstitial fluid, and the plasma of the blood. The lymphatic system returns to the bloodstream the excess interstitial fluid, which includes proteins and fluid derived from the blood.

9-10. STRUCTURES OF THE HUMAN LYMPHATIC SYSTEM

See figure 9-7 for an illustration of the human lymphatic system.

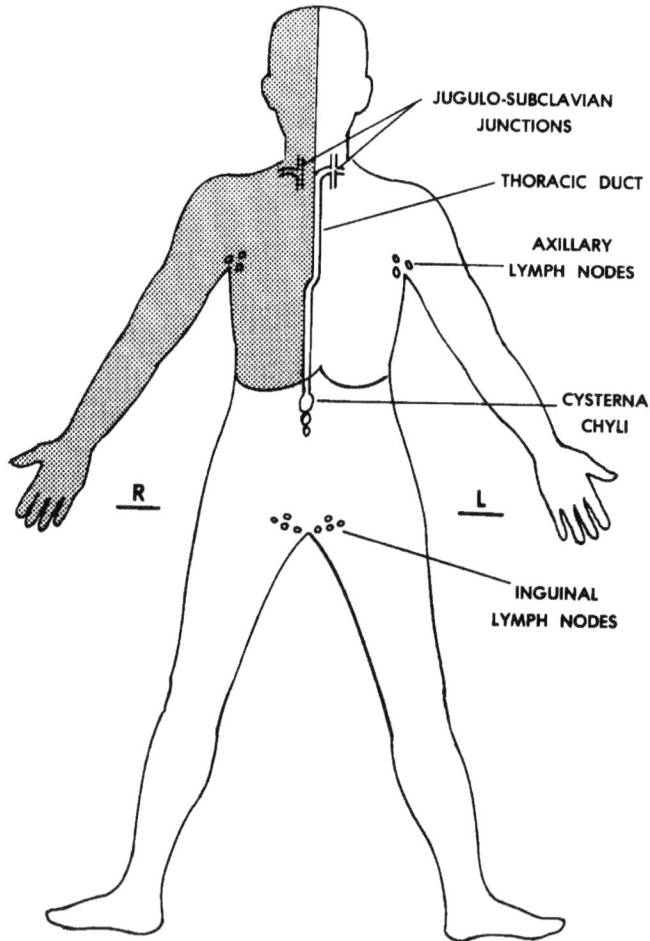

Figure 9-7. The human lymphatic system.

a. **Lymphatic Capillaries**. Lymphatic capillaries are located in the interstitial spaces. Here, they absorb the excess fluids.

b. **Lymph Vessels**. A tributary system of vessels collects these excess fluids, now called <u>lymph</u>. Like veins, lymphatic vessels are supplied with <u>valves</u> to help maintain a flow of lymph in one direction only. The lymphatic vessels, to a greater or lesser extent, parallel the venous vessels along the way. The major lymph vessel in the human body is called the <u>thoracic duct</u>. The thoracic duct passes from the abdomen up through the thorax and into the root of the neck in front of the vertebral column. The thoracic duct there empties into the junction of the left subclavian and jugular veins.

c. **Lymph Nodes**. Along the way, lymphatic vessels are interrupted by special structures known as lymph nodes. These lymph nodes serve as special filters for the lymph fluid passing through.

d. **Tonsils**. Tonsils are special collections of lymphoid tissue, very similar to a group of lymph nodes. These are protective structures and are located primarily at the entrances of the respiratory and digestive systems.

Continue with Exercises

EXERCISES, LESSON 9

REQUIREMENT. The following exercises are to be answered by completing the incomplete statement or by writing the answer in the space provided at the end of the question.

After you have completed all the exercises, turn to "Solutions to Exercises," at the end of the lesson and check your answers.

1.   The four basic components of any circulatory system are a _____, _____s, a _____ _____, and _____s. The vehicle is the substance which actually _____. A conduit is a _____ through which a vehicle _____s. If we say that a force is motive, we mean that it _____ _____. Systems providing a motive force are often known as _____. Exchange areas exist so that materials being transported may be eventually _____.

2.   The human cardiovascular system is a collection of interacting _____s designed to supply _____ and _____ to living _____s and to remove _____and other wastes. Its four major components are the _____, _____, _____ and _____. The vehicle is the _____. The conduits are the _____. The primary motive force is provided by the _____. The exchange areas are provided by minute vessels called _____.

3.   The major subdivisions of blood are the _____ and the _____. Plasma makes up about ___ percent of the total blood volume. Plasma is mainly composed of _____. Among the most important materials dissolved in plasma are _____s. After the blood clots, the clear fluid remaining is _____, which does not contain the proteins used for _____. Otherwise, it is very similar to _____.

4.   The formed elements of the blood make up about ___ percent of the total blood volume. While red blood cells and white blood cells are cells, the platelets are only _____ of cells.

What is the shape of an RBC? B_____ d_____.

In a cubic millimeter of normal adult blood, there are about how many RBCs?

RBCs contain a protein called _____ which transports most of the oxygen carried by the blood.

5.   The most common types of white blood cells are _____and _____.
Neutrophils p_____ foreign particles and organisms. Lymphocytes produce
_____s.

In a cubic millimeter of normal adult blood, there are about how many
WBCs?

6.   The main function of platelets is to aid in clotting by ____ing and by releasing
c_____ f_____s related to clotting.

In a cubic millimeter of normal blood, there are about how many platelets?

7.   Four general functions of blood are:

a.   _____.

b.   _____.

c.   _____.

d.   _____.

8.   The inner, smooth epithelial layer of a blood vessel is called the i_____.
The middle layer of smooth muscle tissue is called the m_____. The outer
layer of FCT is the a_____.

9.   The three types of blood vessels are _____, _____,
and _____. The arteries carry blood away from _____. The veins carry blood
toward the _____. Capillaries have extremely thin walls so that exchanges can take
place between the _____ and _____.

10.   What are the heart chambers?

What are the atria?

Each atrium has an ear-like projection known as an _____.

What are the ventricles? _____.

Between the two atria is a common wall known as the _____.
Between the two ventricles is a common wall known as the _____.

MD0006   9-19

11. The three layers in the walls of the heart chambers are the _____m, the _____m, and the _____m. The inner layer is a smooth e_____. The middle layer is made up of cardiac _____ tissue. The outer layer is another e_____.

12. THIN OR THICK? The atrial walls are relatively _____. The right ventricular wall is much _____er than the atrial walls. The left ventricular wall is three to five times _____er than the right ventricular wall.

13. The valve between the atrium and ventricle of each side is the _____ (__) valve. The right A-V valve is known as the _____ valve. The left A-V valve is known as the _____ valve. The fibrous cords attached to the underside of the A-V valves are called _____. They are attached to the inner walls of the ventricles by _____ muscles. The valve at the base of the pulmonary trunk and the valve at the base of the aortic arch are both _____ valves, each with cusps. They are often called the _____ valve and the _____ valve.

14. Extrinsic nervous control of the heart is exerted by nerves of the _____ nervous system. Speeding the heart up are the _____ cardiac nerves. Slowing the heart down is the v_____ p_____ nerve. Intrinsic "nervous" control is built within the _____. It consists of the s_____ (__) node, the a_____ (__) nodes, and the s_____b_____. For humoral control, there appears to be _____ which have varying effects upon the functioning of the heart.

15. The coronary arteries supply "_____" blood to the heart walls. The coronary arteries arise from the base of the _____ and are spread over the surface of the heart. This blood is collected by the _____ veins, which empty into the right _____ of the heart. If a coronary artery becomes closed, the receiving area of the heart will probably _____.

16. The pericardium is a special serous sac surrounding the _____ and reducing the _____l forces upon its moving surfaces.

17. The human cardiovascular system is closed because at no place is whole blood ever _____. It is two-cycle because the blood passes through the heart twice with each complete _____. In the pulmonary cycle, the blood passes from the _____ heart, through the _____, and to the _____ heart. In the systemic cycle, the blood passes from the _____ heart, through the _____, and returns to the _____ heart.

18.   In the case of collateral circulation, if one blood vessel to an area is damaged, then _____. However, when an end artery is damaged, the receiving area will usually _____.

19.   PULMONARY CYCLE:
In which chamber of the heart does the pulmonary cycle begin?

Contraction of the wall of the right ventricle forces the _____ valve to close. This keeps blood from flowing back into the _____. The pressure forces blood past the _____ valve into the _____. Upon relaxation of the right ventricle, back pressure of the blood in the pulmonary trunk closes the _____ valve. The blood then passes into the _____ through the pulmonary arterial system. Gases are exchanged between the _____ of the lungs and the blood in the _____ next to the alveoli. The oxygenated blood is collected by the _____ and carried to the _____ of the heart. This completes the pulmonary cycle.

20.   SYSTEMIC CYCLE:
Oxygenated blood is moved from the left atrium into the _____. Contraction of the wall of the left ventricle closes the _____ valve, which prevents blood from returning to the _____. The pressure forces blood past the _____ valve into the _____. Upon relaxation of the left ventricular wall, back pressure of the blood in the aortic arch closes the _____ valve. The blood then passes through the various _____ to the _____. Materials are exchanged between the blood and cells of the body in the _____. The blood returns to the _____ of the heart in vessels called _____.

21.   The head is supplied by the _____ arteries. The neck and upper members are supplied by the _____ arteries. The aortic arch continues as a large single vessel known as the _____. At the lower end of the trunk, the aorta divides into the right and left _____ arteries, supplying the pelvic region and lower members.

22.   Running parallel to the arteries is the system of _____ veins. Immediately beneath the skin is a network of _____ veins. These veins collect and then join the deep veins in the _____ (armpits) and the _____ (groin). Collecting the blood from the head, neck, and upper members is the superior _____ _____. Collecting the blood from the rest of the body is the _____ _____ _____. Thus, the final major veins, emptying the returned blood into the right atrium of the heart, are the _____ _____. Except the veins from the head, veins are generally supplied with _____s to assist in making blood flow toward the heart. Carrying absorbed substances from the gut to the liver is the _____. After being specially treated and conditioned, this blood is returned to the general circulation by the _____ veins.

23.   Located in the interstitial spaces, where they absorb excess interstitial fluid, are the l_____s. A tributary system collects this fluid, now called _____. To help maintain lymph flow in one direction, lymphatic vessels are supplied with _____.   The major lymph vessel (which passes from the abdomen, up through the thorax, and into the root of the neck) is the _____. Lymph nodes are special structures which interrupt _____ vessels and serve as special f_____s for the _____ f_____ passing through. Tonsils are special collections of_____d tissue. They are _____ve structures located primarily at the _____s of the _____y and _____e systems.

Check Your Answers on Next Page

SOLUTIONS TO EXERCISES, LESSON 9

1. The four basic components of any circulatory system are a <u>vehicle</u>, <u>conduit</u>s, a <u>motive force</u>, and <u>exchange area</u>s. The vehicle is the substance which actually <u>carries the materials being transported</u>. A conduit is a <u>channel, pipe, or tube</u> through which a <u>vehicle travel</u>s. If we say that a force is motive, we mean that it <u>produces movement</u>. Systems providing a motive force are often known as <u>pumps</u>. Exchange areas exist so that materials being transported may be eventually <u>exchanged with a part of the body</u>. (para 9-2)

2. The human cardiovascular system is a collection of interacting <u>structure</u>s designed to supply <u>oxygen</u> and <u>nutrients</u> to living <u>cell</u>s and to remove <u>carbon dioxide</u> and other wastes. Its four major components are the <u>blood</u>, <u>blood vessels</u>, <u>heart</u>, and <u>capillaries</u>. The vehicle is the <u>blood</u>. The conduits are the <u>blood vessels</u>. The primary motive force is provided by the <u>heart</u>. The exchange areas are provided by minute vessels called <u>capillaries</u>. (para 9-4)

3. The major subdivisions of blood are the <u>plasma</u> and the <u>formed elements</u>. Plasma makes up about <u>55</u> percent of the total blood volume. Plasma is mainly composed of <u>water</u>. Among the most important materials dissolved in plasma are <u>proteins</u>. After the blood clots, the clear fluid remaining is <u>serum</u>, which does not contain the proteins used for <u>clotting</u>. Otherwise, it is very similar to <u>plasma</u>. (para 9-5)

4. The formed elements of the blood make up about <u>45</u> percent of the total blood volume. While red blood cells and white blood cells are cells, the platelets are only <u>fragments</u> of cells. What is the shape of an RBC? <u>Biconcave</u> <u>disc</u>. In a cubic millimeter of normal blood, there are about <u>5,000,000</u> RBCs. RBCs contain a protein called <u>hemoglobin</u>, which transports most of the oxygen carried by the blood. (para 9-5b)

5. The most common types of white blood cells are <u>neutrophils</u> and <u>lymphocytes</u>. Neutrophils <u>phagocytize</u> foreign particles and organisms. Lymphocytes produce <u>antibodie</u>s. In a cubic millimeter of normal adult blood, there are about <u>5,000 to 11,000</u> WBCs. (para 9-5b(2))

6. The main function of platelets is to aid in clotting by <u>clumping together</u> and by releasing <u>chemical factor</u>s related to clotting. In a cubic millimeter of normal blood, there are about <u>150,000 - 350,000</u> platelets. (para 9-5b(3))

7. Four general functions of blood are:

   a. <u>Serving as a vehicle</u>.
   b. <u>Aiding in temperature control</u>.
   c. <u>Protecting our bodies by providing immunity</u>.
   d. <u>Blood clotting</u>. (para 9-5c)

8. The inner, smooth epithelial layer of a blood vessel is called the intima. The middle layer of smooth muscle tissue is called the media. The outer layer of FCT is the adventitia. (para 9-6a)

9. The three types of blood vessels are arteries, veins, and capillaries. The arteries carry blood away from the chambers of the heart. The veins carry blood toward the chambers of the heart. Capillaries have extremely thin walls so that exchanges can take place between the blood and tissue cells. (para 9-6b)

10. The heart chambers are the four cavities into which the heart is divided. The atria are the upper two chambers of the heart. Each atrium has an ear-like projection known as an auricle. The ventricles are the lower two chambers of the heart. Between the two atria is a common wall known as the interatrial septum. Between the two ventricles is a common wall known as the interventricular septum. (para 9-7a(1))

11. The three layers in the walls of the heart chambers are the endocardium, the myocardium, and the epicardium. The inner layer is a smooth epithelium. The middle layer is made up of cardiac muscle tissue. The outer layer is another epithelium. (para 9-7a(2))

12. The atrial walls are relatively thin. The right ventricular wall is much thicker than the atrial walls. The left ventricular wall is three to five times thicker than the right ventricular wall. (para 9-7a(3))

13. The valve between the atrium and ventricle of each side is the atrioventricular (A-V) valve. The right A-V valve is known as the tricuspid valve. The left A-V valve is known as the mitral valve. The fibrous cords attached to the underside of the A-V valves are called chordae tendineae. They are attached to the inner walls of the ventricles by papillary muscles. (para 9-7a(4)(a))

The valve at the base of the pulmonary trunk and the valve at the base of the aortic arch are both semilunar valves, each with three cusps. They are often called the pulmonary valve and the aortic valve. (para 9-7a(4)(b))

14. Extrinsic nervous control of the heart is exerted by nerves of the autonomic nervous system. Speeding the heart up are the sympathetic cardiac nerves. Slowing the heart down is the vagus parasympathetic nerve. (para 9-7b(1))

Intrinsic "nervous" control is built within the heart. It consists of the sinoatrial (S-A) node, the atrioventricular (A-V) node, and the septal bundles. (para 9-7b(2))

For humoral control, there appears to be substances in the blood itself which have varying effects upon the functioning of the heart. (para 9-7b(3))

15. The coronary arteries supply "<u>nutritive</u>" blood to the heart walls. The coronary arteries arise from the base of the <u>aortic arch</u> and are spread over the surface of the heart. This blood is collected by the <u>cardiac</u> veins, which empty into the right <u>atrium</u> of the heart. If a coronary artery becomes closed, the receiving area of the heart will probably <u>die</u>. (para 9-7c)

16. The pericardium is a special serous sac surrounding the <u>heart</u> and reducing the <u>frictional</u> forces upon its moving surfaces. (para 9-7d)

17. The human cardiovascular system is closed because at no place is whole blood ever <u>outside the system</u>. It is two-cycle because the blood passes through the heart twice with each complete <u>circuit of the body</u>. In the pulmonary cycle, the blood passes from the <u>right</u> heart, through the <u>lungs</u>, and to the <u>left</u> heart. In the systemic cycle, the blood passes from the <u>left</u> heart, through the <u>body in general</u>, and returns to the <u>right</u> heart. (para 9-8a)

18. In the case of collateral circulation, if one blood vessel to an area is damaged, then <u>another blood vessel will continue the supply</u>. However, when an end artery is damaged, the receiving area will usually <u>die</u>. (para 9-8a(3))

19. PULMONARY CYCLE: The pulmonary cycle begins in the <u>right ventricle</u>. Contraction of the wall of the right ventricle forces the <u>tricuspid</u> valve to close. This keeps blood from flowing back into the <u>right atrium</u>. The pressure forces blood past the <u>pulmonary semilunar</u> valve into the <u>pulmonary trunk</u>. Upon relaxation of the right ventricle, back pressure of the blood in the pulmonary trunk closes the <u>pulmonary semilunar</u> valve. The blood then passes into the <u>lungs</u> through the pulmonary arterial system. Gases are exchanged between the <u>alveoli</u> of the lungs and the blood in the <u>capillaries</u> next to the alveoli. The oxygenated blood is collected by the <u>pulmonary veins</u> and carried to the <u>left atrium</u> of the heart. (para 9-8b)

20. SYSTEMIC CYCLE: Oxygenated blood is moved from the left atrium into the <u>left ventricle</u>. Contraction of the wall of the left ventricle closes the <u>mitral</u> valve, which prevents blood from returning to the <u>left atrium</u>. The pressure forces blood past the <u>aortic semilunar</u> valve into the <u>aortic arch</u>. Upon relaxation of the left ventricular wall, back pressure of the blood in the aortic arch closes the <u>aortic semilunar</u> valve. The blood then passes through the various <u>arteries</u> to the <u>tissues of the body</u>. Materials are exchanged between the blood and cells of the body in the <u>capillary beds</u>. The blood returns to the <u>right atrium</u> of the heart in vessels called <u>veins</u>. (para 9-8c)

21. The head is supplied by the <u>carotid</u> arteries. The neck and upper members are supplied by the <u>subclavian</u> arteries. The aortic arch continues as a large single vessel known as the <u>aorta</u>. At the lower end of the trunk, the aorta divides into the right and left <u>iliac</u> arteries, supplying the pelvic region and lower members. (para 9-8c(2))

22. Running parallel to the arteries is the system of <u>deep</u> veins. Immediately beneath the skin is a network of <u>superficial</u> veins. These veins collect and then join the deep veins in the <u>axillae</u> (armpits) and the <u>inguinal region</u> (groin). (paras 9-8c(4)(a)-(b))

Collecting the blood from the head, neck, and upper members is the superior <u>vena cava</u>. Collecting the blood from the rest of the body is the <u>inferior vena cava</u>. Thus, the final major veins, emptying the returned blood into the right atrium of the heart, are the <u>venae cavae</u>. (para 9-8c(4)(c))

Except the veins from the head, veins are generally supplied with <u>valves</u> to assist in making blood flow toward the heart. (para 9-8c(4)(d))

Carrying absorbed substances from the gut to the liver is the <u>hepatic portal venous system</u>. After being specially treated and conditioned, this blood is returned to the general circulation by the <u>hepatic</u> veins. (para 9-8c(4)(e))

23. Located in the interstitial spaces, where they absorb excess interstitial fluid, are the <u>lymphatic capillaries</u>. A tributary system collects this fluid, now called <u>lymph</u>. To help maintain lymph flow in one direction, lymphatic vessels are supplied with <u>valves</u>. The major lymph vessel (which passes from the abdomen, up through the thorax, and into the root of the neck) is the <u>thoracic duct</u>. Lymph nodes are special structures which interrupt <u>lymphatic</u> vessels and serve as special <u>filters</u> for the <u>lymph fluid</u> passing through. Tonsils are special collections of <u>lymphoid</u> tissue. They are <u>protective</u> structures located primarily at the <u>entrances</u> of the <u>respiratory</u> and <u>digestive</u> systems. (para 9-10)

End of Lesson 9

LESSON ASSIGNMENT

LESSON 10   The Human Endocrine System.

TEXT ASSIGNMENT   Paragraphs 10-1 through 10-18.

LESSON OBJECTIVES   After completing this lesson, you should be able to:

    10-1. Define <u>endocrine glands</u>, <u>hormones</u>, <u>target organs</u>, and <u>feedback mechanism</u>.

    10-2. Briefly describe three different control systems of the human body.

    10-3. Briefly describe the endocrine system and name six better known endocrine organs.

    10-4. Describe the pituitary body, including its location, its major subdivisions, and the origins and hormones of each subdivision.

    10-5. Describe the location, structure, and hormone(s) for each of the following:

        a. The thyroid gland.
        b. The parathyroid glands.
        c. The pancreatic islets.
        d. The suprarenal glands.

    10-6. Name the primary sex organs and the sex hormones for each gender.

SUGGESTION   After completing the assignment, complete the exercises at the end of this lesson. These exercises will help you to achieve the lesson objectives.

LESSON 10

THE HUMAN ENDOCRINE SYSTEM

Section I. INTRODUCTION

10-1. DEFINITIONS

ENDO = internal
CRINE = secrete

a. The endocrine glands are glands of internal secretion (rather than external, as seen with the sweat glands and digestive glands).

b. This internal secretion results from the fact that these glands have no ducts. Thus, they are often referred to as the ductless glands.

c. The secretions produced by the endocrine glands are called hormones.

d. Hormones are carried by the bloodstream to specific organs or tissues, which are then called the target organs.

e. The activity of the target organ, in turn, affects the activity of the endocrine organ. Thus, it is a reverse or feedback mechanism.

10-2. GENERAL

a. **Control "Systems" of the Human Body**. The structure and function of the human body is controlled and organized by several different "systems."

(1) Heredity/environment. The interaction of heredity and environment is the fundamental control "system." Genes determine the range of potentiality and environment develops it. For example, good nutrition will allow a person to attain his full body height and weight within the limits of his genetic determination. Genetics is the study of heredity.

(2) Hormones. The hormones of the endocrine system serve to control the tissues and organs in general. (Vitamins have a similar role.) Both hormones and vitamins are chemical substances required only in small quantities.

(3) Nervous system. More precise and immediate control of the structures of the body is carried out by the nervous system.

b. **The Endocrine System**. In the human body, the endocrine system consists of a number of ductless glands producing their specific hormones. Because these hormones are carried to their target organs by the bloodstream, the endocrine organs (glands) are richly supplied with blood vessels.

c. **Better Known Endocrine Organs of Humans**. The better known endocrine organs are the:

(1) Pituitary body.

(2) Thyroid gland.

(3) Parathyroid glands.

(4) Pancreatic islets (islands of Langerhans).

(5) Suprarenal (adrenal) glands.

(6) Gonads (female--ovaries; male--testes).

In addition, there are several other endocrine organs, less well understood, and other organs suspected to be of the endocrine type. See figure 10-1, which shows the better known endocrine glands and their locations.

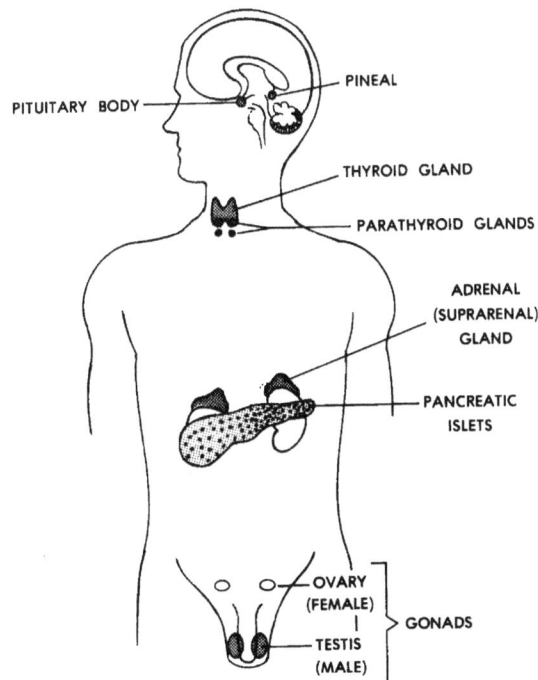

Figure 10-1. The endocrine glands of the human body and their locations.

Section II. THE PITUITARY BODY

10-3. GENERAL

a. **Location**. The pituitary body is a small pea-sized and pea- shaped structure. It is attached to the base of the brain in the region of the hypothalamus (see paragraph 11-9). In addition, it is housed within a hollow of the bony floor of the cranial cavity. This hollow is called the sella turcica ("Turk's saddle").

b. **Major Subdivisions**. The pituitary body is actually two glands-- the posterior pituitary gland and the anterior pituitary gland. Initially separate, these glands join together during development of the embryo.

10-4. POSTERIOR PITUITARY GLAND

The posterior pituitary gland is the portion which comes from and retains a direct connection with the base of the brain. The hormones of the posterior pituitary gland are actually produced in the hypothalamus of the brain. From the hypothalamus, the hormones are delivered to the posterior pituitary gland, where they are released into the bloodstream. At present, we recognize two hormones of the posterior pituitary gland.

a. **ADH (Antidiuretic Hormone)**. ADH is involved with the resorption or salvaging of water within the kidneys. ADH is produced under thirst conditions.

b. **Oxytocin**. Oxytocin is concerned with contractions of smooth muscle in the uterus and with milk secretion.

10-5. ANTERIOR PITUITARY GLAND

a. The anterior pituitary gland originates from the roof of the embryo's mouth. It then "attaches" itself to the posterior pituitary gland.

b. The anterior pituitary gland is indirectly connected to the hypothalamus by means of a venous portal system. By "portal," we mean that the veins carry substances from the capillaries at one point to the capillaries at another point (hypothalamus to the anterior pituitary gland).

c. In the hypothalamus, certain chemicals known as releasing factors are produced. These are carried by the portal system to the anterior pituitary gland. Here, they stimulate the cells of the anterior pituitary gland to secrete their specific hormones.

d. The anterior pituitary gland produces many hormones. In general, they stimulate the target organs to develop or produce their own products. This stimulating effect is referred to as trophic.

e. Of the many hormones produced by the anterior pituitary gland, we will examine:

(1) <u>Somatotrophic hormone (growth hormone)</u>. The target organs of this hormone are the growing structures of the body. This hormone influences such structures to grow.

(2) <u>ACTH (adrenocorticotrophic hormone)</u>. This hormone of the anterior pituitary gland stimulates the cortex of the suprarenal (adrenal) gland to produce its hormones. We will later see that the hormones of the suprarenal cortex are involved with anti-inflammatory reactions of the body.

(3) <u>Thyrotropin (TSH)</u>. This hormone stimulates the thyroid gland to produce its hormones.

(4) <u>Luteinizing hormone (LH)</u>. LH stimulates ovulation and luteinization of ovarian follicles in females and promotes testosterone production in males.

(5) <u>Follicle-stimulating hormone (FSH)</u>. FSH stimulates ovarian follicle growth in females and stimulates spermatogenesis in males.

(6) <u>Prolactin</u>. Prolactin stimulates milk production and maternal behavior in females.

Section III. THE THYROID GLAND

10-6. LOCATION

The thyroid gland is in the neck region just below the larynx and surrounds the trachea.

10-7. ANATOMY

a. The right and left thyroid <u>lobes</u> are the masses on either side of the trachea. The <u>isthmus</u> is found across the front of the trachea and connects the two lobes.

b. Each lobe of the thyroid gland is supplied by arteries from above and below (<u>superior</u> and <u>inferior thyroid arteries</u>).

10-8. HORMONES

The primary hormone of the thyroid gland is <u>thyroxin</u>. Thyroxin affects the basal metabolic rate (BMR), the level of activity of the body. Since iodine is a necessary element in the production of thyroxin, one can observe malformations of the thyroid gland (called goiters) where there is little or no iodine available. A second hormone, calcito-nin, is produced by the thyroid gland and it is involved with calcium metabolism in the body.

Section IV. THE PARATHYROID GLANDS

10-9. LOCATION AND STRUCTURE

Located on the posterior aspects of the thyroid lobes are two pairs of small round masses of tissue, known as the parathyroid glands.

10-10. HORMONE

The hormone produced by these glands is called parathyroid hormone, or parathormone. It is involved with calcium metabolism.

Section V. THE PANCREATIC ISLETS (ISLANDS OF LANGERHANS)

10-11. LOCATION AND STRUCTURE

Within the substance of the pancreas are distributed small groups of cells known as islets. Although the pancreas is a ducted gland of the digestive system, these isolated islets are, in fact, ductless glands.

10-12. HORMONES

Insulin and glucagon are the two most commonly recognized hormones of the islets. These hormones are involved with glucose metabolism.

Section VI. THE SUPRARENAL (ADRENAL) GLANDS

10-13. LOCATION AND STRUCTURE

Embedded in the fat above each kidney is a suprarenal gland. Both suprarenal glands have an internal medulla and an external cortex.

10-14. HORMONES OF THE SUPRARENAL MEDULLA

The medullary portion of each suprarenal gland produces a pair of hormones--epinephrine (adrenalin) and norepinephrine (noradrenalin). These hormones are involved in the mobilization of energy during the stress reaction ("fight or flight").

10-15. HORMONES OF THE SUPRARENAL CORTEX

Each suprarenal cortex produces a variety of hormones which can be grouped into three categories:

a. **Mineralocorticoids** (for example, aldosterone), which are concerned with the electrolytes of the body.

b. **Glucocorticoids** (for example, cortisol), which are concerned with many metabolic functions and are anti-inflammatory in nature.

c. **Sex hormones**. Adrenal androgens and estrogens.

Section VII. THE GONADS

10-16. GENERAL

In humans, the primary sex organs are known as gonads (lesson 8). The gonads produce sex cells (gametes) and sex hormones. These sex hormones are in addition to those produced by the suprarenal cortex (see para 10-15c).

10-17. FEMALE SEX HORMONES

In the female, the ovaries produce two types of sex hormones during the menstrual cycle. During the first half of the cycle (days 1 - 14), the estrogens are produced. During the last half of the cycle (days 15 - 28), progesterone is produced. These hormones are concerned with female sexuality and with the preparation of female sex organs for reproduction.

10-18. MALE SEX HORMONES

In the male, certain cells of the testes produce the male sex hormones known as androgens (for example, testosterone). Androgens are concerned with male sexuality.

Continue with Exercises

EXERCISES, LESSON 10

REQUIREMENT. The following exercises are to be answered by completing the incomplete statement or by writing the answer in the space provided at the end of the question.

After you have completed all the exercises, turn to "Solutions to Exercises," at the end of the lesson and check your answers.

1. Endocrine glands are glands of _____l secretion. These glands are also called _____ less glands. Hormones are the secretions produced by _____ glands. Target organs are the specific organs or tissues to which _____s are carried by the _____. This is a feedback mechanism because the activity of the target organ affects the activity of the _____.

2. The fundamental control "system" is the interaction of _____ and _____. Genes determine the range of _____. Environment _____s it. Controlling the tissues and organs in general are the _____s of the _____ system. Providing more precise and immediate control of the body structures is the _____ system.

3. Why are endocrine organs (glands) richly supplied with blood vessels?

4. Name six of the better known endocrine organs.

   a. _____.

   b. _____.

   c. _____.

   d. _____.

   e. _____.

   f. _____.

5. The pituitary body is a small _____-sized and ____-shaped structure. It is attached to the base of the brain in the region of the h_____. In addition, it is housed within a hollow of the bony floor of the _____ cavity. The pituitary body is actually two glands: the _____ pituitary gland and the _____ pituitary gland.

6. The posterior pituitary gland is that portion of the pituitary body which comes from and retains its connection with the _____. The hormones of the posterior pituitary gland are actually produced in the h_____ of the brain. The two recognized hormones of the posterior pituitary gland are _____ (a hormone) and _____. The first is involved with the _____ of water within the kidneys; it is produced under _____ conditions. The second is concerned with contractions of smooth muscle in the _____ and with _____ production.

7. The anterior pituitary gland originates from the roof of the embryo's _____. It then attaches itself to the _____ gland. By means of a venous portal system, the anterior pituitary gland is connected to the h_____. Here, certain chemicals known as r_____ f_____ are produced. These are carried to the anterior pituitary by the ____ _____ system. They stimulate the anterior pituitary gland's cells to secrete their specific _____. In turn, these hormones stimulate the target organs to produce their own products. This stimulating effect is referred to as _____. Two hormones produced by the anterior pituitary gland are _____trophic hormone and _____ (_____trophic hormone). The target organs of the first are the _____ing structures of the body. The second stimulates the cortex of the _____ (____) gland to produce its hormones.

8. The thyroid gland is in the _____ region just below the _____ and surrounds the _____. The masses on either side of the trachea are the right and left thyroid _____. The tissue connecting the two lobes is called the _____. It is found across the front of the _____. Each lobe of the thyroid gland is supplied by the superior and inferior _____ arteries. The primary hormone of the thyroid gland is _____, which affects the _____ _____ ____ (____), the level of activity of the body.

9. Where are the parathyroid glands located?

The hormone produced by these glands is called _____ hormone or _____. It is involved with _____ metabolism.

10.   Within the pancreas are distributed small groups of cells known as _____.
The two most commonly recognized hormones of the islets are _____ and
_____. These hormones are involved with _____ metabolism.

11.   The suprarenal glands are embedded in the fat above the _____
on each side. Each suprarenal gland has an internal _____ and an external
_____. The inner portion produces a pair of hormones:
e_____ (_____) and n_____ (_____). These
are involved in the mobilization of _____ during the stress reaction ("_____ or
_____"). Each suprarenal cortex produces hormones which can be grouped into
three different categories:

        a.   M_____s (for example, aldosterone), which are
concerned with the _____ of the body.

        b.   G_____s (for example, cortisol), which are concerned with
many metabolic functions and are anti-_____ in nature.

        c.   _____ hormones.

12.   In humans, the primary sex organs are known as _____s. These organs
produce _____ cells (_____) and sex _____s.

13.   During the first half of the menstrual cycle, the ovaries produce _____s.
During the second half, they produce _____e. These hormones are concerned
with female _____y and with the preparation of female sex _____s
for reproduction.

14.   The testes produce the male sex hormones known as _____(for
example, _____). These hormones are concerned with male _____.

Check Your Answers on Next Page

SOLUTIONS TO EXERCISES, LESSON 10

1. Endocrine glands are glands of <u>internal</u> secretion. These glands are also called <u>duct</u>less glands. Hormones are the secretions produced by <u>endocrine</u> glands. Target organs are the specific organs or tissues to which <u>hormones</u> are carried by the <u>bloodstream</u>. This is a feedback mechanism because the activity of the target organ affects the activity of the <u>endocrine organ</u>. (para 10-1)

2. The fundamental control "system" is the interaction of <u>heredity</u> and <u>environment</u>. Genes determine the range of <u>potentiality</u>. Environment <u>develops</u> it. Controlling the tissues and organs in general are the <u>hormones</u> of the <u>endocrine</u> system. Providing more precise and immediate control of the body structures is the <u>nervous</u> system. (para 10-2a)

3. Endocrine organs are richly supplied with blood vessels <u>because hormones must be carried to their target organs by the bloodstream.</u> (para 10-2b)

4. a. <u>Pituitary body</u>.
    b. <u>Thyroid gland</u>.
    c. <u>Parathyroid glands</u>.
    d. <u>Pancreatic islets</u>.
    e. <u>Suprarenal (adrenal) glands</u>.
    f. <u>Gonads (female--ovaries, male--testes)</u>. (para 10-2c)

5. The pituitary body is a small <u>pea</u>-sized and <u>pea</u>-shaped structure. It is attached to the base of the brain in the region of the <u>hypothalamus</u>. In addition, it is housed within a hollow of the bony floor of the <u>cranial</u> cavity. The pituitary body is actually two glands: the <u>posterior</u> pituitary gland and the <u>anterior</u> pituitary gland. (para 10-3)

6. The posterior pituitary gland is that portion of the pituitary body which comes from and retains its connection with the <u>base of the brain</u>. The hormones of the posterior pituitary gland are actually produced in the <u>hypothalamus</u> of the brain. The two recognized hormones of the posterior pituitary gland are <u>ADH</u> (<u>antidiuretic hormone</u>) and <u>oxytocin</u>. The first is involved with the <u>resorption or salvaging</u> of water within the kidneys; it is produced under <u>thirst</u> conditions. The second is concerned with contraction of smooth muscle in the <u>uterus</u> and with <u>milk</u> production. (para 10-4)

7. The anterior pituitary gland originates from the roof of the embryo's mouth. It then attaches itself to the posterior pituitary gland. By means of a venous portal system, the anterior pituitary gland is connected to the hypothalamus. Here, certain chemicals known as releasing factors are produced. These are carried to the anterior pituitary by the venous portal system. They stimulate the anterior pituitary gland's cells to secrete their specific hormones. In turn, these hormones stimulate the target organs to produce their own products. This stimulating effect is referred to as trophic. Two of the hormones produced by the anterior pituitary gland are somatotrophic hormone and ACTH (adrenocorticotrophic hormone). The target organs of the first are the growing structures of the body. The second stimulates the cortex of the suprarenal (adrenal) gland to produce its own hormones. (para 10-5)

8. The thyroid gland is in the neck region just below the larynx and surrounds the trachea. The masses on either side of the trachea are the right and left thyroid lobes. The tissue connecting the two lobes is called the isthmus. It is found across the front of the trachea. Each lobe of the thyroid gland is supplied by the superior and inferior thyroid arteries. The primary hormone of the thyroid gland is thyroxin, which affects the basal metabolic rate (BMR), the level of activity of the body. (paras 10-6--10-8)

9. The parathyroid glands are located on the posterior aspects of the thyroid lobes. The hormone produced by these glands is called parathyroid hormone or parathormone. It is involved with calcium metabolism. (paras 10-9, 10-10)

10. Within the pancreas are distributed small groups of cells known as islets. The two most commonly recognized hormones of the islets are insulin and glucagon. Theses hormones are involved with glucose metabolism. (paras 10-11, 10-12)

11. The suprarenal glands are embedded in the fat above the kidney on each side. Each suprarenal gland has an internal medulla and an external cortex. The inner portion produces a pair of hormones: epinephrine (adrenalin) and norepinephrine (noradrenalin). These are involved in the mobilization of energy during the stress reaction ("fight or flight"). Each suprarenal cortex produces hormones which can be grouped into three different categories:

    a. Mineralocorticoids (for example, aldosterone), which are concerned with the electrolytes of the body.

    b. Glucocorticoids (for example, cortisol), which are concerned with many metabolic functions and are anti-inflammatory in nature.

    c. Sex hormones. (paras 10-13--10-15)

12. In humans, the primary sex organs are known as gonads. These organs produce sex cells (gametes) and sex hormones. (para 10-16)

13. During the first half of the menstrual cycle, the ovaries produce estrogens. During the second half, they produce progesterone. These hormones are concerned with female sexuality and with the preparation of female sex organs for reproduction. (para 10-17)

14. The testes produce the male sex hormones known as androgens (for example, testosterone). These hormones are concerned with male sexuality. (para 10-18)

End of Lesson 10

LESSON ASSIGNMENT

LESSON 11   The Human Nervous System.

TEXT ASSIGNMENT   Paragraphs 11-1 through 11-39.

LESSON OBJECTIVES   After completing this lesson, you should be able to:

11-1.   Name and identify two types of nervous tissues.

11-2.   Name three functions for which nervous tissues are specialized.

11-3.   Define neuron, dendrite, and axon.

11-4.   When given the shape, diameter, or function, name the corresponding type of neuron.

11-5.   Describe neuron "connections," including the synapse and the neuromuscular junction.

11-6.   Name and identify the three major divisions of the human nervous system; name the two major subdivisions of the CNS.

11-7.   Name and briefly describe the three major subdivisions of the human brain; name and locate the four ventricles and their connecting channels.

11-8.   Describe the spinal cord, including the two enlargements, elements of its cross section, and the surrounding vertebral canal.

11-9.   Describe the meninges and the skeletal coverings of the CNS.

11-10. Name and identify the main arteries and veins of the brain and briefly describe the blood supply of the spinal cord.

11-11. Describe the formation of cerebrospinal fluid (CSF) and the path of CSF flow.

11-12. Define <u>peripheral</u> <u>nervous</u> <u>system</u> (PNS) and <u>nerve</u>; name and briefly describe two categories of PNS nerves; describe the anatomy of a "typical" spinal nerve; define <u>reflex</u> and <u>reflex</u> <u>arc</u>; briefly describe the components of the general reflex arc.

11-13. Define <u>autonomic nervous system</u> (ANS) and <u>visceral organs</u>; briefly describe efferent pathways of the ANS; name the major divisions of the human ANS; briefly describe the major activities of the human ANS for the thoraco-lumbar and cranio-sacral outflows; briefly describe the first and second neurons, innervations, and effects in each case.

11-14. Define <u>pathway</u>, <u>neuraxis</u>, <u>sensor pathway</u>, and <u>motor pathway</u>; briefly describe levels of control, pyramidal and extra-pyramidal motor pathways, and sensory pathways; and give examples of <u>general senses</u> and <u>special</u> <u>senses</u>.

11-15. Briefly describe the sensory receptors and sensory pathways for the special senses of smell and taste.

11-16. Describe the structures of the bulbus oculi, the orbit, and the adnexa.

11-17. Describe the structures of the external ear, the middle ear, and the internal ear.

11-18. Describe the structures of the sacculus, utriculus, semicircular ducts, and the vestibular nerve.

11-19. Describe controls in the human nervous system.

SUGGESTION

After completing the assignment, complete the exercises at the end of this lesson. These exercises will help you to achieve the lesson objectives.

LESSON 11

THE HUMAN NERVOUS SYSTEM

Section I. INTRODUCTION

11-1. NERVOUS TISSUES

There are two types of nervous tissues--the neurons (nerve cells) and glia (neuroglia). See paragraph 2-17. The neuron is the basic structural unit of the nervous system. The glia are cells of supporting tissue for the nervous system. There are several different types of glia, but their general function is support (physical, nutritive, etc.).

11-2. SPECIALIZATION

Nervous tissues are specialized to:

a. **Receive Stimuli**. Cells receiving stimuli are said to be "irritable" (as are all living cells to a degree).

b. **Transmit Information**.

c. **"Store" Information**. The storing of information is called memory.

Section II. THE NEURON AND ITS "CONNECTIONS"

11-3. DEFINITION

A neuron (figure 11-1) is a nerve cell body and all of its processes (branches).

11-4. NEURON CELL BODY

The neuron cell body is similar to that of the "typical" animal cell described in lesson 1.

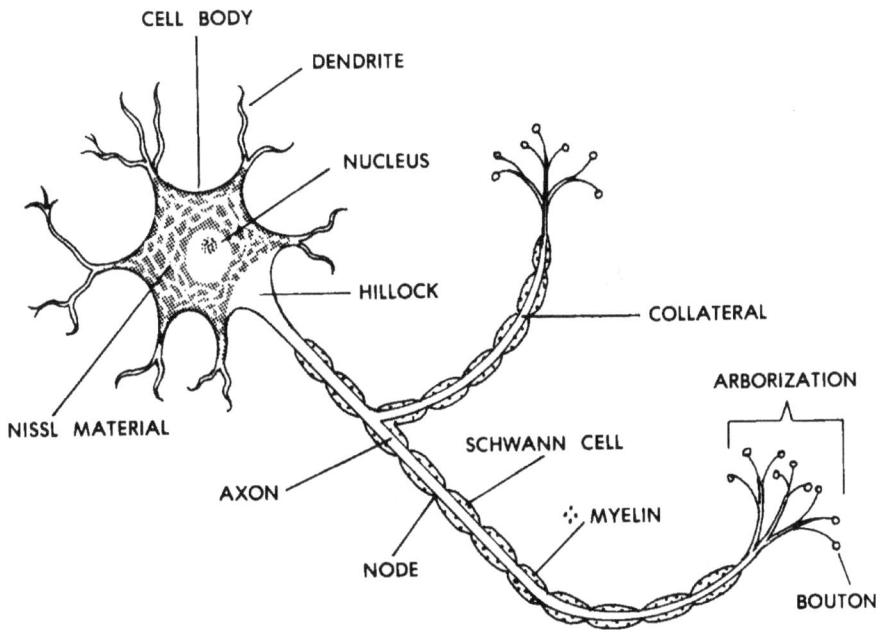

Figure 11-1. A "typical" neuron.

11-5. NEURON PROCESSES

There are two types of neuron processes--dendrites and axons.

a. **Dendrite**. A <u>dendrite</u> is a neuron process which carries impulses <u>toward</u> the cell body. Each neuron may have one or more dendrites. Dendrites receive information and transmit (carry) it to the cell body.

b. **Axon**. An <u>axon</u> is a neuron process which transmits information <u>from</u> the cell body to the next unit. Each neuron has only one axon.

c. **Information Transmission**. Information is carried as electrical impulses along the length of the neuron.

d. **Coverings**. Some neuron processes have a covering which is a series of Schwann cells, interrupted by nodes (thin spots). This gives the neuron process the appearance of links of sausage. The Schwann cells produce a lipid (fatty) material called <u>myelin</u>. This myelin acts as an electrical insulator during the transmission of impulses.

11-6. TYPES OF NEURONS

Neurons may be identified according to shape, diameter of their processes, or function.

a. **According to Shape**. A pole is the point where a neuron process meets the cell body. To determine the type according to shape, count the number of poles.

(1) Multipolar neurons. Multipolar neurons have more than two poles (one axon and two or more dendrites).

(2) Bipolar neurons. Bipolar neurons have two poles (one axon and one dendrite).

(3) Unipolar neurons. Unipolar neurons have a single process which branches into a T-shape. One arm is an axon; the other is a dendrite.

b. **According to Diameter (Thickness) of Processes**. Neurons may be rated according to the thickness of myelin surrounding the axon. In order of decreasing thickness, they are rated A (thickest), B, and C (thinnest). The thickness affects the rate at which impulses are transmitted. The thickest are fastest. The thinnest are slowest.

c. **According to Function**.

(1) Sensory neurons. In sensory neurons, impulses are transmitted from receptor organs (for pain, vision, hearing, etc.) to the central nervous system (CNS).

(2) Motor neurons. In motor neurons, impulses are transmitted from the CNS to muscles and glands (effector organs).

(3) Interneurons. Interneurons transmit information from one neuron to another. An interneuron "connects" two other neurons.

(4) Others. There are other, more specialized types, for example, in the CNS.

11-7. NEURON "CONNECTIONS"

A neuron may "connect" either with another neuron or with a muscle fiber. A phrase used to describe such "connections" is "continuity without contact." Neurons do not actually touch. There is just enough space to prevent the electrical transmission from crossing from the first neuron to the next. This space is called the synaptic cleft. Information is transferred across the synaptic cleft by chemicals called neurotransmitters. Neurotransmitters are manufactured and stored on only one side of the cleft. Because of this, information flows in only one direction across the cleft.

a. **The Synapse**. A synapse (figure 11-2) is a "connection" between two neurons.

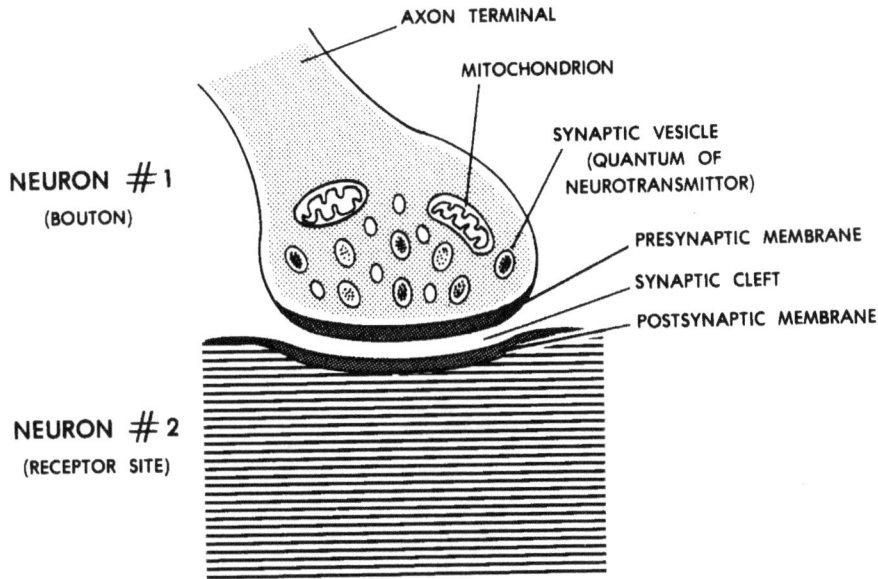

NEURON #1
(BOUTON)

NEURON #2
(RECEPTOR SITE)

AXON TERMINAL

MITOCHONDRION

SYNAPTIC VESICLE
(QUANTUM OF
NEUROTRANSMITTOR)

PRESYNAPTIC MEMBRANE

SYNAPTIC CLEFT

POSTSYNAPTIC MEMBRANE

Figure 11-2. A synapse.

(1) First neuron. An axon terminates in tiny branches. At the end of each branch is found a terminal bulb. Synaptic vesicles (bundles of neurotransmitter) are located within each terminal bulb. That portion of the terminal bulb which faces the synaptic cleft is thickened and is called the presynaptic membrane. This is the membrane through which neurotransmitters pass to enter the synaptic cleft.

(2) Synaptic cleft. The synaptic cleft is the space between the terminal bulb of the first neuron and the dendrite or cell body of the second neuron.

(3) Second neuron. The terminal bulb of the first neuron lies near a site on a dendrite or the cell body of the second neuron. The membrane at this site on the second neuron is known as the postsynaptic membrane. Within the second neuron is a chemical that inactivates the used neurotransmitter.

b. **The Neuromuscular Junction**. A neuromuscular junction (figure 11-3) is a "connection" between the terminal of a motor neuron and a muscle fiber. The neuromuscular junction has an organization identical to a synapse. However, the bulb is larger. The postsynaptic membrane is also larger and has foldings to increase its surface area.

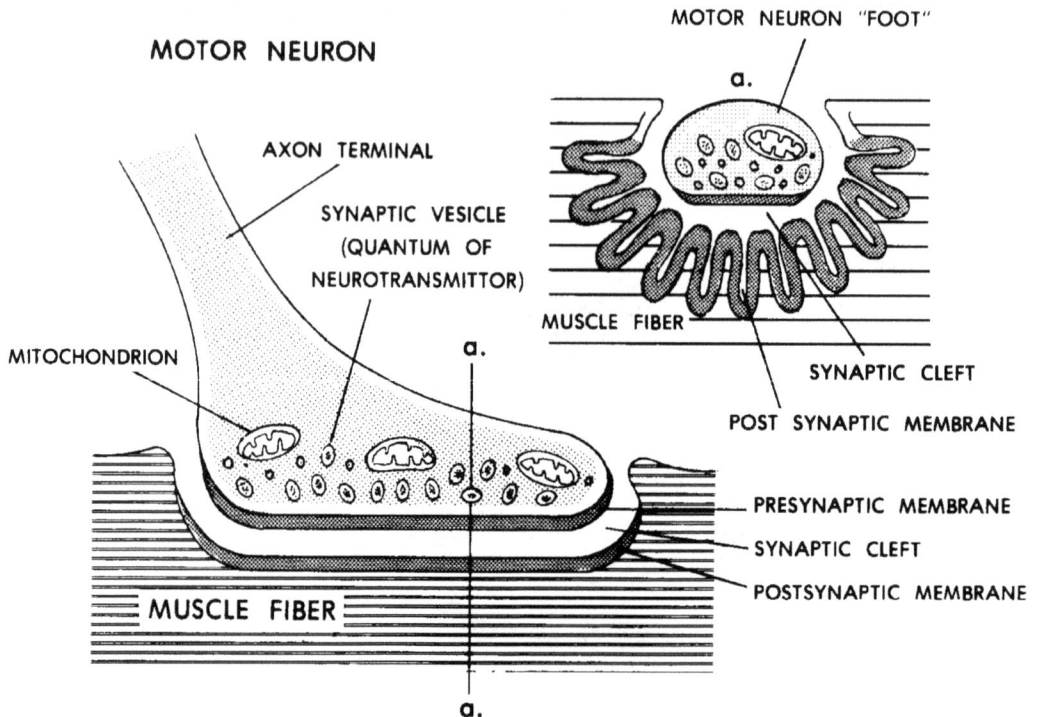

MOTOR NEURON

MOTOR NEURON "FOOT"

a.

AXON TERMINAL

SYNAPTIC VESICLE
(QUANTUM OF
NEUROTRANSMITTOR)

MUSCLE FIBER

SYNAPTIC CLEFT

POST SYNAPTIC MEMBRANE

MITOCHONDRION

a.

PRESYNAPTIC MEMBRANE

SYNAPTIC CLEFT

POSTSYNAPTIC MEMBRANE

MUSCLE FIBER

a.

Figure 11-3. A neuromuscular junction.

(1) <u>Motor neuron</u>. The axon of a motor neuron ends as it reaches a striated muscle fiber (of a skeletal muscle). At this point, it has a <u>terminal bulb</u>. Within this bulb are <u>synaptic vesicles</u> (bundles of neurotransmitter). The <u>presynaptic membrane</u> lines the surface of the terminal bulb and lies close to the muscle fiber.

(2) <u>Synaptic cleft</u>. The <u>synaptic cleft</u> is a space between the terminal bulb of the motor neuron and the membrane of the muscle fiber.

(3) <u>Muscle fiber</u>. The terminal bulb of the motor neuron protrudes into the surface of the muscle fiber. The membrane lining the synaptic space has foldings and is called the <u>postsynaptic membrane</u>. Beneath the postsynaptic membrane is a chemical which inactivates the used neurotransmitter.

Section III. THE HUMAN CENTRAL NERVOUS SYSTEM

11-8. GENERAL

The major divisions of the human nervous system are the central nervous system (CNS), the peripheral nervous system (PNS), and the autonomic nervous system (ANS). The CNS is made up of the brain and spinal cord. Both the PNS and the ANS carry information to and from the central nervous system. The PNS is generally concerned with the innervation of skeletal muscles and other muscles made up of striated muscle tissue, as well as sensory information from the periphery of the body. The ANS is that portion of the nervous system concerned with control of smooth muscle, cardiac muscle, and glands. The CNS (figure 11-4) is known as <u>central</u> because its anatomical location is along the central axis of the body and because the CNS is central in function. If we use a computer analogy to understand that it is central in function, the CNS would be the central processing unit and other parts of the nervous system would supply inputs and transmit outputs.

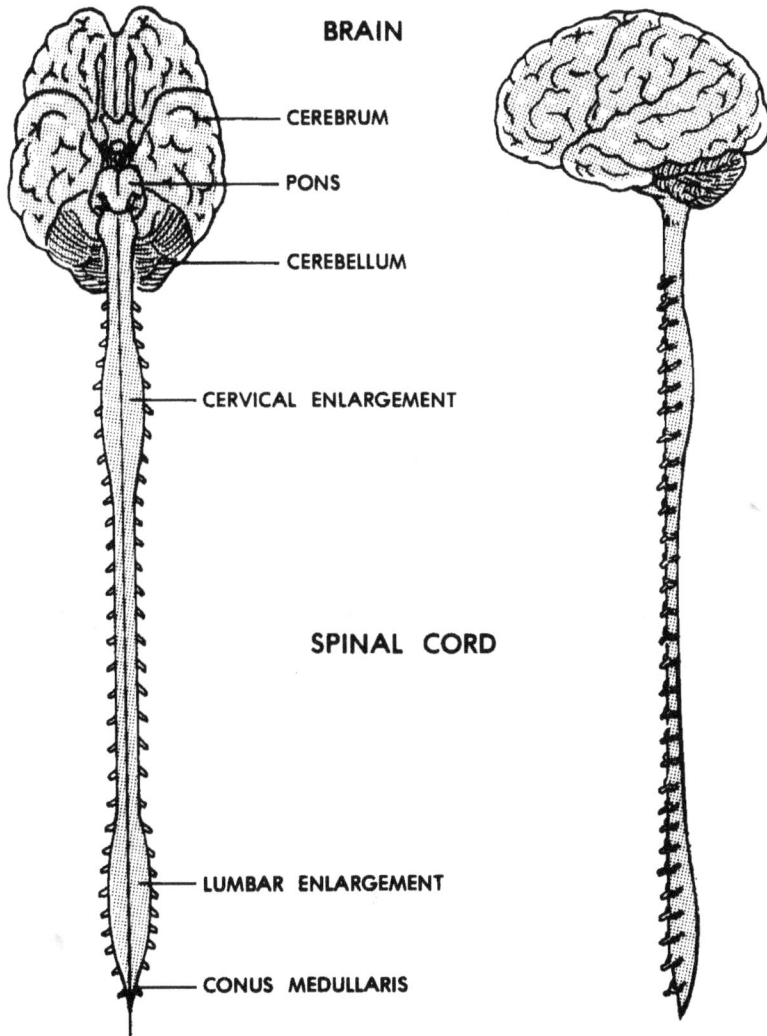

BRAIN

CEREBRUM

PONS

CEREBELLUM

CERVICAL ENLARGEMENT

SPINAL CORD

LUMBAR ENLARGEMENT

CONUS MEDULLARIS

Figure 11-4. The human central nervous system.

a. **Major Subdivisions of the CNS**. The major subdivisions of the CNS are the brain and the spinal cord.

b. **Coverings of the CNS**. The coverings of the CNS are skeletal and fibrous.

c. **Cerebrospinal Fluid (CSF)**. The CSF is a liquid thought to serve as a cushion and circulatory vehicle within the CNS.

11-9. THE HUMAN BRAIN

The human brain has three major subdivisions: brainstem, cerebellum, and cerebrum. The CNS is first formed as a simple tubelike structure in the embryo. The concentration of nervous tissues at one end of the human embryo to produce the brain and head is referred to as cephalization. When the embryo is about four weeks old, it is possible to identify the early forms of the brainstem, cerebellum, and cerebrum, as well as the spinal cord. As development continues, the brain is located within the cranium (para 4-13c(1)) in the cranial cavity. See figures 11-5A and 11-5B for illustrations of the adult brain.

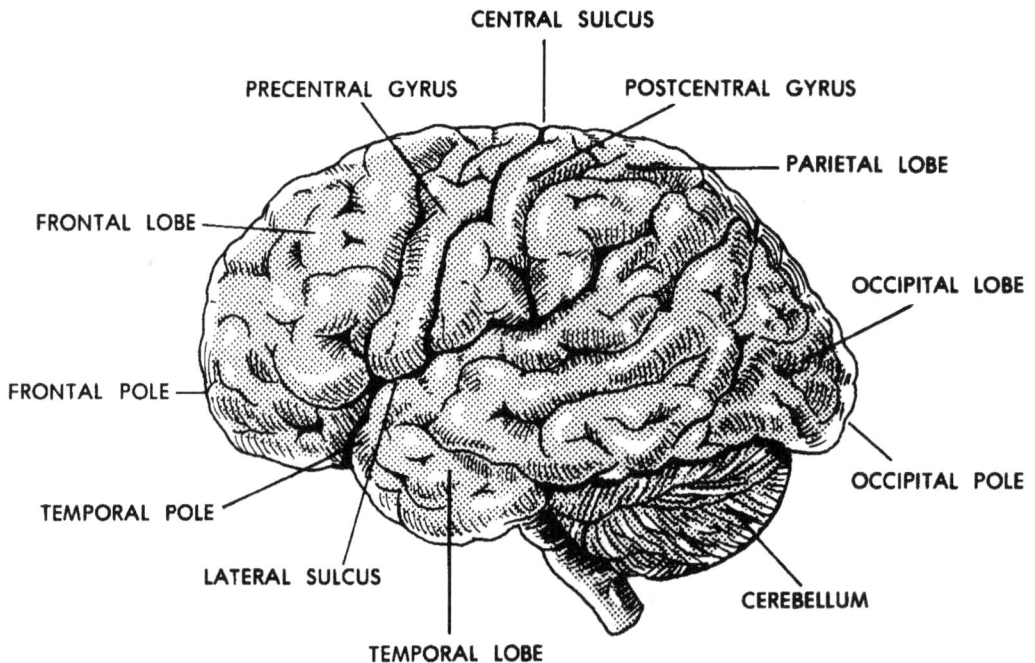

Figure 11-5A. Human brain (side view).

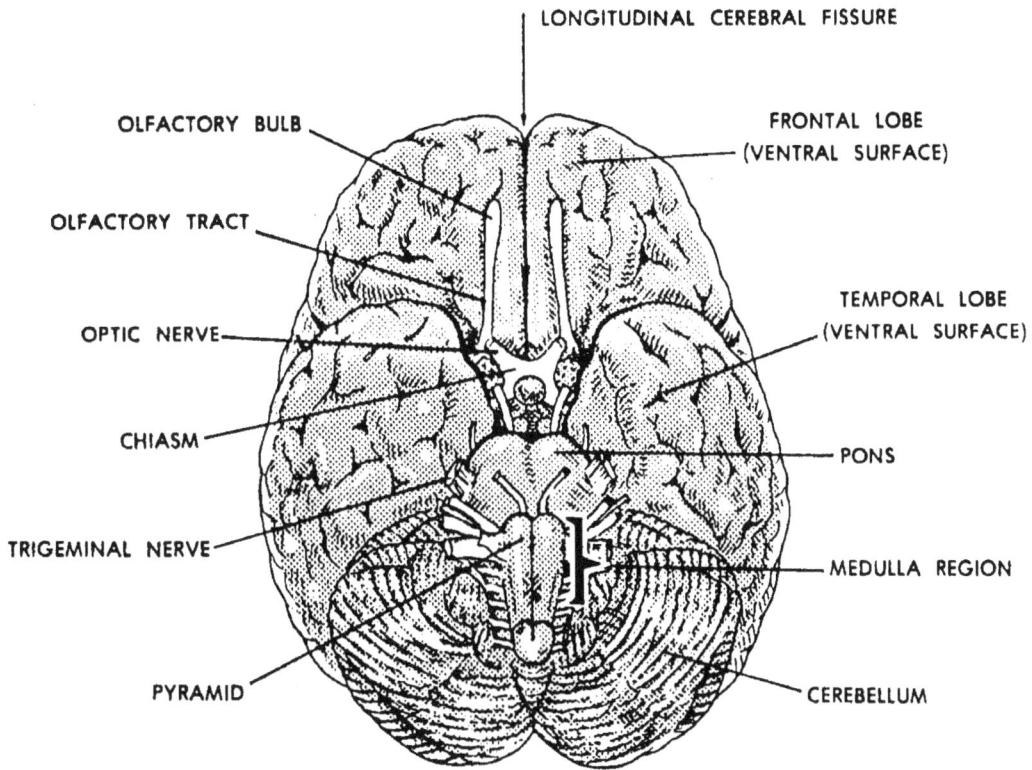

Figure 11-5B. Human brain (bottom view).

a. **The Brainstem**. The term brainstem refers to that part of the brain that would remain after removal of the cerebrum and cerebellum. The brainstem is the basal portion (portion of the base) of the brain. The brainstem can be divided as follows:

FOREBRAINSTEM: thalamus
                                 hypothalamus

MIDBRAINSTEM: corpora quadrigemina
                                 cerebral peduncles

HINDBRAINSTEM: pons
                                 medulla

(1) The brainstem is continuous with the spinal cord. Together, the brainstem and the spinal cord are sometimes known as the neuraxis.

(2) The brainstem provides major relays and controls for information passing up or down the neuraxis.

(3) The 12 pairs of cranial nerves connect at the sides of the brainstem.

b. **Cerebellum**. The cerebellum is a spherical mass of nervous tissue attached to and covering the hindbrainstem. It has a narrow central part called the vermis and right and left cerebellar hemispheres.

(1) Peduncles. A peduncle is a stem-like connecting part. The cerebellum is connected to the brainstem with three pairs of peduncles.

(2) General shape and construction. A cross section of the cerebellum reveals that the outer cortex is composed of gray matter (cell bodies of neurons) with many folds and sulci (shallow grooves). More centrally located is the white matter (myelinated processes of neurons).

(3) Function. The cerebellum is the primary coordinator/integrator of motor actions of the body.

c. **Cerebrum**. The cerebrum consists of two very much enlarged hemispheres connected to each other by a special structure called the corpus callosum. Each cerebral hemisphere is connected to the brainstem by a cerebral peduncle. The surface of each cerebral hemisphere is subdivided into areas known as lobes. Each lobe is named according to the cranial bone under which it lies: frontal, parietal, occipital, and temporal.

(1) The space separating the two cerebral hemispheres is called the longitudinal fissure. The shallow grooves in the surface of the cerebrum are called sulci (sulcus, singular). The ridges outlined by the sulci are known as gyri (gyrus, singular).

(2) The cerebral cortex is the gray outer layer of each hemisphere. The occurrence of sulci and gyri helps to increase the amount of this layer. Deeper within the cerebral hemispheres, the tissue is white. The "gray matter" represents cell bodies of the neurons. The "white matter" represents the axons.

(3) The areas of the cortex are associated with groups of related functions.

(a) For example, centers of speech and hearing are located along the lateral sulcus, at the side of each hemisphere.

(b) Vision is centered at the rear in the area known as the occipital lobe.

(c) Sensory and motor functions are located along the central sulcus, which separates the frontal and parietal lobes of each hemisphere. The motor areas are located along the front side of the central sulcus, in the frontal lobe. The sensory areas are located along the rear side of the central sulcus, in the parietal lobe.

d. **Ventricles**. Within the brain, there are interconnected hollow spaces filled with cerebrospinal fluid (CSF). These hollow spaces are known as ventricles. The right and left lateral ventricles are found in the cerebral hemispheres. The lateral ventricles are connected to the third ventricle via the interventricular foramen (of Monroe). The third ventricle is located in the forebrainstem. The fourth ventricle is in the hindbrainstem. The cerebral aqueduct (of Sylvius) is a short tube through the midbrainstem which connects the third and fourth ventricles. The fourth ventricle is continuous with the narrow central canal of the spinal cord.

11-10. THE HUMAN SPINAL CORD

a. **Location and Extent**. Referring to figure 4-4, you can see that the typical vertebra has a large opening called the vertebral (or spinal) foramen. Together, these foramina form the vertebral (spinal) canal for the entire vertebral column. The spinal cord, located within the spinal canal, is continuous with the brainstem. The spinal cord travels the length from the foramen magnum at the base of the skull to the junction of the first and second lumbar vertebrae.

(1) Enlargements. The spinal cord has two enlargements. One is the cervical enlargement, associated with nerves for the upper members. The other is the lumbosacral enlargement, associated with nerves for the lower members.

(2) Spinal nerves. A nerve is a bundle of neuron processes which carry impulses to and from the CNS. Those nerves arising from the spinal cord are spinal nerves. There are 31 pairs of spinal nerves.

b. **A Cross Section of the Spinal Cord (figure 11-6)**. The spinal cord is a continuous structure which runs through the vertebral canal down to the lumbar region of the column. It is composed of a mass of central gray matter (cell bodies of neurons) surrounded by peripheral white matter (myelinated processes of neurons). The gray and white matter are thus considered columns of material. However, in a cross section, this effect of columns is lost.

(1) Central canal. A very narrow canal, called the central canal, is located in the center of the spinal cord. The central canal is continuous with the fourth ventricle of the brain.

(2) The gray matter. In the cross section of the spinal cord, one can see a central H-shaped region of gray matter. Each arm of the H is called a horn, resulting in two posterior horns and two anterior horns. The connecting link is called the gray commissure. Since the gray matter extends the full length of the spinal cord, these horns are actually sections of the gray columns.

(3) The white matter. The peripheral portion of the spinal cord cross section consists of white matter. Since a column of white matter is a large bundle of processes, it is called a funiculus. In figure 11-6, note the anterior, lateral, and posterior funiculi.

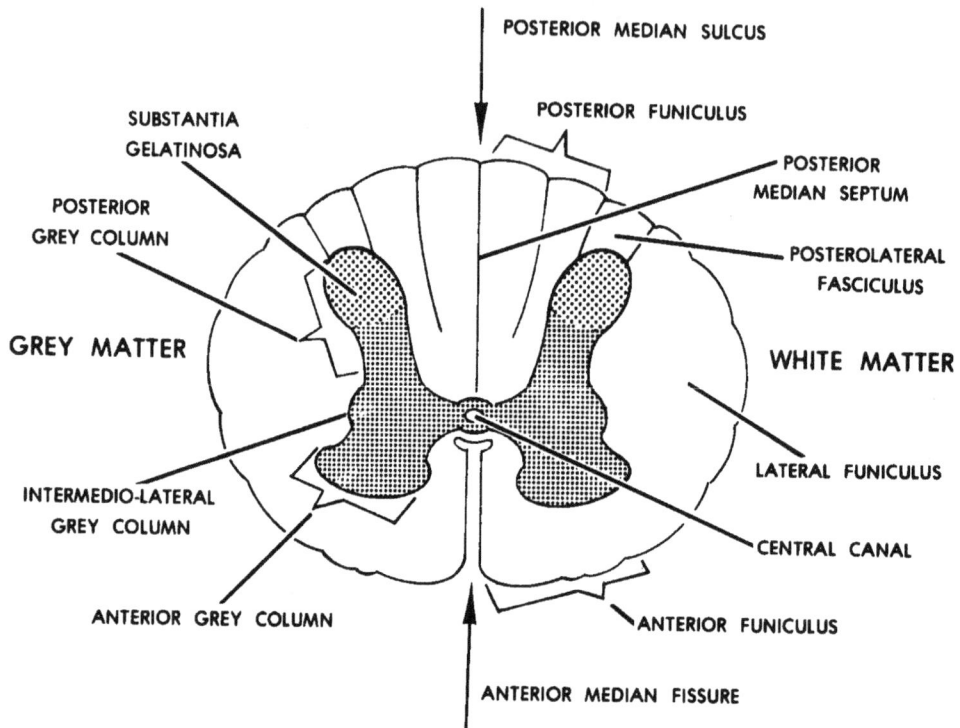

Figure 11-6. A cross-section of the spinal cord.

11-11. COVERINGS OF THE CNS

The coverings of the CNS are skeletal and fibrous.

a. **Skeletal Coverings**.

(1) <u>Brain</u>. The bones of the cranium form a spherical case around the brain. The <u>cranial cavity</u> is the space inclosed by the bones of the cranium.

(2) <u>Spinal cord</u>. The vertebrae, with the vertebral foramina, form a cylindrical case around the spinal cord. The overall skeletal structure is the <u>vertebral column</u> (spine). The <u>vertebral (spinal) canal</u> is the space inclosed by the foramina of the vertebrae.

b. **Meninges (Fibrous Membranes)**. The brain and spinal cord have three different membranes surrounding them called meninges (figure 11-7). These coverings provide protection.

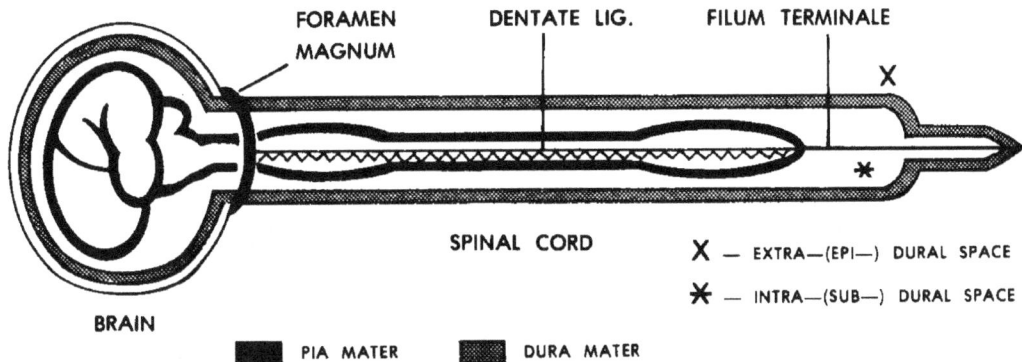

Figure 11-7. A schematic diagram of the meninges, as seen in side view of the CNS.

(1) Dura mater. The dura mater is a tough outer covering for the CNS. Beneath the dura mater is the subdural space, which contains a thin film of fluid.

(2) Arachnoid mater. To the inner side of the dura mater and subdural space is a fine membranous layer called the arachnoid mater. It has fine spiderweb-type threads which extend inward through the subarachnoid space to the pia mater. The subarachnoid space is filled with cerebrospinal fluid (CSF).

ARACHNOID = spider-like

(3) Pia mater. The pia mater is a delicate membrane applied directly to the surface of the brain and the spinal cord. It carries a network of blood vessels to supply the nervous tissues of the CNS.

11-12. BLOOD SUPPLY OF THE CNS

a. **Blood Supply of the Brain**. The paired internal carotid arteries and the paired vertebral arteries supply blood rich in oxygen to the brain. Branches of these arteries join to form a circle under the base of the brain. This is called the cerebral circle (of Willis). From this circle, numerous branches supply specific areas of the brain.

(1) A single branch is often the only blood supply to that particular area. Such an artery is called an end artery. If it fails to supply blood to that specific area, that area will die (stroke).

(2) The veins and venous sinuses of the brain drain into the paired internal jugular veins, which carry the blood back toward the heart.

b. **Blood Supply of the Spinal Cord**. The blood supply of the spinal cord is by way of a combination of three longitudinal arteries running along its length and reinforced by segmental arteries from the sides.

11-13. CEREBROSPINAL FLUID (CSF)

A clear fluid called cerebrospinal fluid (CSF) is found in the cavities of the CNS. CSF is found in the ventricles of the brain (para 11-9d), the subarachnoid space (para 11-11b(2)), and the central canal of the spinal cord (para 11-10b(1)). CSF and its associated structures make up the circulatory system for the CNS.

a. **Choroid Plexuses**. Choroid plexuses are special collections of arterial capillaries found in the roofs of the third and fourth ventricles of the brain. The choroid plexuses continuously produce CSF from the plasma of the blood.

b. **Path of the CSF Flow**. Blood flows through the arterial capillaries of the choroid plexuses. As CSF is produced by the choroid plexuses, it flows into all four ventricles. CSF from the lateral ventricles flows into the third ventricle and then through the cerebral aqueduct into the fourth ventricle. By passing through three small holes in the roof of the fourth ventricle, CSF enters the subarachnoid space. From the subarachnoid space, the CSF is transported through the arachnoid villi (granulations) into the venous sinuses. Thus, the CSF is formed from arterial blood and returned to the venous blood.

Section IV. THE PERIPHERAL NERVOUS SYSTEM (PNS)

11-14. GENERAL

a. **Definitions**.

(1) The peripheral nervous system (PNS) is that portion of the nervous system generally concerned with commands for skeletal muscles and other muscles made up of striated muscle tissue, as well as sensory information from the periphery of the body. The sensory information is carried to the CNS where it is processed. The PNS carries commands from the CNS to musculature.

(2) A nerve is a collection of neuron processes, together and outside the CNS. (A fiber tract is a collection of neuron processes, together and inside the CNS.)

b. **General Characteristics of the Peripheral Nerves**. The PNS is made up of a large number of individual nerves. These nerves are arranged in pairs. Each pair includes one nerve on the left side of the brainstem or spinal cord and one nerve on the right side. The nerve pairs are in a series, each pair resembling the preceding, from top to bottom.

c. **Categories of PNS Nerves**. PNS nerves include cranial nerves and spinal nerves.

(1) <u>Cranial nerves</u>. The 12 pairs of nerves attached to the right and left sides of the brainstem are called cranial nerves. Each cranial nerve is identified by a Roman numeral in order from I to XII and an individual name. For example, the Vth ("fifth") cranial nerve is known as the trigeminal nerve (N.).

TRI = three

GEMINI = alike

TRIGEMINAL = having three similar major branches

(2) <u>Spinal nerves</u>. Attached to the sides of the spinal cord are 31 pairs of spinal nerves. The spinal nerves are named by:

(a) The <u>region</u> of the spinal cord with which the nerve is associated.

(b) An <u>Arabic numeral</u> within the region. For example, T-5 is the fifth spinal nerve in the thoracic region.

11-15. A "TYPICAL" SPINAL NERVE

In the human body, every spinal nerve has essentially the same construction and components. By learning the anatomy of one spinal nerve, you can understand the anatomy of all spinal nerves.

a. **Parts of a "Typical" Spinal Nerve (figure 11-8)**. Like a tree, a typical spinal nerve has roots, a trunk, and branches (rami).

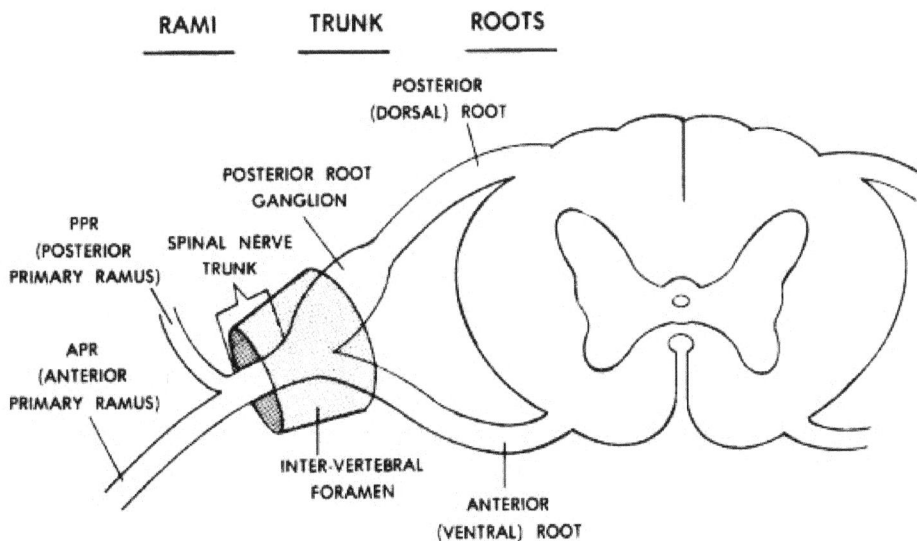

Figure 11-8. A "typical" spinal nerve with a cross section of the spinal cord.

(1) Coming off of the posterior and anterior sides of the spinal cord are the posterior (dorsal) and anterior (ventral) roots of the spinal nerve. An enlargement on the posterior root is the posterior root ganglion. A ganglion is a collection of neuron cell bodies, together, outside the CNS.

(2) Laterally, the posterior and anterior roots of the spinal nerve join to form the spinal nerve trunk. The spinal nerve trunk of each spinal nerve is located in the appropriate intervertebral foramen of the vertebral column. (An intervertebral foramen is a passage formed on either side of the junction between two vertebrae.)

(3) Where the spinal nerve trunk emerges laterally from the intervertebral foramen, the trunk divides into two major branches. These branches are called the anterior (ventral) and posterior (dorsal) primary rami (ramus, singular). The posterior primary rami go to the back. The anterior primary rami go to the sides and front of the body and also to the upper and lower members.

b. **Neurons of a "Typical" Spinal Nerve**. A nerve is defined above as a collection of neuron processes. Thus, neuron processes are the components that make up a nerve. These processes may belong to any of several different types of neurons: afferent (sensory), efferent (motor), and visceral motor neurons of the ANS.

(1) The afferent neuron and the efferent neuron are the two types we will consider here. An afferent neuron is one which carries information from the periphery to the CNS.

A = toward

FERENT = to carry

An efferent neuron is one which carries information from the CNS to a muscle or gland.

E = away from

FERENT = to carry

(2) The afferent neuron is often called the sensory neuron because it carries information about the senses to the CNS. The efferent neuron is often called the motor neuron because it carries commands from the CNS to cause a muscle to act.

(3) A stimulus acts upon a sensory receptor organ in the skin or in another part of the body. The information is carried by an afferent (sensory) neuron through merging branches of the spinal nerve to the posterior root ganglion. The afferent (sensory) neuron's cell body is located in the posterior root ganglion. From this point, information continues in the posterior root to the spinal cord. The efferent (motor) neuron carries command information from the spinal cord to the individual muscle of the human body.

(4) Visceral motor neurons of the ANS (see section V), which innervate visceral organs of the body's periphery, are distributed along with the peripheral nerves.

c. **The General Reflex Arc (figure 11-9).**

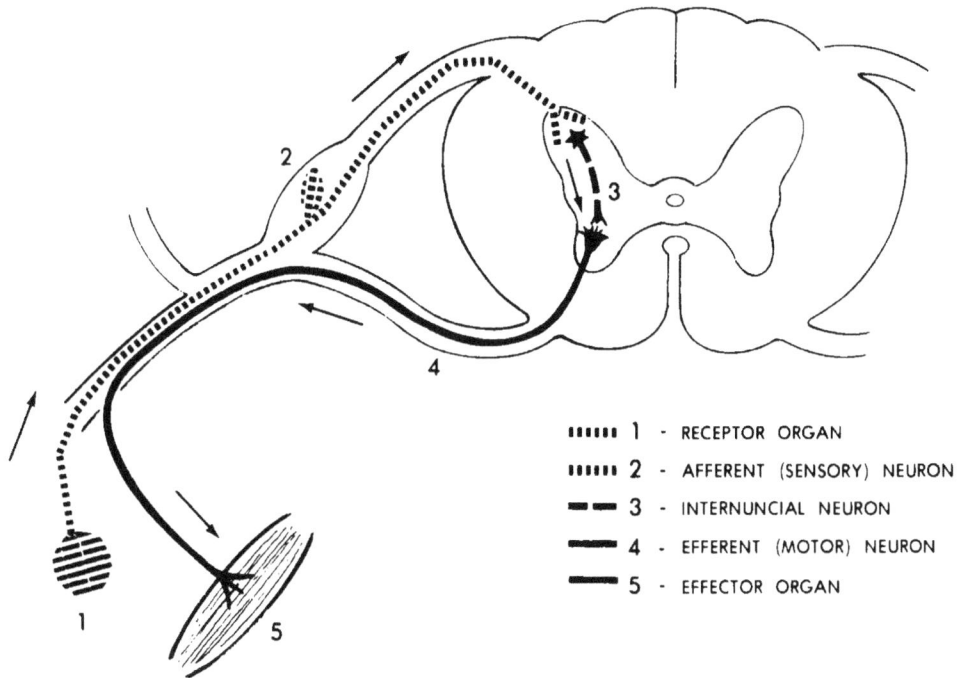

IIIII 1 - RECEPTOR ORGAN
IIIII 2 - AFFERENT (SENSORY) NEURON
━ ━ 3 - INTERNUNCIAL NEURON
━━ 4 - EFFERENT (MOTOR) NEURON
━━ 5 - EFFECTOR ORGAN

Figure 11-9. The general reflex arc.

(1) Definitions.

(a) An automatic reaction to a stimulus (without first having conscious sensation) is referred to as a reflex. (As an example: The withdrawal of the hand from a hot object.)

(b) The pathway from the receptor organ to the reacting muscle is called the reflex arc.

(2) Components of the general reflex arc. The pathway of a general reflex arc involves a minimum of five structures.

(a) The stimulus is received by a receptor organ.

(b) That information is transmitted to the CNS by the afferent (sensory) neuron.

(c) Within the spinal cord, there is a special neuron connecting the afferent neuron to the efferent neuron. This special connecting neuron is called the internuncial neuron, or interneuron.

INTER = between

NUNCIA = messenger

INTERNUNCIAL = the carrier of information between

(d) The efferent (motor) neuron carries the appropriate command from the spinal cord to the reacting muscle.

(e) The reacting muscle is called the effector organ.

Section V. THE AUTONOMIC NERVOUS SYSTEM (ANS)

11-16. GENERAL

The autonomic nervous system (ANS) is that portion of the nervous system generally concerned with commands for smooth muscle tissue, cardiac muscle tissue, and glands.

a. **Visceral Organs**.

(1) Definition. The term visceral organs may be used to include:

(a) The various hollow organs of the body whose walls have smooth muscle tissue in them. Examples are the blood vessels and the gut.

(b) The glands.

(2) Distribution. The visceral organs are located in the central cavity of the body (example: stomach) and throughout the periphery of the body (example: sweat glands of the skin).

(3) Control. It has always been thought that the control of visceral organs was "automatic" and not conscious. However, recent researches indicate that proper training enables a person to consciously control some of the visceral organs.

b. **Efferent Pathways**. Earlier, we said that each neuron in the PNS extended the entire distance from the CNS to the receptor or effector organ. In the ANS, there are always two neurons (one after the other) connecting the CNS with the visceral organ. The cell bodies of the second neurons form a collection outside the CNS, called a ganglion.

(1) The first neuron extends from the CNS to the ganglion and is therefore called the preganglionic neuron.

(2) Cell bodies of the second neuron make up the ganglion. The second neuron's processes extend from the ganglion to the visceral organ. Thus, the second neuron is called the post-ganglionic neuron.

c. **Major Divisions of the Human ANS**. The efferent pathways of the ANS fall into two major divisions:

(1) The thoraco-lumbar outflow (sympathetic nervous system).

(2) The cranio-sacral outflow (parasympathetic nervous system).

d. **Major Activities of the Human ANS.**

(1) The ANS maintains visceral activities in a balanced or stable state. This is called homeostasis.

(2) When subjected to stress, such as a threat, the body responds with the "fight-or-flight reaction." That is, those activities of the body necessary for action in an emergency are activated and those not necessary are deactivated. This is the primary function of the sympathetic portion of the ANS.

11-17. THE THORACO-LUMBAR OUTFLOW (SYMPATHETIC NERVOUS SYSTEM)

a. Refer to paragraph 11-10b(2) which describes the H-shaped region of gray matter in the cross section of the spinal cord. Imagine extending the cross link of the H slightly to the left and right of the vertical arms; the extended ends would correspond to the intermediolateral gray columns. Cell bodies of the first neurons of the sympathetic NS make up those columns between the T-1 and L-2 levels of the spinal cord, a total of 14 levels. Here, we are speaking of preganglionic sympathetic neurons.

b. Cell bodies of the second neurons make up various sympathetic ganglia of the body. These ganglia include the trunk or chain ganglia and the pre-aortic or "central" ganglia. Here, we are speaking of post- ganglionic sympathetic neurons.

c. The sympathetic NS innervates:

(1) Peripheral visceral organs (example: sweat glands).

(2) Central visceral organs (examples: lungs and stomach).

d. The neurons innervating the peripheral visceral organs are distributed to them by being included in the nerves of the PNS.

e. The sympathetic NS <u>activates</u> those visceral organs needed to mobilize energy for action (example: heart) and <u>deactivates</u> those not needed (example: gut).

11-18. THE CRANIO-SACRAL OUTFLOW (PARASYMPATHETIC NERVOUS SYSTEM)

a. Cell bodies of the <u>first</u> neurons of the parasympathetic NS make up the <u>inter-mediolateral gray columns</u> in the sacral spinal cord at the S-2, S-3, and S-4 levels. See paragraph 11-17a above for the position of the intermediolateral gray columns. Cell bodies of the <u>first</u> neurons also make up four pairs of nuclei in the brainstem; these nuclei are associated with cranial nerves III, VII, IX, and X. Here, we are speaking of <u>preganglionic parasympathetic neurons</u>.

b. Cell bodies of the <u>second</u> neurons make up intramural ganglia within the walls of the visceral organs. These second neurons innervate the central visceral organs. They do NOT innervate peripheral visceral organs. Here, we are speaking of the <u>post-ganglionic parasympathetic neurons</u>.

c. The parasympathetic NS has the opposite effect on visceral organs from that of the sympathetic NS. (Example: The heart is accelerated by the sympathetic NS and decelerated by the parasympathetic NS.)

Section VI. PATHWAYS OF THE HUMAN NERVOUS SYSTEM

11-19. GENERAL

a. **Definitions**.

(1) A <u>pathway</u> is the series of nervous structures utilized in the transmission of an item of information. An example of a pathway is the reflex arc discussed in para-graph 11-15c.

(2) The brainstem is continuous with the spinal cord. Together, the brainstem and the spinal cord are sometimes known as the <u>neuraxis</u>.

b. **General Categories of Neural Pathways**.

(1) <u>Sensory pathways</u>. A <u>sensory pathway</u> is a series of nervous structures used to transmit information from the <u>body to the CNS</u>. Upon arrival in the CNS, these pathways ascend (go up) the neuraxis to the brain.

(2) <u>Motor pathways</u>. A <u>motor pathway</u> is a series of nervous structures used to transmit information from the <u>CNS to the body</u>. The commands for motor action originate in the brain and descend (go down) the neuraxis to the appropriate spinal levels. From this point, the commands pass through the nerves to the effector organs.

c. **Controls**. The human nervous system has several levels for control. The lowest level is the simple reflex arc (see para 11-15c). The highest level of control is the conscious level. From the lowest to the highest levels are several progressively higher levels, such as the righting reflex. Thus, the processing of information and the transmission of commands are not haphazard but very carefully monitored and controlled. All information input and all information output are monitored and evaluated.

11-20. THE MOTOR PATHWAYS

Motor pathways begin in the brain. They descend the neuraxis in bundles of a number of specific neuron processes called <u>motor fiber tracts</u>. Commands originating in the <u>right</u> half of the brain leave the CNS through peripheral nerves on the <u>left</u> side. Commands from the left half of the brain leave the CNS on the right side. Therefore, the right half of the brain controls the left side of the body and the left half of the brain controls the right side of the body. For example, the actions of the right hand are controlled by the left half of the brain. (In those people who are right-handed, we refer to the left half of the brain as being <u>dominant</u>.)

a. **Pyramidal Motor Pathways**. A pyramidal motor pathway is primarily con-cerned with volitional (voluntary) control of the body parts, in particular the fine movements of the hands. Because control is volitional, the pathways can be used for neurological screening and testing. These pathways are called <u>pyramidal</u> because their neuron processes contribute to the makeup of a pair of structures in the base of the brain known as the pyramids.

b. **Extrapyramidal Motor Pathways**. An extrapyramidal pathway is primarily concerned with automatic (nonvolitional) control of body parts for purposes of coordination. Extrapyramidal pathways use many intermediate relays before reaching the effector organs. The cerebellum of the brain plays a major role in extrapyramidal pathways; the cerebellum helps to integrate patterned movements of the body.

11-21. THE SENSORY PATHWAYS

a. The body is continuously bombarded by types of information called <u>stimuli</u> (stimulus, singular). Those few stimuli which are consciously perceived (in the cerebral hemispheres) are called <u>sensations</u>.

b. Those stimuli received throughout the body are called the <u>general</u> <u>senses</u>. Stimuli received by only single pairs of organs in the head (for example, the eyes) are called <u>special senses</u> (for example, smell and taste).

c. The general senses in humans include pain, temperature (warm and cold), touch (light and deep), and proprioception ("body sense": posture, tone, tension).

d. The special senses in humans include smell (olfaction), taste (gustation), vision, hearing (auditory), and equilibrium.

e. The input from each special sensory receptor goes to its own specific area of the opposite cerebral hemisphere. The general sensory pathway is from the receptor organ, via the PNS nerves, to the CNS. This general pathway then ascends fiber tracts in the neuraxis. The pathway ends in the central area of the cerebral hemisphere (on the side opposite to the input).

Section VII. THE SPECIAL SENSE OF SMELL (OLFACTION)

11-22. SENSORY RECEPTORS

Molecules of various materials are dispersed (spread) throughout the air we breathe. A special olfactory epithelium is located in the upper recesses of the nasal chambers in the head. Special hair cells in the olfactory epithelium are called chemore-ceptors, because they receive these molecules in the air.

11-23. OLFACTORY SENSORY PATHWAY

The information received by the olfactory hair cells is transmitted by way of the olfactory nerves (cranial nerves I). It passes through these nerves to the olfactory bulbs and then into the opposite cerebral hemisphere. Here, the information becomes the sensation of smell.

Section VIII. THE SPECIAL SENSE OF TASTE (GUSTATION)

11-24. SENSORY RECEPTORS

Molecules of various materials are also dispersed or dissolved in the fluids (saliva) of the mouth. These molecules are from the food ingested (taken in). Organs known as taste buds are scattered over the tongue and the rear of the mouth. Special hair cells in the taste buds are chemoreceptors to react to these molecules.

11-25. SENSORY PATHWAY

The information received by the hair cells of the taste buds is transmitted to the opposite side of the brain by way of three cranial nerves (VII, IX, and X). This information is interpreted by the cerebral hemispheres as the sensation of taste.

Section IX. THE SPECIAL SENSE OF VISION (SIGHT)

11-26. GENERAL

a. **Stimulus**. Rays of light stimulate the receptor tissues of the eyeballs (bulbus oculi) to produce the special sense of vision. This includes both the sensation of vision or seeing and a variety of reactions known as the light reflexes. The actual reception of the light energy is a chemical reaction which in turn stimulates the neuron endings.

b. **Optical Physics**. To appreciate the functioning of the bulbus oculi, some simple principles of optical physics must be understood.

(1) By means of a lens system, light rays are bent and brought to the focal point for acute vision. This process is referred to as focusing.

(2) The focal length is the distance from the focal point to the center of the lens. The amount of bending or focusing depends upon the exact curvatures of the lens system.

c. **Sense Organ**. The eyeball is the special sense organ which contains the receptor tissues. The eyeball is suspended in the orbit. The orbit is a skeletal socket of the skull which helps protect the eyeball. Various structures associated with the functioning of the eyeball are called the adnexa. The adnexa include the eyelids, the lacrimal system, etc.

11-27. THE EYEBALL (FIGURE 11-10)

a. **Shape**. In the main, the eyeball is a spherical bulb-like structure. Its anterior surface, transparent and more curved, is known as the cornea of the eyeball.

b. **Wall of the Eyeball**. The eyeball is a hollow structure. Its wall is made up of three layers known as coats or tunics.

(1) Sclera. The outermost layer is white and very dense FCT (fibrous connective tissue). It is known as the sclera, scleral coat, or fibrous tunic. Its anterior portion is called the cornea. As already mentioned, the cornea is transparent and more curved than the rest of the sclera. The fixed curvature of the cornea enables it to serve as the major focusing device for the eyeball.

(2) Choroid. The middle layer of the wall of the eyeball is known as the choroid, the choroid coat, or the vascular tunic. This layer is richly supplied with blood vessels. It is also pigmented with a black material. The black color absorbs light rays and prevents them from reflecting at random.

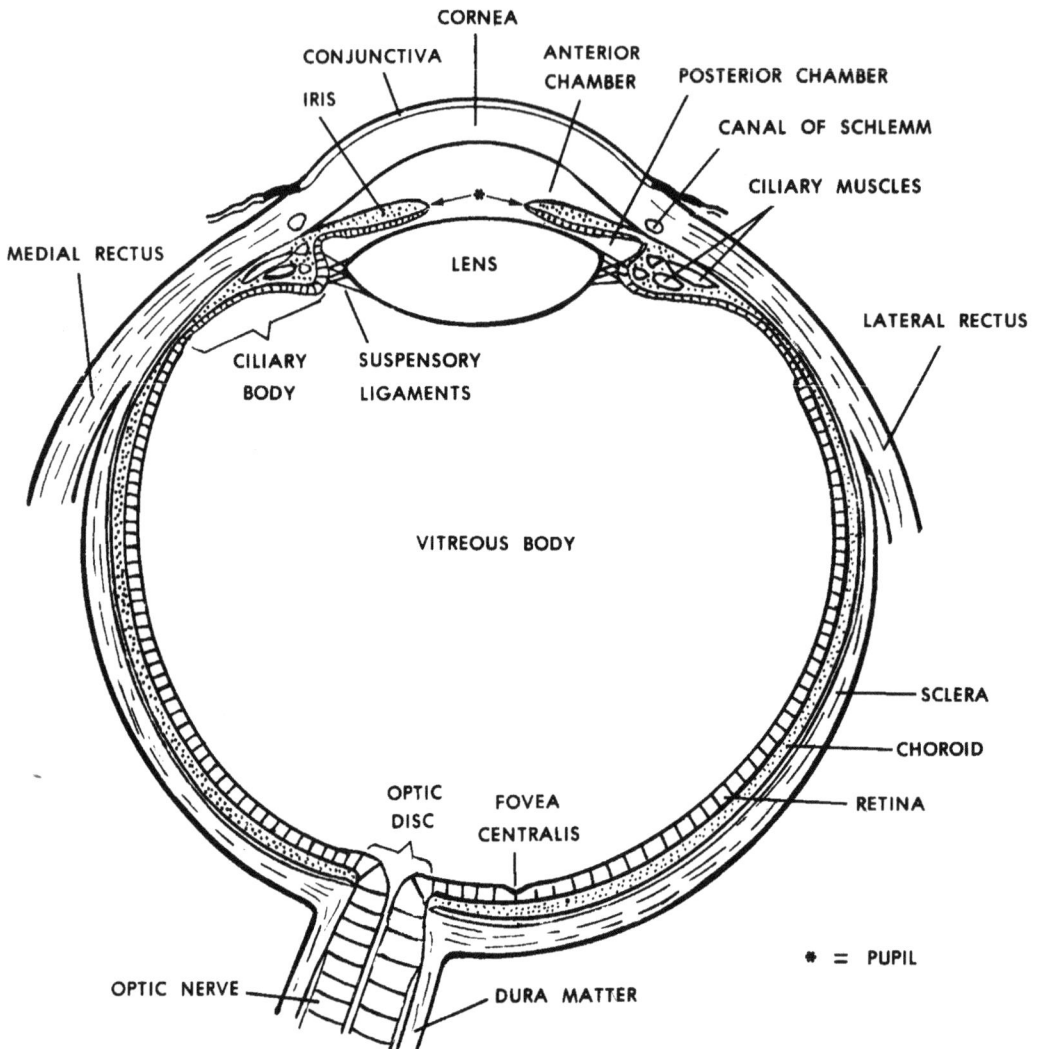

Figure 11-10. A horizontal section of the eyeball.

(3) <u>Retina</u>. The inner layer of the wall of the eyeball is known as the <u>retina</u>, <u>retinal coat</u>, or <u>internal tunic</u>. The actual photoreceptor elements are located in the retina at the back and sides of the eyeball. These elements are the rods and cones. They constitute the nervous portion of the retina. In the anterior part of the eyeball, the retina continues as a nonnervous portion.

c. **Internal Structures of the Eyeball**.

   (1) <u>The nervous retina</u>.

        (a) The photoreceptors of the nervous portion of the retina (figure 11-11) contain chemicals known as <u>visual pigments</u> (rhodopsin). The <u>cones</u> are more concentrated in the center at the back of the eyeball. The cones can register colors and are used for acute vision. However, cones require more intense light than do rods. The <u>rods</u> are distributed more toward the sides of the nervous retina. Although the rods are capable of registering less intense light, rods perceive only black and white.

INSIDE

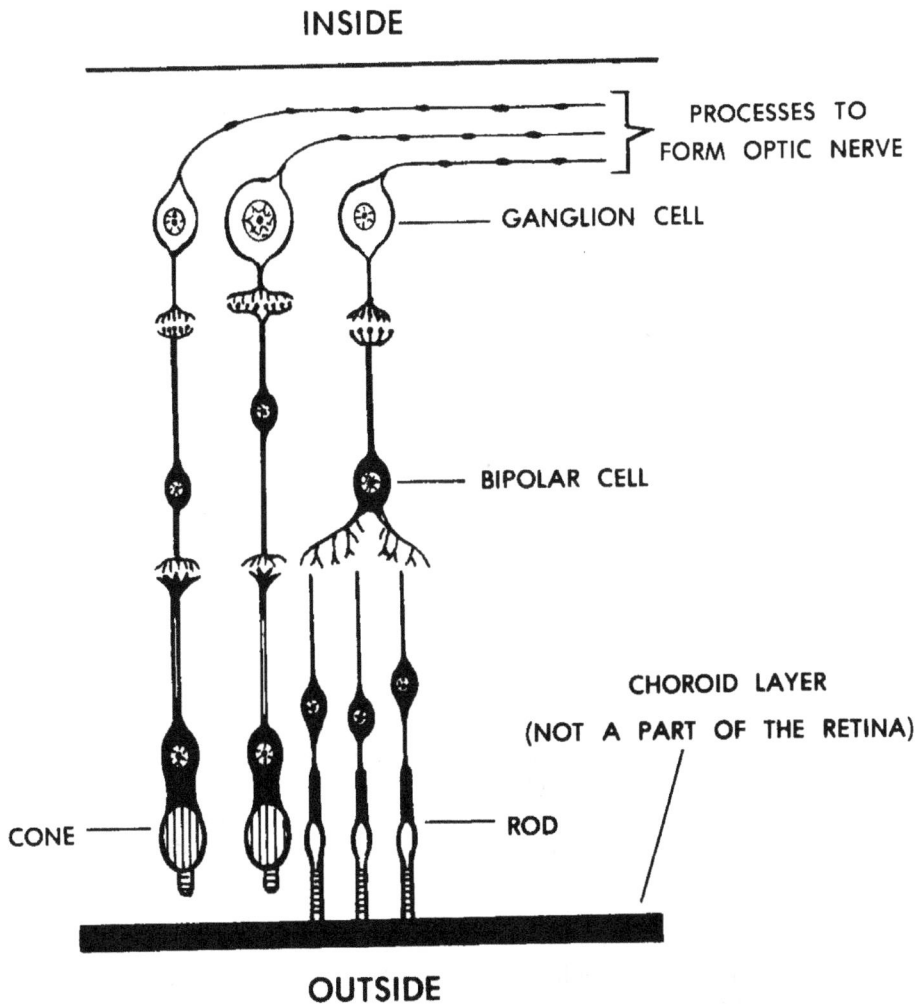

PROCESSES TO FORM OPTIC NERVE

GANGLION CELL

BIPOLAR CELL

CHOROID LAYER

(NOT A PART OF THE RETINA)

CONE

ROD

OUTSIDE

Figure 11-11. Cellular detail of the retina.

(b) If you look directly at an object, light from the object will fall in a small depression of the retina called the fovea centralis. The fovea centralis is at the posterior end of the eyeball, exactly opposite the centers of the cornea, pupil, and lens. The fovea centralis is found in a small yellow area of the retina called the macula lutea. The macula lutea is the area of the retina where vision is sharpest.

FOVEA = small depression

CENTRALIS = center

MACULA = spot

LUTEA = yellow

(c) Associated with the rods and cones are the beginnings of neurons of the optic nerve. These neurons pass out of the eyeball at the posterior end (in a point medial and superior to the fovea centralis). At the point of exit, there are no rods or cones. Therefore, it is called the blind spot (optic disc).

(2) Ciliary body. The anterior end of the choroid layer thickens to form a circular "picture frame" around the lens of the eyeball. This is also near the margin of the base of the cornea. The framelike structure is called the ciliary body. It includes mostly radial muscle fibers, which form the ciliary muscle.

(3) Ligaments. The lens is suspended in place by ligaments (fibers of the ciliary zonule). These ligaments connect the margin (equator) of the lens with the ciliary body.

(4) Lens. The lens is located in the center of the anterior of the eyeball, just behind the cornea.

(a) The lens is biconvex. This means that it has two outwardly curved surfaces. The anterior surface is flatter (less curved) than the posterior surface.

(b) The lens is transparent and elastic. (As one grows older, the lens becomes less and less elastic.) The ligaments maintain a tension upon the lens. This tension keeps the lens flatter and allows the lens to focus on distant objects. When the ciliary muscle contracts, the tension on the lens is decreased. The decreased tension allows the lens to thicken. The greater thickness increases the anterior curvature and allows close objects to be seen clearly.

(c) The process of focusing the lens for viewing close objects clearly is called accommodation. The process of accommodation is accompanied by a reduction in the pupil size as well as a convergence of the two central lines of sight (axes of eyeball).

(5) Iris. Another structure formed from the anterior portion of the choroid layer is the iris. The iris is located between the lens and the cornea.

(a) The pupil is the hole in the middle of the iris. The size of the pupil is controlled by radial and circular muscles in the iris. The radial muscles are dilators. The circular muscles are constrictors. By changing the size of the pupil, the iris controls the amount of light entering the eyeball.

(b) The iris may have many different colors. The actual color is determined by multiple genes.

(6) Chambers. The space between the cornea and the lens is called the anterior cavity. The space between the cornea and the iris is called the anterior chamber. The space between the iris and the lens is called the posterior chamber (see fig 11-10). Both chambers of the anterior cavity are filled with a fluid called the aqueous humor. The aqueous humor is secreted into the chambers by the ciliary body. It drains into the encircling canal of Schlemm, located in the angle between the cornea and the iris. This angle is called the iridiocornealis angle.

(7) Vitreous body. Behind the lens is a jellylike material called the vitreous body.

11-28. THE ORBIT

The orbit is the cavity in the upper facial skull which contains the eyeball and its adnexa. The orbit is open anteriorly.

a. The floor of the orbit is generally horizontal. Its medial wall is generally vertical and straight from front to back. Since the lateral wall and roof converge to the rear, the orbit is a conelike cavity.

b. In the facial skull, the orbit is surrounded by a number of specific spaces. Superiorly, the roof of the orbit is also the floor of the anterior cranial cavity, where the frontal portion of the brain is. Just medial to the medial wall are the structures of the nasal chamber. Inferiorly, the floor of the orbit is also the roof of the maxillary sinus. Laterally, the wall of the orbit is the inner wall of the temporal fossa, a depression on each side of the skull where a fan-shaped chewing muscle (temporalis M.) is attached.

11-29. THE ADNEXA

The adnexa are the various structures associated with the eyeball.

a. **Extrinsic Ocular Muscles**. Among the adnexa are the extrinsic ocular muscles, which move the eyeball within the orbit. Each eyeball has associated with it six muscles made up of striated muscle fibers.

(1) <u>Four recti</u>. Four of these muscles are straight from the rear of the orbit to the eyeball. They are therefore known as the <u>recti</u> muscles (RECTUS = straight). Each name indicates the position of the muscles in relationship to the eyeball as follows:

lateral rectus M. (on the outer side)

superior rectus M. (above)

medial rectus M. (on the inner side)

inferior rectus M. (below)

(2) <u>Two obliques</u>. Two muscles approach the eyeball from the medial side and are known as the <u>superior oblique</u> and <u>inferior oblique</u> muscles.

b. **Eyelids**. Attached to the margins of the orbit, in front of the eyeball, are the upper and lower eyelids (palpebra (Latin), blepharon (Greek)). These have muscles for opening and closing the eyelids. The <u>eyelashes</u> (cilia) are special hairs of the eyelids which help protect the eyeball. The margins of the eyelids have special oil to prevent the loss of fluids from the area. The inner lining of the eyelids is continuous with the conjunctiva, a membrane over the anterior surface of the eyeball.

c. **Lacrimal Apparatus**. The conjunctiva must be kept moist and clean at all times. To do this, a lacrimal apparatus is associated with the eyelids. In the upper outer corner of the orbit is a <u>lacrimal gland</u>, which secretes a <u>lacrimal fluid</u> (tears) into the junction between the upper eyelid and the conjunctiva. By the motion of the eyeball and the eyelids (blinking), this fluid is moved across the surface of the conjunctiva to the medial inferior aspect. Here, the lacrimal fluid is collected and delivered into the nasal chamber by the <u>nasolacrimal duct</u>.

d. **Eyebrow**. The eyebrow (supercilium) is a special group of hairs above the orbit. The eyebrow serves to keep rain and sweat away from the eyeball.

e. **Optic Nerve (Cranial Nerve II)**. Neurons carry information from the photoreceptors of the nervous retina. They leave the eyeball at the blind spot. At the optic nerve, or second cranial nerve, the neurons pass to the rear of the orbit. There, the optic nerve exits through the <u>optic canal</u> into the cranial cavity. Beneath the brain, the optic nerves from both sides join to form the <u>optic chiasma</u>, in which half of the neurons from each optic nerve cross to the opposite side. From the optic chiasma, the right and left optic tracts proceed to the brain proper.

Section X. THE SPECIAL SENSE OF HEARING (AUDITORY)

11-30. GENERAL

The human ear serves two major special sensory functions--hearing (auditory) and equilibrium (balance). The stimulus for hearing is sound waves. The stimulus for equilibrium is gravitational forces.

a. **Methods of Sound Transmission**. The sound stimulus is transmitted in a variety of ways. Regardless of the actual transmission method, the sound stimulus is unchanged. Sound may be transmitted as:

(1) Airborne waves. These airborne waves have frequency (pitch) and amplitude (loudness or intensity).

(2) Mechanical oscillations (vibrations) of structures.

(3) Fluid-borne pressure pulses.

(4) Electrical impulses along the neurons to and in the brain.

b. **Sections of the Human Ear (figure 11-12)**. The human ear has three major parts. Each part serves a specific function in the transmission and reception of the sound stimulus. The three parts are known as the external (outer) ear, the middle ear, and the internal (inner) ear.

11-31. THE EXTERNAL EAR

The external ear begins on the outside of the head in the form of a funnel-shaped auricle (pinna). Actually serving as a funnel, the auricle directs airborne sound waves into the external auditory meatus. The external auditory meatus is a tubular canal extending into the temporal portion of the skull.

11-32. THE MIDDLE EAR

a. **Tympanic Membrane**. At the inner end of the external auditory meatus is the tympanic membrane. The tympanic membrane (eardrum) is a circular membrane separating the external auditory meatus from the middle ear cavity. The tympanic membrane vibrates (mechanically oscillates) in response to airborne sound waves.

b. **Middle Ear Cavity**. On the medial side of the tympanic membrane is the middle ear cavity. The middle ear cavity is a space within the temporal bone.

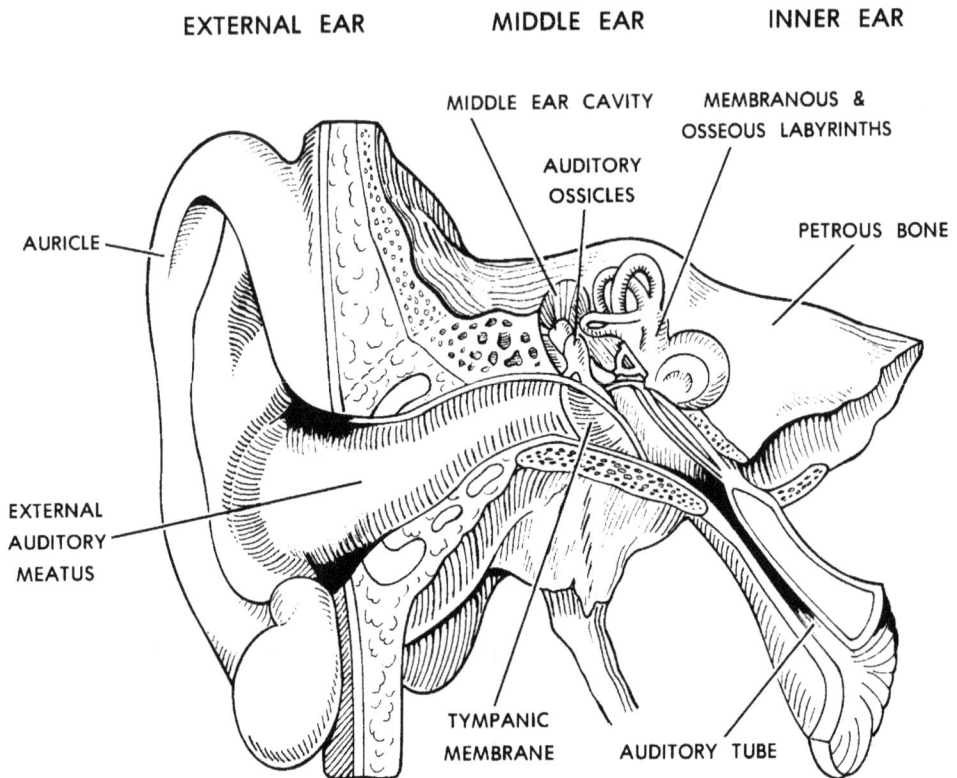

Figure 11-12. A frontal section of the human ear.

c. **Auditory Ossicles**. The <u>auditory ossicles</u> (OSSICLE = small bone) are three very small bones which form a chain across the middle ear cavity. They join the tympanic membrane with the medial wall of the middle ear cavity. In order, the ossicles are named as follows: <u>malleus</u>, <u>incus</u>, and <u>stapes</u>. The malleus is attached to the tympanic membrane. A sound stimulus is transmitted from the tympanic membrane to the medial wall of the middle ear cavity by way of the ossicles. The ossicles vibrate (mechanically oscillate) in response to the sound stimulus.

d. **Auditory (Eustachian) Tube**. The <u>auditory tube</u> is a passage connecting the middle ear cavity with the nasopharynx. The auditory tube maintains equal air pressure on the two sides of the tympanic membrane.

e. **Association With Other Spaces**. The middle ear cavity is associated with other spaces in the skull. The thin roof of the middle ear cavity is the floor of part of the cranial cavity. The middle ear cavity is continuous posteriorly with the mastoid air cells via the antrum (an upper posterior recess of the middle ear cavity).

11-33. THE INTERNAL EAR

a. **Labyrinths (Figure 11-13).**

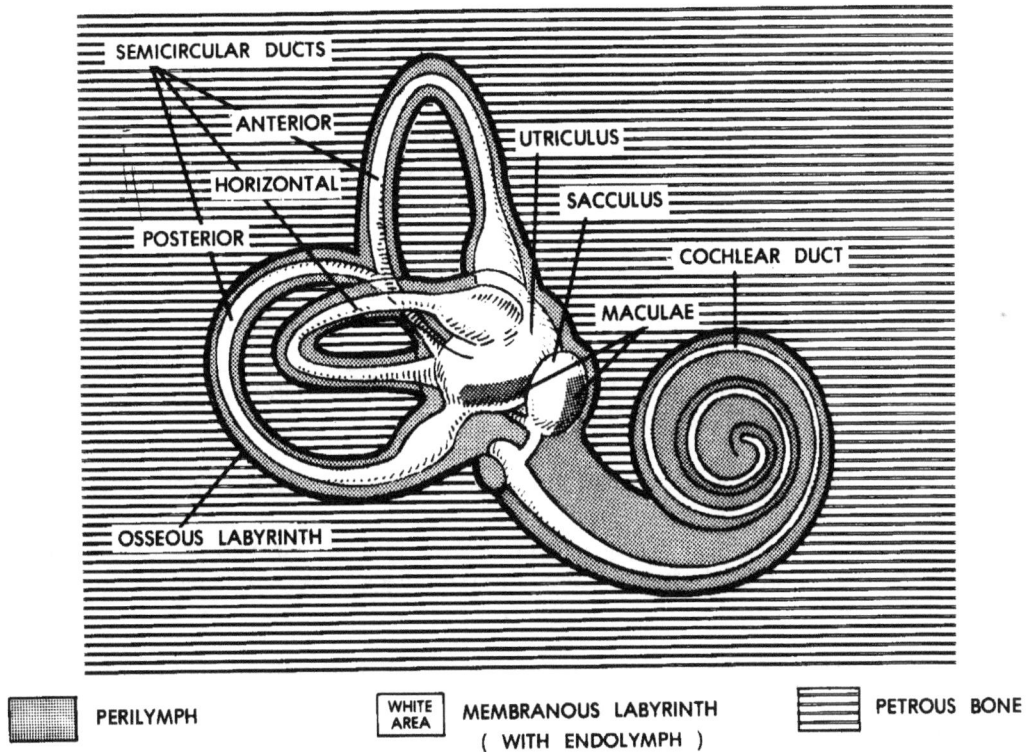

Figure 11-13. The labyrinths of the internal ear.

(1) <u>Bony labyrinth</u>. The <u>bony labyrinth</u> (LABYRINTH = a maze) is a complex cavity within the temporal bone. It has three semicircular canals, a vestibule (hallway), and a snail-shaped cochlear portion.

(2) <u>Membranous labyrinth</u>. The <u>membranous labyrinth</u> is a hollow tubular structure suspended within the bony labyrinth.

b. **Fluids of the Internal Ear**. The <u>endolymph</u> is a fluid filling the space within the membranous labyrinth. The <u>perilymph</u> is a fluid filling the space between the membranous labyrinth and the bony labyrinth. These fluids are continuously formed and drained away.

ENDO = within

PERI = around

c. **The Cochlea**. The cochlea is a spiral structure associated with hearing. It has 2-1/2 turns. Its outer boundaries are formed by the snail- shaped portion of the bony labyrinth.

(1) The central column or axis of the cochlea is called the modiolus. Extending from this central column is a spiral shelf of bone called the spiral lamina. A fibrous membrane called the basilar membrane (or basilar lamina) connects the spiral lamina with the outer bony wall of the cochlea. The basilar membrane forms the floor of the cochlear duct, the spiral portion of the membranous labyrinth. Within the cochlear duct, there is a structure on the basilar membrane called the organ of Corti. The organ of Corti has hairs which are the sensory receptors for the special sense of hearing.

LAMINA = thin plate

(2) Within the bony cochlea, the space above the cochlear duct is known as the scala vestibuli and the space below is known as the scala tympani. (See figure 11-14.) Since the scalae are joined at their apex, they form a continuous channel and the connection between them is called the helicotrema.

(3) Between the scalae and the middle ear cavity are two windows.

(a) Fenestra vestibuli (oval window). Between the middle ear cavity and the scala vestibuli is an oval window called the fenestra vestibuli. It is filled with the foot plate of the stapes.

(b) Fenestra cochleae (round window). Between the middle ear cavity and the scala tympani is a round window called the fenestra cochleae. It is covered or closed by a membrane.

d. **Transmission**.

(1) The sound stimulus is transferred from the stapes to the perilymph of the scala vestibuli. Here the stimulus is transmitted as a pressure pulse in the fluid.

(2) In response, the basilar membrane of the cochlea vibrates (mechanically oscillates). Only selected portions of the basilar membrane vibrate at any one time, depending on the frequency of the sound stimulus.

(3) The hair cells of the organ of Corti at that particular location are mechanically stimulated. This stimulation is transferred to the neurons of the acoustic nerve (cranial nerve VIIIa). The acoustic nerve passes out of the modiolus into the internal auditory meatus of the temporal bone. From here, it enters into the cranial cavity and goes to the brain.

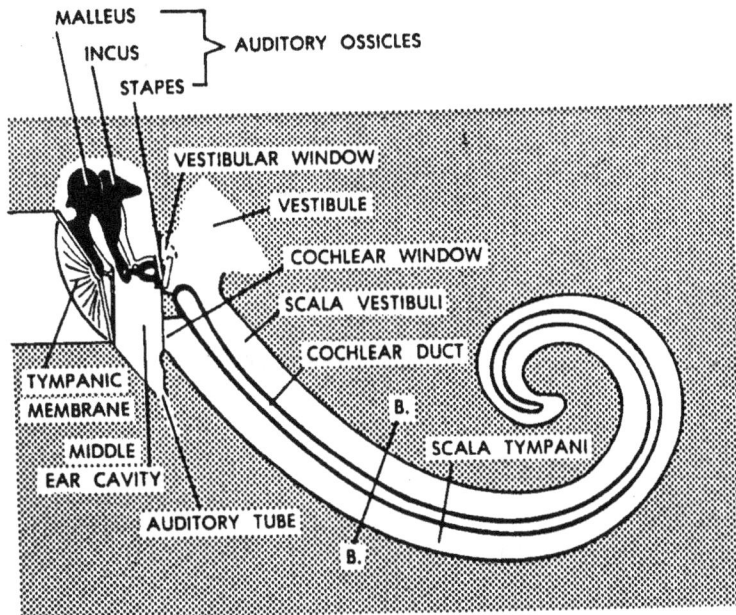

A - schematic relationships

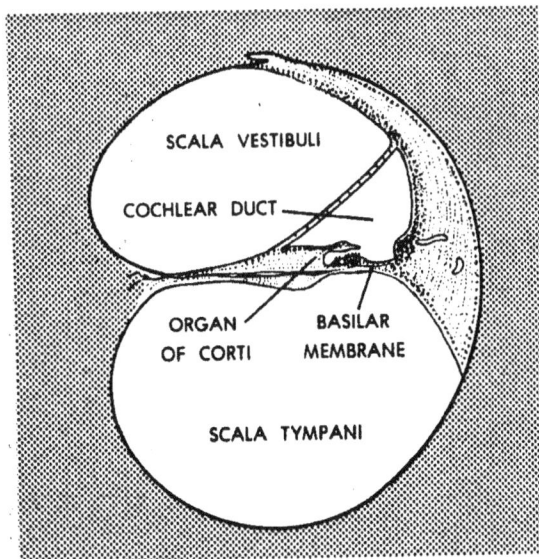

B - cross-section

Figure 11-14. Diagram of the scalae.

Section XI. THE SPECIAL SENSE OF EQUILIBRIUM (BALANCE)

11-34. GENERAL

a. **Posture**. Posture is the specific alinement of the body parts at any given time. Humans can assume an infinite variety of postures. However, the truly erect posture is unique to humans.

b. **Equilibrium**. Equilibrium is the state of balance of the body. An erect standing human has a highly unstable equilibrium and therefore can easily fall. Through a variety of sensory inputs (visual, etc.) and postural reflexes, the body is maintained in its erect posture.

c. **Stimulus-Gravitational Forces**. A primary sensory input for equilibrium consists of gravitational forces. This input is received by the membranous labyrinth within the internal ear. The gravitational forces are of two types: static, when the body is standing still, and kinetic, when the body is moving in either linear (straight) or angular directions.

d. **Membranous Labyrinth**. The specific portions of the membranous labyrinth involved are the two sac-like structures--the sacculus and the utriculus. Each of these two structures has an area of special hair cells called the macula. In addition, there are three semicircular ducts located within the osseous semicircular canals of the temporal bone of the skull. Each semicircular duct has a crista, a little ridge of hair cells across the axis of the duct.

e. **"Body Sense."** All of the various sensory inputs related to the maintenance of equilibrium and posture are integrated within the brain as "body sense." Correct information is sent to the muscles of the body by means of specific postural reflexes in order to maintain the proper posture.

11-35. SACCULUS AND UTRICULUS

a. The sacculus and the utriculus are two sac-like portions of the membranous labyrinth. They are filled with endolymph.

b. On the wall of each sac is a collection of special hair cells known as the macula, which serves as a receptor organ for static and linear kinetic gravitational forces. The saccular macula and the utricular macula are oriented at more or less right angles to each other. For the pair of maculae in the membranous labyrinth of the right side, there is a corresponding pair in the labyrinth of the left side. Information from all of these maculae is sent into the brain for continuous sensing of the position of the head in space.

11-36. SEMICIRCULAR DUCTS (FIGURE 11-15)

Extending from and opening into the utriculus are three hollow structures called the semicircular ducts. Since the utriculus completes the circle for each duct, the ducts act as if they were complete circles.

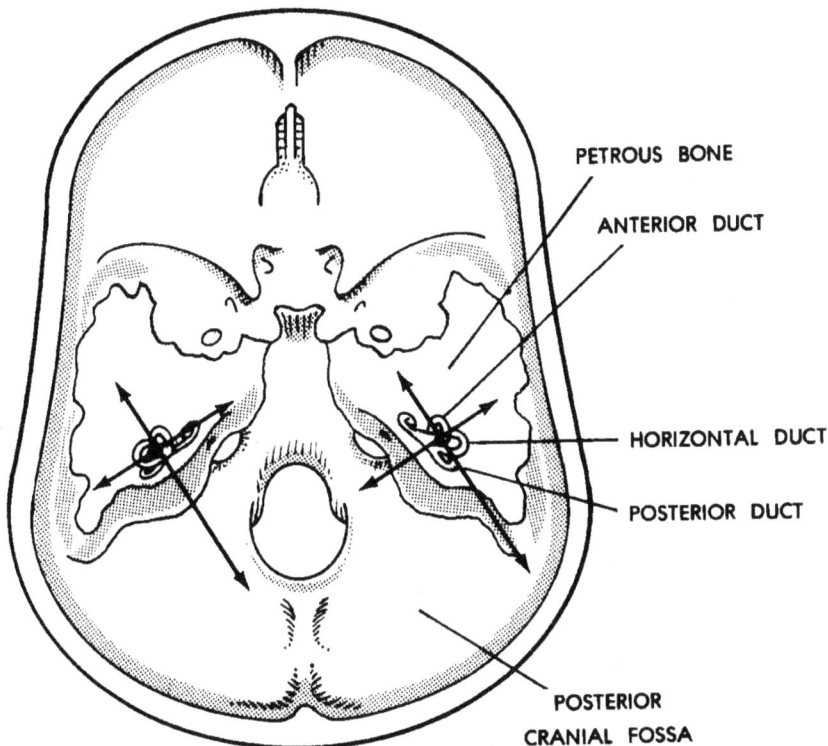

Figure 11-15. Diagram of semicircular duct orientation.

a. **Orientation**. Two of the ducts are <u>vertically</u> oriented (one <u>anterior</u> and one <u>posterior</u>). The third duct is essentially <u>horizontal</u>. The three ducts are all oriented at right angles to each other. In addition, the three ducts of one membranous labyrinth are matched or paired by the three ducts of the opposite membranous labyrinth.

b. **Ampullae and Cristae**. Each semicircular duct ends with an enlargement where it opens into the utriculus. This enlargement or swelling is called an <u>ampulla</u>. The crista is at a right angle to the axis of the duct. Movement of the endolymph within the duct--caused by movement of the head in space--deforms (bends) the hairs of the crista in specific directions. These are responses to linear and/or angular kinetic gravitational forces.

11-37. THE VESTIBULAR NERVE

The vestibular nerve (cranial nerve VIII) carries all this information from the maculae and cristae to the brain. The vestibular and auditory nerves are contained in the same fibrous sheath from the membranous labyrinth to the brain. Within the brain, the vestibular and auditory nerves separate into different pathways.

Section XII. CONTROLS IN THE HUMAN NERVOUS SYSTEM

11-38. GENERAL CONCEPT

The human nervous system can be thought of as a series of steps or levels. Each level is more complex than the level just below. No level is completely overpowered by upper levels, but each level is controlled or guided by the next upper level as it functions.

11-39. LEVELS OF CONTROL

a. **Reflex Arc**. The simplest and lowest level of control is the reflex arc (see para 11-15c). The reflex arc operates essentially on the level of the sensory input.

b. **Segmental Reflexes**. Segmental reflexes produce a wider reaction to a stimulus than the reflex arc. For this purpose, the nervous system is organized more complexly. Thus, information spreads to a wider area of the CNS. We can observe a greater reaction to the stimulus.

c. **Medullary Hindbrain**. In the hindbrainstem are to be found a number of nuclei (collections of neuron cell bodies) which monitor and control the activities of the visceral functions of the body, such as respiration, heartbeat, etc.

d. **Reticular Formation**. Within the substance of the brainstem is a diffuse system called the reticular formation.

RETICULAR = network

This reticular formation has a facilitatory (excitatory) area and an inhibitory area. These areas monitor and control general body functions, including sleep.

e. **Thalamus**. In the forebrainstem is a major collection of nuclei, all together called the thalamus. The thalamus is a primary relay for information going to and from the cerebrum and cerebellum. In the lowest animals, the thalamus represents the highest level of nervous control.

f. **Cerebellum**. The cerebellum has been greatly developed with many functional subdivisions. All together, it is one of the most important integrators of motor activity of the body.

g. **Cerebrum**. In humans, the highest level of nervous control is localized in the cerebrum. It is at this level that conscious sensation and volitional motor activity are localized. Even so, we can clearly designate three levels of control within the cerebrum:

(1) Visceral (vegetative) level. This level is concerned primarily with visceral activities of the body as related to fight-or-flight, fear, and other emotions.

(2) Patterned (stereotyped) motor actions. Here, activities of the body are standardized and repetitive in nature. An example of a stereo- typed pattern of muscle activity would be the sequence of muscle actions involved in walking.

(3) Volitional level. The volitional level is the highest and newest level of control. Here, unique, brand-new solutions can be created.

Continue with Exercises

EXERCISES, LESSON 11

REQUIREMENT. The following exercises are to be answered by completing the incomplete statement or by writing the answer in the space provided at the end of the question.

After you have completed all the exercises, turn to "Solutions to Exercises," at the end of the lesson and check your answers.

1.   Two types of nervous tissues are _____and _____.

What role does the first play in the nervous system?

What role does the second play?

2.   Nervous tissues are specialized to:

a.   _____ stimuli.

b.   _____ information.

c.   _____ information.

3.   A neuron is a nerve cell body and all of its _____s.

4.   A dendrite carries impulses (toward) (away from) the cell body.

5.   What is an axon?

6.   Each item below indicates the number of poles for a type of neuron. Give the name which corresponds to each.

a.   More than two poles: _____.

b.   Two poles: _____.

c.   One pole: _____.

7.   Each item below refers to the thickness of the myelin surrounding an axon. Give the letter indicating the type of neuron.

     a.   Thickest: _____.

     b.   Medium: _____.

     c.   Thinnest: _____.

8.   Each item below indicates the route over which impulses are transmitted. Give the type of neuron corresponding to each route.

     a.   From receptor organs to the CNS: _____.

     b.   From the CNS to muscles and glands: _____.

     c.   From one neuron to another: _____.

9.   What is meant by the term "continuity without contact" as related to neuron "connections"?

10.   What is a synapse?

An axon terminates in tiny branches. What is at the end of each branch?

Where is neurotransmitter stored?

What is the presynaptic membrane?

What is the synaptic cleft?

What is the postsynaptic membrane?

11. What is a neuromuscular junction?

   Compare the neuromuscular junction to a synapse.

12. The major divisions of the human nervous system are the_____
nervous system (_____), the _____ nervous system (_____), and the
_____ nervous system (_____). The CNS is made up of the _____ and
the _____ _____.

13. The three major subdivisions of the human brain are the_____,
the _____, and the _____.

   What is the brainstem?

14. The cerebellum is a spherical mass of nervous tissue attached to and
covering the _____. Its three major parts are the _____ and right
and left _____ hemispheres. In addition, the cerebellum has three pairs of
stem-like connecting parts called _____. The outer cortex is composed of
_____ matter, which is the _____s of neurons. More central is the
_____ matter, which is the myelinated processes of_____.
The cerebellum is the primary _____/_____ of motor actions of the body.

15. The cerebrum consists of two very much enlarged _____s
connected to each other by a special structure called the c_____c_____.
Each cerebral hemisphere is connected to the brainstem by a c_____p_____.
The surface of each cerebral hemisphere is subdivided into areas known as l_____.
The names of the four lobes are f_____, p_____, o_____, and t_____.

16. The space separating the two cerebral hemispheres is called the longitudinal
_____. The shallow grooves in the surface of the cerebrum are called _____.
The ridges outlined by the grooves are called _____.

17. The gray outer layer of each hemisphere is the _____ _____.
Deeper within the cerebral hemispheres, the tissue is colored _____. The "gray
matter" represents the _____ _____s of the neurons. The "white matter" represents
the _____.

18.   Groups of related functions are associated with specific areas of the cerebral cortex. For example, centers of speech and hearing are located along the lateral _____. Vision is centered in the _____ lobe. Sensory and motor functions are located along the central_____.

19.   The ventricles of the brain are interconnected hollow spaces filled with _____. The right and left lateral ventricles are found in the cerebral _____s. The lateral ventricles are connected to the third ventricle by the i_____ f_____. The third ventricle is located in the f_____. The third and fourth ventricles are connected by the c_____ a_____. The fourth ventricle is located in the h_____. The fourth ventricle is continuous with the part of the spinal cord known as the c_____ c_____.

20.   The spinal cord, located within the spinal _____l, is continuous with the b_____. The spinal cord has two enlargements. One, associated with nerves for the upper members, is called the _____ enlargement. The other, associated with the nerves for the lower members, is called the _____ enlargement. Nerves arising from the spinal cord are called _____ nerves.

      There are how many pairs of spinal nerves?

21.   In the cross section of the spinal cord, one can see a central region of gray matter shaped like an _____. Each arm of this figure is called a _____. The connecting link is called the gray _____. These horns are actually sections of the gray _____s. Since a column of white matter is a large bundle of processes, it is called a _____.

22.   The skeletal covering for the brain is provided by bones of the _____. The overall skeletal structure covering the spinal cord is the _____ column (spine).

23.   The brain and spinal cord have three different membranes surrounding them called _____. The tough outer covering for the CNS is the _____. Beneath it is the _____ space. The fine second membrane is called the _____. Beneath it is the _____ space, which is filled with _____. The delicate membrane applied directly to the surface of the brain and spinal cord is called the _____.

24.   The two main pairs of arteries supply oxygenated blood to the brain are the internal _____ and _____ arteries. Beneath the brain, branches of these arteries join to form a circle, called the _____ circle (of_____). The main pair of veins carrying blood back toward the heart is the internal _____ veins. The blood supply of the spinal cord is by way of a combination of three l_____ arteries running along its length and reinforced by s_____ arteries from the sides.

25.   Found in the cavities of the CNS is a clear fluid called_____fluid (___). This fluid is found in the _____s of the brain, the sub_____ space, and the spinal cord's _____ canal. Special collections of arterial capillaries found in the roofs of the third and fourth ventricles are called choroid _____s. These structures continuously produce CSF from the _____ of the blood.

26.   As CSF is produced by the choroid plexuses, it flows into all four _____s. CSF from the lateral ventricles flows into the _____ ventricle, and then through the _____ aqueduct into the _____ ventricle. By passing through three small holes in the roof of the fourth ventricle, CSF enters the subarachnoid _____. From here, the CSF is transported through the arachnoid _____ into the venous sinuses.

27.   The peripheral nervous system is that portion of the nervous system which generally provides commands for _____ muscles and other _____ muscles and carries _____y information from the p_____ of the body. A nerve is a collection of neuron _____s, together and _____ the CNS.

28.   The 12 pairs of nerves attached to the right and left sides of the brainstem are called _____ nerves. Each such nerve is identified by a _____ in order from _____ to _____ and an individual name. Attached to the sides of the spinal cord are 31 pairs of_____ nerves. For each, the region is designated by a _____; within each region, a nerve pair is identified by an _____.

29.   Like a tree, a typical spinal nerve has _____s, a ____, and branches (called _____). Coming off of the posterior and anterior sides of the spinal cord are the posterior and anterior ____ of the spinal nerve. An enlargement on the posterior root is the _____. A ganglion is a collection of _____, together, outside the CNS. Laterally, the posterior and anterior roots of the spinal nerve join to form the spinal nerve _____. The spinal nerve trunk of each spinal nerve is located in the corresponding intervertebral _____ of the vertebral column. As the nerve trunk emerges laterally, it divides into the anterior and posterior ____.

30.   If it carries information from the periphery to the CNS, it is an _____t (_____) neuron. If it carries information from the CNS to a muscle or gland, it is an _____t (_____) neuron.

31.   An automatic reaction to a stimulus is referred to as a _____.
The pathway from the receptor organ to the reacting muscle is called the _____ _.

32.   The pathway of a general reflex arc involves a minimum of ____ structures.
The stimulus is received by a _____ organ. That information is transmitted to the CNS by the _____t (_____) neuron. Within the spinal cord, there is a special neuron connecting the afferent neuron to the efferent neuron; this special connecting neuron is called the _____. Carrying the appropriate command from the spinal cord to the reacting muscle is the _____t (_____) neuron. The reacting muscle is called the e_____ organ.

33.   The autonomic nervous system is that portion of the nervous system generally concerned with commands for s_____ muscle, c_____ muscles, and _____s.

34.   In the ANS, the number of neurons connecting the CNS with a visceral organ is always _____. The cell bodies of the second neuron form a collection outside the CNS, called a _____. The first neuron extends from the CNS to the ganglion and is therefore called the _____ neuron. Cell bodies of the second neurons make up the _____. The second neuron's processes extend from the ganglion to the _____. Thus, the second neuron is called the _____ neuron.

35.   The efferent pathways of the ANS fall into two major divisions. The one most active during a "fight-or-flight" reaction is the _____-_____ outflow (_____ nervous system). The other is the ____-_____ outflow (_____ nervous system).

36.   The intermediolateral gray columns from the T-1 to the L-2 levels of the spinal cord are made up of the cell bodies of the ___-ganglionic sympathetic neurons. The sympathetic ganglia are made up of the cell bodies of the _____-ganglionic sympathetic neurons. The sympathetic NS activates those visceral organs needed to _____. It deactivates those which are _____.

37. Four pairs of nuclei in the brainstem and the intermediolateral gray columns at the S-2 through S-4 levels of the spinal cord are made up of the cell bodies of the p_____ p_____ neurons. The intramural ganglia within the walls of the _____ organs are made up of the cell bodies of the p_____ p_____ neurons. As compared to that of the sympathetic NS, the parasympathetic NS has the (same) (opposite) effect on visceral organs.

38. What is a pathway?

39. What is the neuraxis?

.

40. What is a sensory pathway?

.

41. What is a motor pathway?

.

42. The human nervous system has several levels of control. The lowest level is the _____ _____ _____. The highest level is the _____ level. Between, there are several progressively _____ levels. All information input and all information output are _____d and _____d.

43. The right half of the brain controls the _____ side of the body. The left half of the brain controls the _____ side of the body.

44. A pyramidal pathway is primarily concerned with _____ (_____) control of body parts, particularly the _____ movements of _____s. These pathways are called pyramidal because their neuron processes help to make up structures in the base of the brain called _____.

45. An extrapyramidal pathway is primarily concerned with _____ (_____) control of body parts for purposes of _____.

46. Name examples of general senses.

    a.   _____.

    b.   _____.

    c.   _____.

    d.   _____.

47. Name examples of special senses.

    a.   _____.

    b.   _____.

    c.   _____.

    d.   _____.

    e.   _____.

48. The general sensory pathway is from the _____ organ, via the ___ nerves, to the _____. This general pathway then ascends fiber tracts in the _____. The pathway ends in the central area of the opposite _____ hemisphere.

49. The receptors for the sense of smell are special hair cells called c_____s. These are found in the o_____ e_____, high in the n_____ c_____s in the head. The information received is transmitted by way of the o_____ nerves to the _____y bulbs and then into the opposite _____l hemisphere.

50. Describe the sensory receptors for the special sense of taste.

The information received is transmitted to the opposite side of the brain by three _____ nerves.

51. What is the eyeball?

The eyeball is shaped like a _____.

52. The outermost layer of the eyeball is colored _____ and is made up of very dense _____; it is known as the _____. Its anterior portion is called the _____. The major focusing device for the eyeball is the _____.

53. The middle layer of the wall of the eyeball is known as the _____. This layer is richly supplied with _____ and pigmented with a _____ material.

54. The inner layer of the wall of the eyeball is known as the _____. The actual photoreceptor elements are located at the _____ and the _____s. These elements are the _____s and the _____s.

55. The elements which register colors are the _____. However, _____ require more intense light than do _____. Rods register only _____.

56. What are the fovea centralis and macula lutea?

57. What is the blind spot?

58. The thickening of the choroid layer around the edge of the lens is called the _____. It includes radial muscle fibers making up the _____ muscle.

59. Describe the lens and the process of accommodation.

60. The space between the cornea and the iris is called the _____ _____. The space between the iris and the lens is called the _____ _____. Together, these make up the space between the cornea and the lens, called the _____ _____ and filled with the _____ _____. This drains into the encircling _____, located in the angle between the _____ and the _____. Behind the lens is a jellylike material called the _____. It fills the _____ cavity of the eyeball.

61.　The orbit is the cavity in the upper facial skull which contains the _____ and its _____. The orbit is shaped roughly like a _____.

62.　Examples of the adnexa are the:

    a.　　_____.

    b.　　_____.

    c.　　_____.

    d.　　_____.

    e.　　_____.

63.　Of the six extrinsic ocular muscles, four are called _____ muscles. Two are _____ muscles. The lateral rectus M. is on the _____ side of the eyeball. The superior rectus M. is _____ the eyeball. The medial rectus M. is on the _____ side of the eyeball. The inferior rectus M. is _____ the eyeball. The superior oblique and inferior oblique muscles approach the eyeball from the _____ side.

64.　Attached to the margins of the orbit are the upper and lower _____. These have special hairs called _____. The inner lining of the eyelids is continuous with the _____, a membrane over the anterior surface of the eyeball.

65.　In the upper outer corner of the orbit is a lacrimal _____d, which secretes a lacrimal _____d, which is ultimately collected and delivered into the nasal chamber by the _____ duct.

66.　Neurons carry information from the photoreceptors located in the nervous _____. They leave the eyeball at the _____. Passing to the rear of the orbit, the neurons now belong to the _____ nerve (cranial nerve __). The optic nerve enters the cranial cavity by passing through the _____ canal. Beneath the brain, the optic nerves from both sides join to form the _____, in which half of the neurons from each optic nerve _____. From the optic chiasma, the right and left optic _____s proceed to the brain proper.

67.　The human ear has two major special sensory functions: _____ (_____y) and _____ (_____e). The three parts of the human ear are the _____ (_____) ear, the _____ ear, and the _____ (_____) ear.

68. The external flap of the ear is called the _____ (_____). It directs airborne sound waves into the canal called the external auditory _____, which extends into the _____ portion of the skull.

69. Where is the tympanic membrane?

On the medial side of the tympanic membrane, there is a space within the temporal bone called the _____.

What are the auditory ossicles?

The auditory ossicles respond to a sound stimulus by _____. From the lateral to the medial ends, the names of the ossicles are: _____, _____, and _____. The auditory tube connects the middle ear cavity with the _____.

70. What is the bony labyrinth?

It has three _____ canals, a _____ (hallway), and a snail-shaped _____ portion.

What is the membranous labyrinth?

71. Where is the endolymph found?

Where is the perilymph found?

72. The cochlea is a _____ structure associated with _____ing. It has _____ turns. Its outer boundaries are formed by the snail-shaped portion of the _____.

73.   The central column of the cochlea is called the m_____. Extending from this central column is a spiral shelf of bone called the s_____ l_____. Connecting this shelf with the outer bony wall is a fibrous membrane called the b_____ membrane. This membrane forms the floor of the spiral portion of the membranous labyrinth called the c_____ d____. This contains a structure with hairs, sensory receptors of hearing; this structure is called the organ of _____.

74.   Within the bony cochlea, the space above the cochlear duct is known as the _____ _____ and the space below is known as the _____ _____. Between the middle ear cavity and the upper space is an oval window called the fenestra _____. Between the middle ear cavity and the lower space is a round window called the fenestra _____.

75.   A sound stimulus is transferred from the stapes to the fluid _____ of the _____. In response, the b_____ membrane of the cochlea vibrates. The hair cells of the _____ of _____ are mechanically stimulated. This stimulation is transferred to the neurons of the_____ nerve, which passes out of the modiolus into the internal auditory _____ of the temporal bone. From here, the nerve enters the _____ cavity and goes to the _____.

76.   The two sac-like portions of the membranous labyrinth are the _____ and the _____. They are filled with _____. On the wall of each sac is a collection of special hair cells known as the _____, which serves as a receptor organ for _____ and linear _____ gravitational forces. The saccular macula and the utricular macula are oriented at more or less _____° angles to each other.

77.   Extending from and opening into the utriculus are three hollow structures called the _____ ducts. The utriculus completes the circle for each _____. The three ducts are all oriented at ___° angles to each other. Where it opens into the utriculus, each semicircular duct ends in an enlargement called an _____. Movement of the fluid endolymph bends the hairs of the _____ in specific directions. These are responses to _____ and/or _____ kinetic gravitational forces.

78.   Carrying the information from the maculae and the cristae to the brain is the _____ nerve. Contained in the same fibrous sheath from the membranous labyrinth to the brain are the v_____ and a_____ nerves.

79.   The simplest and lowest level of control is the _____ _____. Producing wider reactions to stimuli are s_____ reflexes. A number of nuclei in the hindbrain monitor and control v_____l functions of the body, including r_____ and h_____b_____. The facilitatory and inhibitory areas of the reticular formation monitor and control general body functions, including _____. The thalamus is a primary relay for information going to and from the _____ and _____. One of the most important integrators of motor activity of the body is the _____.

80.   In humans, the highest level of control is in the _____. Here, we can clearly designate three levels of control:

a.   The first level is concerned with _____ activities of the body, as related to _____, fear, and other emotions.

b.   At the second level, activities of the body are s_____d and repetitive in nature. An example is the sequence of muscle actions involved in w_____ing.

c.   At the third level, brand new solutions can be created. This is the v_____ level.

Check Your Answers on Next Page

SOLUTIONS TO EXERCISES, LESSON 11

1. Two types of nervous tissues are <u>neurons (nerve cells)</u> and <u>glia (neuroglia)</u>. The neuron is <u>the basic structural unit of the nervous system</u>. The glia are cells of <u>supporting tissue for the nervous system</u>. (para 11-1)

2. Nervous tissues are specialized to:

    a. <u>Receive stimuli</u>.
    b. <u>Transmit information</u>.
    c. <u>Store information</u>. (para 11-2)

3. A neuron is a nerve cell body and all of its <u>processes</u>. (para 11-3)

4. A dendrite carries impulses <u>toward</u> the cell body. (para 11-5a)

5. An axon is <u>a neuron process which transmits information from the cell body to the next unit</u>. (para 11-5b)

6. More than two poles: <u>multipolar neuron</u>.
    Two poles: <u>bipolar neuron</u>.
    One pole: <u>unipolar neuron</u>.
    (para 11-6a)

7. Thickest: <u>A</u>.
    Medium: <u>B</u>.
    Thinnest: <u>C</u>. (para 11-6b)

8. From receptor organs to the CNS: <u>sensory neurons</u>.
    From the CNS to muscles and glands: <u>motor neurons</u>.
    From one neuron to another: <u>interneurons</u>. (para 11-6c)

9. The term "continuity without contact" <u>refers to the fact that neurons do not actually touch. Thus, there is no electrical transmission of impulses from one neuron to the next. In fact, information is transferred across the synaptic cleft by chemicals called neurotransmitters</u>. (para 11-7)

10. A synapse is <u>a "connection" between two neurons</u>. An axon terminates in tiny branches. At the end of each branch is a <u>terminal bulb</u>. Neurotransmitters are stored in bundles called <u>synaptic vesicles located within each terminal bulb</u>. The presynaptic membrane is the <u>thickened layer of the terminal bulb which faces the synaptic cleft and through which pass the neurotransmitters before entering the synaptic cleft</u>. The synaptic cleft is <u>the space between the terminal bulb of the first neuron and the dendrite or cell body of the second neuron</u>. The postsynaptic membrane is <u>that portion of the membrane of the second neuron which lies near the terminal bulb of the first neuron</u>. (para 11-7a)

11. A neuromuscular junction is a "connection" between the terminal of a motor neuron and a muscular fiber. Comparison: The neuromuscular junction has an organization identical to a synapse. However, the bulb is larger and protrudes into the surface of the muscle fiber. The postsynaptic membrane is also larger and has foldings. (para 11-7b)

12. The major divisions of the human nervous system are the central nervous system (CNS), the peripheral nervous system (PNS), and the autonomic nervous system (ANS). The CNS is made up of the brain and the spinal cord. (para 11-8)

13. The three major subdivisions of the human brain are the brainstem, the cerebellum, and the cerebrum. The brainstem is that part of the brain remaining after removal of the cerebrum and cerebellum. It is the basal portion. Together with the spinal cord, it is known as the neuraxis. (para 11-9a)

14. The cerebellum is a spherical mass of nervous tissue attached to and covering the hindbrainstem. Its three major parts are the vermis and right and left cerebellar hemispheres. In addition, the cerebellum has three pairs of stem-like connecting parts called peduncles. The outer cortex is composed of gray matter, which is the cell bodies of neurons. More central is the white matter, which is the myelinated processes of neurons. The cerebellum is the primary coordinator/ integrator of motor actions of the body. (para 11-9b)

15. The cerebrum consists of two very much enlarged hemispheres connected to each other by a special structure called the corpus callosum. Each cerebral hemisphere is connected to the brainstem by a cerebral peduncle. The surface of each cerebral hemisphere is subdivided into areas known as lobes. The names of the four lobes are frontal, parietal, occipital, and temporal. (para 11-9c)

16. The space separating the two cerebral hemispheres is called the longitudinal fissure. The shallow grooves in the surface of the cerebrum are called sulci. The ridges outlined by the sulci are called gyri. (para 11-9c(1))

17. The gray outer layer of each hemisphere is the cerebral cortex. Deeper within the cerebral hemispheres, the tissue is colored white. The "gray matter" represents the cell bodies of the neurons. The "white matter" represents the axons. (para 11-9c(2))

18. Groups of related functions are associated with specific areas of the cerebral cortex. For example, centers of speech and hearing are located along the lateral sulcus. Vision is centered in the occipital lobe. Sensory and motor functions are located along the central sulcus. (para 11-9c(3))

19. The ventricles of the brain are interconnected hollow spaces filled with CSF. The right and left lateral ventricles are found in the cerebral hemispheres. The lateral ventricles are connected to the third ventricle by the interventricular foramen. The third ventricle is located in the forebrainstem. The third and fourth ventricles are connected by the cerebral aqueduct. The fourth ventricle is located in the hindbrainstem. The fourth ventricle is continuous with the part of the spinal cord known as the central canal. (para 11-9d)

20. The spinal cord, located within the spinal canal, is continuous with the brainstem. The spinal cord has two enlargements. One, associated with nerves for the upper members, is called the cervical enlargement. The other, associated with nerves for the lower members, is called the lumbosacral enlargement. Nerves arising from the spinal cord are called spinal nerves. There are 31 pairs of spinal nerves. (para 11-10a)

21. In the cross section of the spinal cord, one can see a central region of gray matter shaped like an H. Each arm of this figure is called a horn. The connecting link is called the gray commissure. These horns are actually sections of the gray columns. Since a column of white matter is a large bundle of processes, it is called a funiculus. (para 11-10b)

22. The skeletal covering for the brain is provided by bones of the cranium. The overall skeletal structure covering the spinal cord is the vertebral column (spine). (para 11-11a)

23. The brain and spinal cord have three different membranes surrounding them called meninges. The tough outer covering for the CNS is the dura mater. Beneath it is the subdural space. The fine second membrane is called the arachnoid mater. Beneath it is the subarachnoid space, which is filled with CSF. The delicate membrane applied directly to the surface of the brain and spinal cord is called the pia mater. (para 11-11b)

24. The two main pairs of arteries supplying oxygenated blood to the brain are the internal carotid and the vertebral arteries. Beneath the brain, branches of these arteries join to form a circle, called the cerebral circle (of Willis). The main pair of veins carrying blood back toward the heart is the internal jugular veins. The blood supply of the spinal cord is by way of a combination of three longitudinal arteries running along its length and reinforced by segmental arteries from the sides. (para 11-12)

25. Found in the cavities of the CNS is a clear fluid called cerebrospinal fluid (CSF). This fluid is found in the ventricles of the brain, the subarachnoid space, and the spinal cord's central canal. Special collections of arterial capillaries found in the roofs of the third and fourth ventricles are called choroid plexuses. These structures continuously produce CSF from the plasma of the blood. (para 11-13)

26. As CSF is produced by the choroid plexuses, it flows into all four ventricles. CSF from the lateral ventricles flows into the third ventricle and then through the cerebral aqueduct into the fourth ventricle. By passing through three small holes in the roof of the fourth ventricle, CSF enters the subarachnoid space. From here, the CSF is transported through the arachnoid villi into the venous sinuses. (para 11-13b)

27. The peripheral nervous system is that portion of the nervous system which generally provides commands for skeletal muscles and other striated muscles and carries sensory information from the periphery of the body. A nerve is a collection of neuron processes, together and outside the CNS. (para 11-14a)

28. The 12 pairs of nerves attached to the right and left sides of the brainstem are called cranial nerves. Each such nerve is identified by a Roman numeral in order from I to XII and an individual name. Attached to the sides of the spinal cord are 31 pairs of spinal nerves. For each, the region is designated by a letter; within each region, a nerve pair is identified by an Arabic numeral. (para 11-14c)

29. Like a tree, a typical spinal nerve has roots, a trunk, and branches (called rami). Coming off of the posterior and anterior sides of the spinal cord are the posterior and anterior roots of the spinal nerve. An enlargement on the posterior root is the posterior root ganglion. A ganglion is a collection of neuron cell bodies, together, outside the CNS. Laterally, the posterior and anterior roots of the spinal nerve join to form the spinal nerve trunk. The spinal nerve trunk of each spinal nerve is located in the corresponding intervertebral foramen of the vertebral column. As the nerve trunk emerges laterally, it divides into the anterior and posterior rami. (para 11-15a)

30. If it carries information from the periphery to the CNS, it is an afferent (sensory) neuron. If it carries information from the CNS to a muscle or gland, it is an efferent (motor) neuron. (para 11-15b)

31. An automatic reaction to a stimulus is referred to as a reflex. The pathway from the receptor organ to the reacting muscle is called the reflex arc. (para 11-15c(1))

32. The pathway of a general reflex arc involves a minimum of five structures. The stimulus is received by a receptor organ. The information is transmitted to the CNS by the afferent (sensory) neuron. Within the spinal cord, there is a special neuron connecting the afferent neuron to the efferent neuron; this special connecting neuron is called the interneuron (or internuncial neuron). Carrying the appropriate command from the spinal cord to the reacting muscle is efferent (motor) neuron. The reacting muscle is called the effector organ. (para 11-15c(2))

33. The autonomic nervous system is that portion of the nervous system generally concerned with commands for smooth muscle, cardiac muscle, and glands. (para 11-16)

34. In the ANS, the number of neurons connecting the CNS with a visceral organ is always <u>two</u>. The cell bodies of the second neurons form a collection outside the CNS, called a <u>ganglion</u>. The first neuron extends from the CNS to the ganglion and is therefore called the <u>preganglionic</u> neuron. Cell bodies of the second neurons make up the <u>ganglion</u>. The second neuron's processes extend from the ganglion to the <u>visceral organ</u>. Thus, the second neuron is called the <u>post-ganglionic</u> neuron. (para 11-16b)

35. The efferent pathways of the ANS fall into two major divisions. The one most active during a "fight-or-flight" reaction is the <u>thoraco- lumbar</u> outflow (<u>sympathetic</u> nervous system). The other is the <u>cranio- sacral</u> outflow (<u>parasympathetic</u> nervous system). (para 11-16c)

36. The intermediolateral gray columns from the T-1 to the L-2 levels of the spinal cord are made up of the cell bodies of the <u>preganglionic</u> sympathetic neurons. The sympathetic ganglia are made up of the <u>post-</u> ganglionic sympathetic neurons. The sympathetic NS activates those visceral organs needed to <u>mobilize energy for action</u>. It deactivates those which are <u>not needed</u>. (para 11-17)

37. Four pairs of nuclei in the brainstem and the intermediolateral gray columns at the S-2 through S-4 levels of the spinal cord are made up of the cell bodies of the <u>preganglionic parasympathetic</u> neurons. The intramural ganglia within the walls of the <u>central visceral</u> organs are made up of the cell bodies of the <u>post-ganglionic parasympathetic</u> neurons. As compared to that of the sympathetic NS, the parasympathetic NS has the <u>opposite</u> effect on visceral organs. (para 11-18)

38. A pathway is <u>the series of nervous structures utilized in the transmission of an item of information</u>. (para 11-19a(1))

39. The neuraxis is <u>the brainstem and the spinal cord, considered together as one structure</u>. (para 11-19a(2))

40. A sensory pathway is <u>a series of nervous structures used to transmit information from the body to the CNS</u>. (para 11-19b(1))

41. A motor pathway is <u>a series of nervous structures used to transmit information from the CNS to the body</u>. (para 11-19b(2))

42. The human nervous system has several levels of control. The lowest level is the <u>simple reflex arc</u>. The highest level is the <u>conscious</u> level. Between, there are several progressively <u>higher</u> levels. All information input and all information output are <u>monitored</u> and <u>evaluated</u>. (para 11-19c)43.The right half of the brain controls the <u>left</u> side of the body. The left half of the brain controls the <u>right</u> side of the body. (para 11-20)

44. A pyramidal motor pathway is primarily concerned with volitional (voluntary) control of body parts, particularly the fine movements of hands. These pathways are called pyramidal because their neuron processes help to make up structures in the base of the brain called pyramids. (para 11-20a)

45. An extrapyramidal pathway is primarily concerned with automatic (nonvolitional) control of body parts for purposes of coordination. (para 11-20b)

46. Examples of general senses are:

    a.   Pain.
    b.   Temperature (warm and cold).
    c.   Touch (light and deep).
    d.   Proprioception ("body sense"). (para 11-21c)

47. Examples of special senses are:

    a.   Smell (olfaction).
    b.   Taste (gustation).
    c.   Vision.
    d.   Hearing (auditory).
    e.   Equilibrium. (para 11-21d)

48. The general sensory pathway is from the receptor organ, via the PNS nerves, to the CNS. This general pathway then ascends fiber tracts in the neuraxis. The pathway ends in the central area of the opposite cerebral hemisphere. (para 11-21e)

49. The receptors for the sense of smell are special hair cells called chemoreceptors. These are found in the olfactory epithelium, high in the nasal chambers in the head. The information received is transmitted by way of the olfactory nerves to the olfactory bulbs and then into the opposite cerebral hemisphere. (paras 11-22, 11-23)

50. Special hair cells (chemoreceptors) are found in the taste buds, scattered over the tongue and the rear of the mouth. These cells, which react to dispersed or dissolved food molecules, are the sensory receptors for the special sense of taste. The information received is transmitted to the opposite side of the brain by three cranial nerves. (paras 11-24, 11-25)

51. The eyeball is the sense organ containing the receptor tissues for the special sense of vision. The eyeball is shaped like a bulb (or sphere). (paras 11-26c, 11-27a)

52. The outermost layer of the eyeball is colored <u>white</u> and is made up of very dense <u>FCT</u>; it is known as the <u>sclera, scleral coat, or fibrous</u> tunic. Its anterior portion is called the <u>cornea</u>. The major focusing device for the eyeball is the <u>cornea</u>. (para 11-27b(1))

53. The middle layer of the wall of the eyeball is known as the <u>choroid, choroid coat, or vascular tunic</u>. This layer is richly supplied with <u>blood vessels</u> and pigmented with a <u>black</u> material. (para 11-27b(2))

54. The inner layer of the wall of the eyeball is known as the <u>retina, retinal coat, or internal tunic</u>. The actual photoreceptor elements are located at the <u>back</u> and the <u>sides</u>. These elements are the <u>rods</u> and the <u>cones</u>. (para 11-27b(3))

55. The elements which register colors are the <u>cones</u>. However, <u>cones</u> require more intense light than do <u>rods</u>. Rods register only <u>black and white</u>. (para 11-27c(1)(a))

56. The fovea centralis is <u>a small depression at the posterior end of the eyeball opposite the pupil</u>. The macula lutea is a small <u>yellow area of the retina where vision is sharpest. It includes the fovea centralis</u>. (para 11-27c(1)(b))

57. The blind spot is <u>the point of exit of the optic nerve, at the posterior end of the eyeball where there are no rods and cones</u>. (para 11-27c(1)(c))

58. The thickening of the choroid layer around the edge of the lens is called the <u>ciliary body</u>. It includes radial muscle fibers making up the <u>ciliary</u> muscle. (para 11-27c(2))

59. The lens is <u>biconvex. The anterior surface is flatter than the posterior surface. The lens is transparent and elastic. Its thickness varies with contraction or relaxation of the ciliary muscle</u>. Accommodation is <u>the process in which close objects are seen more clearly; it involves contraction of the ciliary muscle, reduction in pupil size, and convergence of the lines of sight</u>. (para 11-27c(4))

60. The space between the cornea and the iris is called the <u>anterior chamber</u>. The space between the iris and the lens is called the <u>posterior chamber</u>. Together, these make up the space between the cornea and the lens called the <u>anterior cavity</u> and filled with the <u>aqueous humor</u>. This drains into the encircling <u>canal of Schlemm</u>, located in the angle between the <u>cornea</u> and the <u>iris</u>. Behind the lens is a jellylike material called the <u>vitreous body</u>. It fills the <u>posterior</u> cavity of the eyeball. (para 11-27c(6), (7))

61. The orbit is the cavity in the upper facial skull which contains the <u>eyeball</u> and its <u>adnexa</u>. The orbit is shaped roughly like a <u>cone</u>. (para 11-28a)

62.   Examples of the adnexa are the:

    a.   Extrinsic ocular muscles.
    b.   Eyelids.
    c.   Lacrimal apparatus.
    d.   Eyebrow.
    e.   Optic nerve. (para 11-29)

63.   Of the six extrinsic ocular muscles, four are called recti muscles. Two are oblique muscles. The lateral rectus M. is on the outer side of the eyeball. The superior rectus M. is above the eyeball. The medial rectus M. is on the inner side of the eyeball. The inferior rectus M. is below the eyeball. The superior oblique and inferior oblique muscles approach the eyeball from the medial side. (para 11-29a)

64.   Attached to the margins of the orbit are the upper and lower eyelids. These have special hairs called eyelashes. The inner lining of the eyelids is continuous with the conjunctiva, a membrane over the anterior surface of the eyeball. (para 11-29b)

65.   In the upper outer corner of the orbit is a lacrimal gland, which secretes a lacrimal fluid, which is ultimately collected and delivered into the nasal chamber by the nasolacrimal duct. (para 11-29c)

66.   Neurons carry information from the photoreceptors located in the nervous retina. They leave the eyeball at the blind spot. Passing to the rear of the orbit, the neurons now belong to the optic nerve (cranial nerve II). The optic nerve enters the cranial cavity by passing through the optic canal. Beneath the brain, the optic nerves from both sides join to form the optic chiasma, in which half of the neurons from each optic nerve cross to the opposite side. From the optic chiasma, the right and left optic tracts proceed to the brain proper. (para 11-29e)

67.   The human ear has two major special sensory functions: hearing (auditory) and equilibrium (balance). The three parts of the human ear are the external (outer) ear, the middle ear, and the internal (inner) ear. (para 11-30)

68.   The external flap of the ear is called the auricle (pinna). It directs airborne sound waves into the canal called the external auditory meatus, which extends into the temporal portion of the skull. (para 11-31)

69.   The tympanic membrane is between the external auditory meatus and the middle ear cavity. On the medial side of the tympanic membrane, there is a space within the temporal bone called the middle ear cavity. The auditory ossicles are three very small bones linking the tympanic membrane to the medial wall of the middle ear cavity. The auditory ossicles respond to a sound stimulus by vibrating (mechanically oscillating). From the lateral to the medial ends, the names of the

ossicles are: malleus, incus, and stapes. The auditory tube connects the middle ear cavity with the nasopharynx. (para 11-32)

70. The bony labyrinth is a complex cavity within the temporal bone. It has three semi-circular canals, a vestibule (hallway), and a snail-shaped cochlear portion. The membranous labyrinth is a hollow tubular structure suspended within the bony labyrinth. (para 11-33a)

71. The endolymph fills the space within the membranous labyrinth. The perilymph fills the space between the membranous labyrinth and the bony labyrinth. (para 11-33b)

72. The cochlea is a spiral structure associated with hearing. It has 2-1/2 turns. Its outer boundaries are formed by the snail-shaped portion of the bony labyrinth. (para 11-33c)

73. The central column of the cochlea is called the modiolus. Extending from this central column is a spiral shelf of bone called the spiral lamina. Connecting this shelf with the outer bony wall is a fibrous membrane called the basilar membrane. This membrane forms the floor of the spiral portion of the membranous labyrinth called the cochlear duct. This contains a structure with hairs, sensory receptors of hearing; this structure is called the organ of Corti. (para 11-33c(1))

74. Within the bony cochlea, the space above the cochlear duct is known as the scala vestibuli and the space below is known as the scala tympani. Between the middle ear cavity and the upper space is an oval window called the fenestra vestibuli. Between the middle ear cavity and the lower space is a round window called the fenestra cochleae. (para 11-33c(2), (3))

75. A sound stimulus is transferred from the stapes to the fluid perilymph of the scala vestibuli. In response, the basilar membrane of the cochlea vibrates. The hair cells of the organ of Corti are mechanically stimulated. This stimulation is transferred to the neurons of the acoustic nerve, which passes out of the modiolus into the internal auditory meatus of the temporal bone. From here, the nerve enters the cranial cavity and goes to the brain. (para 11-33d)

76. The two sac-like portions of the membranous labyrinth are the sacculus and the utriculus. They are filled with endolymph. On the wall of each sac is a collection of special hair cells known as the macula, which serves as a receptor organ for static and linear kinetic gravitational forces. The saccular macula and the utricular macula are oriented at more or less 90° angles to each other. (para 11-35)

77. Extending from and opening into the utriculus are three hollow structures called the semicircular ducts. The utriculus completes the circles for each duct. The three ducts are all oriented at 90° angles to each other. Where it opens into the utriculus, each semicircular duct ends in an enlargement called an ampulla.

Movement of the fluid endolymph bends the hairs of the crista in specific directions. These are responses to linear and/or angular kinetic gravitational forces. (para 11-36b)

78. Carrying the information from the maculae and the cristae to the brain is the vestibular nerve. Contained in the same fibrous sheath from the membranous labyrinth to the brain are the vestibular and auditory nerves. (para 11-37)

79. The simplest and lowest level of control is the reflex arc. Producing wider reactions to stimuli are segmental reflexes. A number of nuclei in the hindbrain monitor and control visceral functions of the body, including respiration and heartbeat. The facilitatory and inhibitory areas of the reticular formation monitor and control general body functions, including sleep. The thalamus is a primary relay for information going to and from the cerebrum and cerebellum. One of the most important integrators of motor activity of the body is the cerebellum. (para 11-39)

80. In humans, the highest level of control is in the cerebrum. Here, we can clearly designate three levels of control.

   a. The first level is concerned with visceral activities of the body, as related to fight-or-flight, fear, and other emotions.

   b. At the second level, activities of the body are standardized and repetitive in nature. An example is the sequence of muscle actions involved in walking.

   c. At the third level, brand new solutions can be created. This is the volitional level.
   (para 11-39g)

End of Lesson 11

COMMENT SHEET

SUBCOURSE MD0006 Basic Human Anatomy

EDITION 100

Your comments about this subcourse are valuable and aid the writers in refining the subcourse and making it more usable. Please enter your comments in the space provided. ENCLOSE THIS FORM (OR A COPY) WITH YOUR ANSWER SHEET **ONLY** IF YOU HAVE COMMENTS ABOUT THIS SUBCOURSE..

FOR A WRITTEN REPLY, WRITE A SEPARATE LETTER AND INCLUDE SOCIAL SECURITY NUMBER, RETURN ADDRESS (and e-mail address, if possible), SUBCOURSE NUMBER AND EDITION, AND PARAGRAPH/EXERCISE/EXAMINATION ITEM NUMBER.

PLEASE COMPLETE THE FOLLOWING ITEMS:
(Use the reverse side of this sheet, if necessary.)

1. List any terms that were not defined properly.

_____
_____
_____
_____

2. List any errors.

paragraph   error   correction

_____
_____
_____
_____
_____
_____
_____
_____

3. List any suggestions you have to improve this subcourse.

_____
_____
_____
_____

4. Student Information (optional)

Name/Rank _____
SSN _____
Address _____
_____
E-mail Address _____
Telephone number (DSN) _____
MOS/AOC _____

PRIVACY ACT STATEMENT (AUTHORITY: 10USC3012(B) AND (G))

PURPOSE: To provide Army Correspondence Course Program students a means to submit inquiries and comments.

USES: To locate and make necessary change to student records.

DISCLOSURE: VOLUNTARY. Failure to submit SSN will prevent subcourse authors at service school from accessing student records and responding to inquiries requiring such follow-ups.

U.S. ARMY MEDICAL DEPARTMENT CENTER AND SCHOOL   Fort Sam Houston, Texas 78234-6130

This page intentionally left blank.

Basic Human Physiology

Subcourse MD0007

This page intentionally left blank.

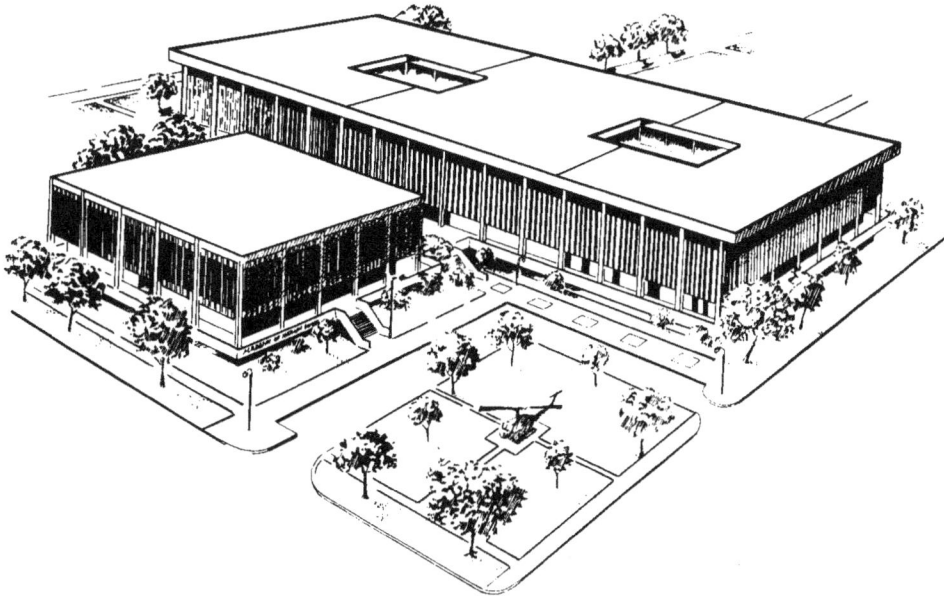

MD0007

BASIC HUMAN PHYSIOLOGY

EDITION 100

DEVELOPMENT

This subcourse reflects the current thought of the Academy of Health Sciences and conforms to printed Department of the Army doctrine as closely as currently possible. Development and progress render such doctrine continuously subject to change.

When used in this publication, words such as "he," "him," "his," and "men" are intended to include both the masculine and feminine genders, unless specifically stated otherwise or when obvious in context.

ADMINISTRATION

Students who desire credit hours for this correspondence subcourse must meet eligibility requirements and must enroll through the Nonresident Instruction Branch of the U.S. Army Medical Department Center and School (AMEDDC&S).

Application for enrollment should be made at the Internet website: http://www.atrrs.army.mil. You can access the course catalog in the upper right corner. Enter School Code 555 for medical correspondence courses. Copy down the course number and title. To apply for enrollment, return to the main ATRRS screen and scroll down the right side for ATRRS Channels. Click on SELF DEVELOPMENT to open the application and then follow the on screen instructions.

In general, eligible personnel include enlisted personnel of all components of the U.S. Army who hold an AMEDD MOS or MOS 18D. Officer personnel, members of other branches of the Armed Forces, and civilian employees will be considered eligible based upon their AOC, NEC, AFSC or Job Series which will verify job relevance. Applicants who wish to be considered for a waiver should submit justification to the Nonresident Instruction Branch at e-mail address: accp@amedd.army.mil.

For comments or questions regarding enrollment, student records, or shipments, contact the Nonresident Instruction Branch at DSN 471-5877, commercial (210) 221-5877, toll-free 1-800-344-2380; fax: 210-221-4012 or DSN 471-4012, e-mail accp@amedd.army.mil, or write to:

NONRESIDENT INSTRUCTION BRANCH
AMEDDC&S
ATTN: MCCS-HSN
2105 11TH STREET SUITE 4191
FORT SAM HOUSTON TX 78234-5064

TABLE OF CONTENTS

TABLE OF CONTENTS (continued)

TABLE OF CONTENTS (continued)

TABLE OF CONTENTS (continued)

LIST OF FIGURES

LIST OF FIGURES (continued)

LIST OF TABLES

CORRESPONDENCE COURSE OF THE
U.S. ARMY MEDICAL DEPARTMENT CENTER AND SCHOOL

SUBCOURSE MD0007

BASIC HUMAN PHYSIOLOGY

INTRODUCTION

In this subcourse, you will study basic human physiology. Anatomy is the study of body structure. Physiology is the study of body functions, particularly at the cellular level. Anatomy and physiology are two subject matter areas that are vitally important to most medical MOSs. Do your best to achieve the objectives of this subcourse. As a result, you will be better able to perform your job or medical MOS.

Subcourse Components:

This subcourse consists of 14 lessons and an examination. The lessons are:

Lesson 1, Introduction to Basic Human Physiology.

Lesson 2, Physiology of Cells and Miscellaneous Tissues.

Lesson 3, Envelopes of the Body.

Lesson 4, The Skeletal System.

Lesson 5, Physiology and Actions of Muscles.

Lesson 6, The Human Digestive System.

Lesson 7, The Human Respiratory System and Breathing.

Lesson 8, The Human Urinary System.

Lesson 9, The Human Reproductive (Genital) System.

Lesson 10, Cardiovascular and Other Circulatory Systems of the Human Body.

Lesson 11, The Human Endocrine System.

Lesson 12, The Human Nervous System.

Lesson 13, The Special Senses.

Lesson 14, Some Elementary Human Genetics.

Credit Awarded:

Upon successful completion of this subcourse, you will be awarded 26 credit hours.

Material Furnished:

In addition to this subcourse booklet, you are furnished an examination answer sheet and an envelope. Answer sheets are not provided for individual lessons in this subcourse because you are to grade your own lessons. Exercises and solutions for all lessons are contained in this booklet.

You must furnish a #2 pencil to be used when marking the examination answer sheet.

Procedures for Subcourse completion:

You are encouraged to complete the subcourse lesson by lesson. When you have completed all of the lessons to your satisfaction, fill out the examination answer sheet and mail it to the AMEDDC&S along with the Student Comment Sheet in the envelope provided. *Be sure that your name, rank, social security number, and address is on all correspondence sent to the AMEDDC&S.* You will be notified by return mail of the examination results. Your grade on the examination will be your rating for the subcourse.

Study Suggestions:

Here are some suggestions that may help you complete this subcourse:

Read and study each lesson assignment carefully.

After reading and studying the first lesson assignment, work the lesson exercises for the first lesson, marking your answers in the lesson booklet. Refer to the text material as needed.

When you have completed the exercises to your satisfaction, compare your answers with the solution sheet located at the end of the lesson. Reread the referenced material for any questions answered incorrectly.

After you have successfully completed one lesson, go to the next lesson and repeat the above procedures.

When you have completed all of the lessons, complete the examination. Reread the subcourse material as needed. We suggest that you mark your answers in the subcourse booklet. When you have completed the examination items to your satisfaction, transfer your responses to the examination answer sheet.

Student Comment Sheet:

Provide us with your suggestions and comments by filling out the Student Comment Sheet found at the back of this booklet and returning it to us with your examination answer sheet.

LESSON ASSIGNMENT

LESSON 1   Introduction to Basic Human Physiology.

LESSON ASSIGNMENT   Paragraphs 1-1 through 1-10.

LESSON OBJECTIVES   After completing this lesson, you should be able to:

1-1.   Define <u>physiology</u>.

1-2.   Describe the levels of function and the relationship between structure and function in the human body.

1-3.   Identify the effects of fundamental laws, concepts, and forces of the Universe.

1-4.   Identify processes which distinguish living from nonliving objects.

1-5.   Match three somatotypes with their descriptions.

1-6.   Identify general body functions and their descriptions.

1-7.   Identify fundamental processes for providing energy to human beings.

SUGGESTION   After completing the assignment, complete the exercises at the end of this lesson. These exercises will help you to achieve the lesson objectives.

LESSON 1

INTRODUCTION TO BASIC HUMAN PHYSIOLOGY

1-1. DEFINITION

Physiology is the study of the functions of the body at the cellular level.

1-2. LEVELS OF FUNCTION

Function in the human body occurs at three general levels:

    a. **Molecular**. The basic functional entity is the molecule. The structure and interaction of the molecules of the body is the subject of the science of <u>biochemistry</u>.

    b. **Cellular**. The individual cell is the basis of the structure and function of the human body. The individual human body consists of great numbers of these cells working together as a total organism. Groups of like cells performing a common function are called <u>tissues</u>. Different tissues collected together form individual <u>organs</u>. Groups of organs performing an overall function are called <u>organ systems</u>, for example, the digestive system, the respiratory system, etc. When these systems are together in a single individual, we refer to that individual as an <u>organism</u>. The cellular level of function is the primary subject matter of <u>physiology</u>.

    c. **Regional**. Here, individual parts of the human body (made up of specific organs) perform activities as a unit. For example, the hand serves as a grasping, tool-holding apparatus. The study of this level of function is called <u>functional anatomy</u>.

1-3. INTERRELATIONSHIPS

There is an inseparable relationship between structure and function in the human body. Every structure is designed to perform a particular function or functions. Likewise, every function has structures designed to perform it.

1-4. LAWS OF NATURE

The Universe has a fundamental order. The Universe is governed by discrete and precise laws of nature. These laws are universal, unchangeable, and omnipresent. The human organism is ultimately controlled by these laws. The organic body of the human being is essentially operated by the laws of physics and chemistry.

    a. **Gravitational Force and Mass**.

        (1) <u>Gravitational force</u>. As you stand upon the surface of the Earth, your body and its parts experience the force called gravity. The measure of this force is

called <u>weight</u>. Gravity is one type of <u>gravitational force</u>, a force which attracts all particles and bodies to each other. Gravity acts upon your body during every instant of your life.

        (2) <u>Mass</u>. If you were standing on the surface of the Moon, you would weigh 1/6 of your weight on Earth, but your <u>mass</u> would remain the same. <u>Mass</u> is an intrinsic property of a particle or object that determines its response to a given force. In a given location, the weight of an object depends upon its mass.

       b. **Space and Time**. Each individual occupies a certain amount of space. We exist over a span of time. During the passage of time, we change--from an infant, to a child, to an adult, to an adult of advanced age.

       c. **Physical States of Matter**. The matter around and in us exists in several states. These various states generally reflect the closeness of the molecules that make up the matter.

        (1) <u>Solid</u>. The most compact organization is the <u>solid</u>, which retains its specific form and shape.

        (2) <u>Liquid</u>. <u>Liquids</u> tend to flow but still stay together.

        (3) <u>Gas</u>. <u>Gases</u> also flow but are widely spread and will readily dissipate in many directions.

       d. **Pressure Gradients**. Substances that flow (gases and liquids) flow in very specific directions. They flow from an area of higher pressure or concentration to an area of lower pressure or concentration as long as the two areas are freely interconnected. The difference in pressures of two interconnected areas is called a <u>pressure gradient</u>. When plotted on graph paper, it is in the form of a slope. The greater the difference, the steeper is the slope and the faster the material flows.

1-5. MECHANICS/BIOMECHANICS

    <u>Machines</u> are devices that do work. The different kinds of machines and their modes of action are the study of applied <u>mechanics</u>. The human body, as already stated, conforms in its structural organization to the laws of physics. The body uses several different kinds of machines, such as levers, pulleys, and valves, in its operation. We refer to these operations as <u>biomechanics</u>.

1-6. LIFE PROCESSES

    The planet upon which we live is composed of inanimate (nonliving) materials such as minerals, water, etc. Living organisms reside upon or in this mass of nonliving material. You can distinguish living from nonliving material by the fact that living material carries on a series of functions known as the life processes. A living thing takes in substances, grows, moves, is irritable, and reproduces. Often, it is difficult to distinguish between living and nonliving materials. But in the ultimate analysis only living materials perform all of these functions.

1-7. VARIATIONS AMONG HUMAN ORGANISMS

The human organism is known scientifically as Homo sapiens, meaning the intelligent human being. There is a more or less common form for human beings. This common form includes one head, two upper members, two lower members, etc., but there are no two individuals exactly alike in detail. (This even includes identical twins. One tends to be left-oriented and the other right-oriented.) As a result, there is a tremendous variation among humans which has been further complicated by selection and propagation of specific traits by humans themselves.

1-8. SOMATOTYPES

Given the variations among human organisms, various methods of categorization have been established to achieve some common order. The method we will use is referred to as somatotyping. See Figure 1-1.

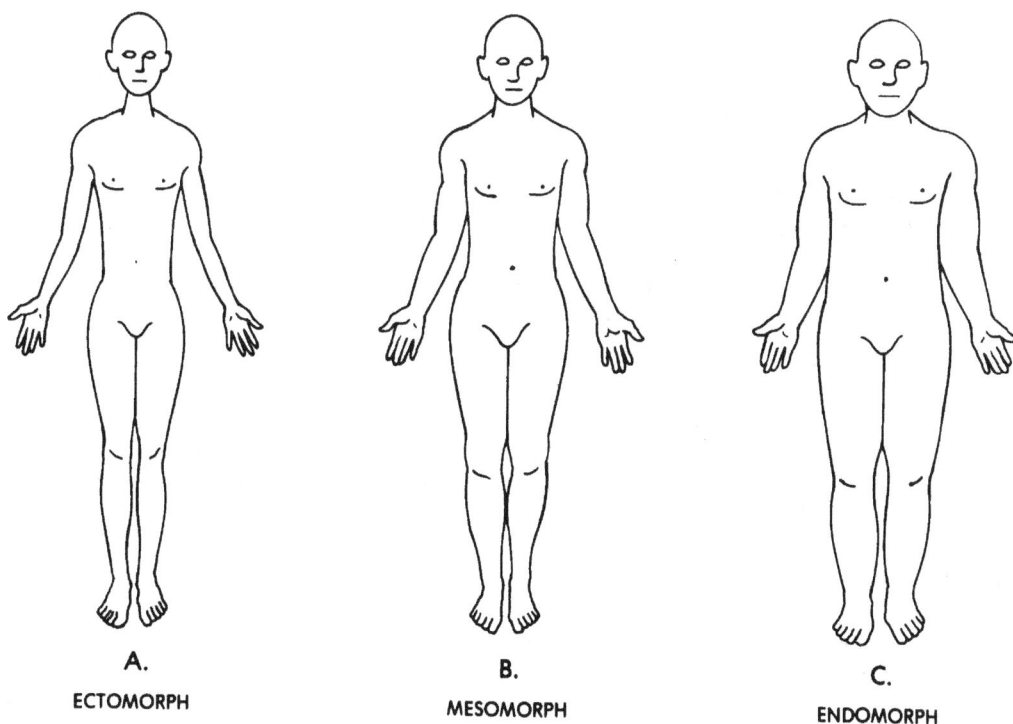

A.
ECTOMORPH

B.
MESOMORPH

C.
ENDOMORPH

Figure 1-1. Human somatotypes.

a. In this method, human beings are categorized into three different groups:

   (1) <u>Ectomorphs</u>, who tend to be thin-bodied individuals.

   (2) <u>Endomorphs</u>, who tend to be broad-bodied individuals.

   (3) <u>Mesomorphs</u>, who have a body form between the other two.

b. It has been demonstrated that there are significant differences among human beings in these categories. These differences exist not only in body form but also in internal anatomy of structures and susceptibility to diseases.

1-9. GENERAL BODY FUNCTIONS

The living human being performs many functions as a part of daily life.

a. **Nutrition**. The body takes in materials for energy, growth, and repair. Since the body cannot produce its own energy, it must continually take in foods to supply that <u>energy</u> to carry on the life processes. This food also provides materials for <u>growth</u> and <u>repair</u> of the cells and tissues.

b. **Motion and Locomotion**. Being an erect, standing organism, the body requires special supporting structures. At the same time, it needs a mechanical arrangement to allow the parts to move (<u>motion</u>) and to move from place to place (<u>locomotion</u>).

c. **Reproduction**. For the species to continue, there must be reproduction, the formation of new human beings belonging to subsequent generations.

d. **Control**. All of this activity is controlled by three major systems of the body--heredity/environment, hormones, and the nervous system. Hormones provide a chemical control system. The <u>nervous system</u> works much like circuitry in a computer. In the final analysis, however, all of the structures and functions of the body are determined by special units called <u>genes</u>, the study of which is <u>genetics</u> and the transmission of which is heredity. <u>Heredity</u> determines the potential range of an organism's characteristics. The <u>environment</u> determines which potential characteristics are developed and to what degree.

1-10. ENERGY

As we have previously mentioned, energy is required to carry on the life processes of each individual human being.

a. One of the laws of nature is <u>conservation of energy</u>. This means that energy cannot be created or destroyed but only transformed. For example, electricity can be transformed into heat. The human body cannot produce energy on its own and must, therefore, continuously take in a fresh supply of energy.

b. Except for a few special situations, all of the energy for living matter on Earth is received from the Sun through solar radiation. Green plants trap and bind this solar energy in molecules of glucose by the process of photosynthesis.

c. Humans take this glucose into their bodies directly by eating green plants or indirectly by eating the flesh of plant-eating animals. The human body releases the trapped energy from glucose by a process known as metabolic oxidation.

d. The released energy is used to form the compound ATP (adenosine triphosphate) from ADP (adenosine diphosphate). ATP is like a charged battery; the "discharged battery" is called ADP. Molecules of ATP are present in all of the living cells of the body. Within each cell, molecules of ATP are "discharged" to release a large quantity of energy to drive the various life processes. Through further metabolic oxidation, the resulting ADP molecules are "recharged" to form ATP molecules once again.

Continue with Exercises

EXERCISES, LESSON 1

REQUIREMENT. The following exercises are to be answered by completing each incomplete statement.

After you have completed all the exercises, turn to "Solutions to Exercises" at the end of the lesson, and check your answers.

1.   Physiology is the study of the _____ s of the body at the _____ level.

2.   Function in the human body occurs at three general levels:
m_____, c_____, and r_____. A science related to the first level is b_____y. The second level is studied in p_____y. The third level is studied in f_____ a_____.

3.   Every structure is designed to perform a particular _____. Every function has _____ s designed to perform it.

4.   As you stand upon the surface of the Earth, your body and its parts experience the forces called _____. The measure of this force is called _____.

If you were standing on the surface of the Moon, you would weigh much less, but your _____ would remain the same.

Matter which retains its specific form and shape is a _____. Matter which flows but stays together is a _____. Matter which flows and dissipates in many directions is a _____.

5.   As long as two areas are freely interconnected, a substance flows from an area where its pressure or concentration is (higher) (lower) to an area where its pressure or concentration is (higher) (lower). The difference in pressure between the two areas is the _____ _____.

6.   A living thing _____ s _____ substances, g_____ s, m_____ s, is i_____ e, and r_____ s.

7.   Ectomorphs are _____-bodied individuals. Endomorphs are _____-bodied individuals. A body form between the other two consists of the _____ s.

8. Important general body functions include n_____ for e_____, g_____, and r_____; m_____ and l_____; r_____; and c_____. Three important control systems are h_____/e_____, h_____s, and the n_____ system. The potential range of an organism's characteristics is determined by h_____. The extent to which these potential characteristics are developed is determined by the e_____.

9. Solar energy is first trapped on Earth by _____s in the process of p_____is. The molecules of g_____ are consumed directly or indirectly by humans. Within the human body, the trapped energy is released by the process of m_____ o_____. The released energy is used to form (ATP) (ADP) from (ATP) (ADP).

Check Your Answers on Next Page

SOLUTIONS TO EXERCISES, LESSON 1

1. Physiology is the study of the <u>functions</u> of the body at the <u>cellular</u> level. (para 1-1)

2. Function in the human body occurs at three general levels: <u>molecular</u>, <u>cellular</u>, and <u>regional</u>. A science related to the first level is <u>biochemistry</u>. The second level is studied in <u>physiology</u>. The third level is studied in <u>functional anatomy</u>. (para 1-2)

3. Every structure is designed to perform a particular <u>function</u>. Every function has <u>structures</u> designed to perform it. (para 1-3)

4. As you stand upon the surface of the Earth, your body and its parts experience the forces called <u>gravity</u>. The measure of this force is called <u>weight</u>.

    If you were standing on the surface of the Moon, you would weigh much less, but your <u>mass</u> would remain the same.

    Matter which retains its specific form and shape is a <u>solid</u>. Matter which flows but stays together is a <u>liquid</u>. Matter which flows and dissipates in many directions is a <u>gas</u>. (para 1-4a thru c)

5. As long as two areas are freely interconnected, a substance flows from an area where its pressure or concentration is <u>higher</u> to an area where its pressure or concentration is <u>lower</u>. The difference in pressure between the two areas is the <u>pressure gradient</u>. (para 1-4d)

6. A living thing <u>takes in</u> substances, <u>grows</u>, <u>moves</u>, is <u>irritable</u>, and <u>reproduces</u>. (para 1-6)

7. Ectomorphs are <u>thin</u>-bodied individuals. Endomorphs are <u>broad-</u> bodied individuals. A body form between the other two consists of the <u>mesomorphs</u>. (para 1-8)

8. Important general body functions include <u>nutrition</u> for <u>energy</u>, <u>growth</u>, and <u>repair</u>; <u>motion</u> and <u>locomotion</u>; <u>reproduction</u>; and <u>control</u>. Three important control systems are <u>heredity/ environment</u>, <u>hormones</u>, and the <u>nervous</u> system. The potential range of an organism's characteristics is determined by <u>heredity</u>. The extent to which these potential characteristics are developed is determined by the <u>environment</u>. (para 1-9)

9. Solar energy is the first trapped on Earth by <u>plants</u> in the process of <u>photosynthesis</u>. The molecules of <u>glucose</u> are consumed directly or indirectly by humans. Within the human body, the trapped energy is released by the process of <u>metabolic oxidation</u>. The released energy is used to form <u>ATP</u> from <u>ADP</u>. (para 1-10)

End of Lesson 1

LESSON ASSIGNMENT

LESSON 2	Physiology of Cells and Miscellaneous Tissues.
LESSON ASSIGNMENT	Paragraphs 2-1 through 2-35.
LESSON OBJECTIVES	After completing this lesson, you should be able to:

2-1. Match the major components of a "typical" animal cell with their functions.

2-2. Identify important functions of ATP and ADP.

2-3. Match the names of the fluid compartments with their descriptions.

2-4. Identify a general requirement for electrolytes, and match terms related to tonicity with their descriptions.

2-5. Identify functions and characteristics of water.

2-6. Identify examples of homeostasis and feedback mechanisms.

2-7. Match terms related to the movement of materials into and out of cells with their descriptions or examples.

2-8. Match terms related to membrane potentials, cell growth, and cell multiplication with their descriptions.

2-9. Match types of tissues with their characteristics.

SUGGESTION   After completing the assignment, complete the exercises at the end of this lesson. These exercises will help you to achieve the lesson objectives.

LESSON 2

PHYSIOLOGY OF CELLS AND
MISCELLANEOUS TISSUES

Section I. CELLS

2-1. THE CELLULAR LEVEL

a. The individual cell is the unit of structure of all living things. An entire organism may consist of a single cell (unicellular) or many cells (multicellular).

b. In human beings and other multicellular organisms, the cells tend to be organized in specific ways. A group of like cells performing a particular function is referred to as a tissue. An organ is a discrete structure composed of several different tissues together. An organ system is a group of organs together performing an overall function. (An example of an organ system is the digestive system.) The individual organism is the combination of all of these things as a discrete and separate entity.

c. Although all living matter is composed of cells, animal cells and plant cells are significantly different from each other. Not only do plant cells contain chlorophyll, a green coloring matter; plant cells also have a cell wall around them which is made up of a very complex carbohydrate known as cellulose. Neither chlorophyll nor a cell wall is present in connection with animal cells.

2-2. THE MAJOR COMPONENTS OF A "TYPICAL" ANIMAL CELL

A "typical" animal cell is illustrated in Figure 2-1.

a. **Cell Membrane.** As its outer boundary, the animal cell has a special structure called the cell or plasma membrane. All of the substances that enter or leave the cell must in some way pass through this membrane.

b. **Protoplasm.** The major substance of the cell is known as protoplasm. It is a combination of water and a variety of materials dissolved in the water. Outside the cell nucleus (see below), protoplasm is called cytoplasm. Inside the cell nucleus, protoplasm is called nucleoplasm.

c. **Organelles.** Within the cytoplasm, certain structures are called organelles. These organelles include structures such as the endoplasmic reticulum, ribosomes, various kinds of vacuoles, the Golgi apparatus, mitochondria, and centrioles.

(1) The endoplasmic reticulum resembles a circulatory system for the individual cell. It is a network composed of unit (single-thickness) membranes.

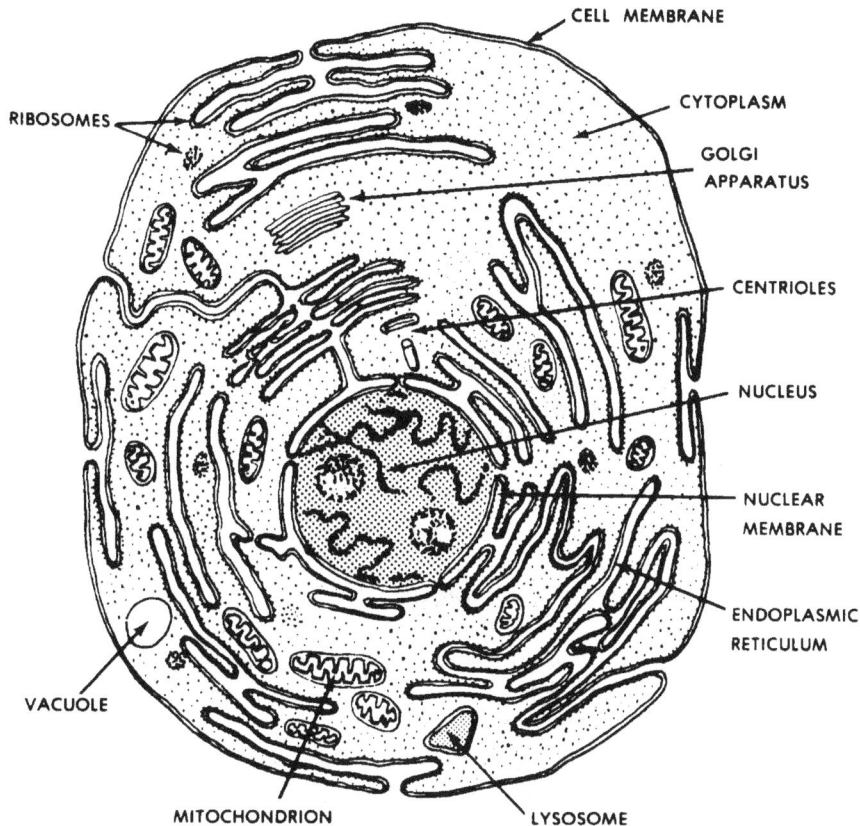

Figure 2-1. A "typical" animal cell.

(2)   The ribosomes are granular particles concerned with protein synthesis. They may be found free, clustered, or attached to the endoplasmic reticulum.

(3)   The vacuoles are small spaces or cavities within the cytoplasm. These serve functions at the cellular level such as digestion, respiration, excretion, and storage.

(4)   The Golgi complex is a portion of the endoplasmic reticulum that aids in the final preparation of certain proteins and mucus-like substances and in the movement of these substances. It is best-developed in secretory cells.

(5)   The mitochondria are the "powerhouses" of the cell. They "recharge" ADP molecules to form ATP molecules.

(6)   There are ordinarily two centrioles. These organelles play a major role in cell division.

d. **Nucleus.** Within the cell is the nucleus. This structure has a <u>nuclear membrane</u> separating it from the cytoplasm. Within the nucleus is the <u>chromatin material</u>, made up of the protein deoxyribonucleic acid (DNA). At the time of cell division, this chromatin material is aggregated into individual structures known as <u>chromosomes</u>. Each chromosome has a set of specific <u>genes</u>, which determine all of the physical and chemical characteristics of the body, which represent its structure and function.

2-3. ENERGY

a. We mentioned in lesson 1 that the human body depended upon external sources for energy. Plants use solar radiation to make glucose and other nutrients. The human body takes glucose and other nutrients directly or indirectly from plants. The body receives oxygen from the air. The energy that was once derived by plants from solar radiation is released within human cells by the process of <u>metabolic oxidation</u>. This involves the combination of glucose and other nutrients with oxygen, releasing the stored energy.

b. The mitochondria of the cells use this released energy to form ATP molecules from ADP molecules. Adenosine diphosphate is converted to ATP by the addition of a "part of a molecule" called a phosphate radical. The binding of this phosphate radical requires a large quantity of energy, which can be released later when the phosphate radical is separated off. Adenosine triphosphate provides energy for cellular processes such as active transport of substances across membranes, synthesis of chemical compounds for the body, and mechanical work (such as muscle contraction). When an Adenosine triphosphate molecule provides energy for such a process, it loses a phosphate radical and becomes ADP. Then, the cycle begins again as ADP is converted into ATP within the mitochondria.

c. Certain cells, such as muscle cells and nerve cells, require great amounts of energy. Such cells have well-developed mitochondria.

Section II. BODY FLUIDS

2-4. INTRODUCTION

Approximately 56 percent of the human body consist of fluids. Soft tissues consist almost completely of fluids. These body fluids are composed largely of water. Thus, water is the major component of living substances.

2-5. FLUID COMPARTMENTS

Regarding the human body, we speak of fluid compartments or spaces. These are intracellular fluid, the interstitial fluid, and the circulating (plasma) fluid. See Figure 2-2 for a scheme of the body fluids and fluid compartments.

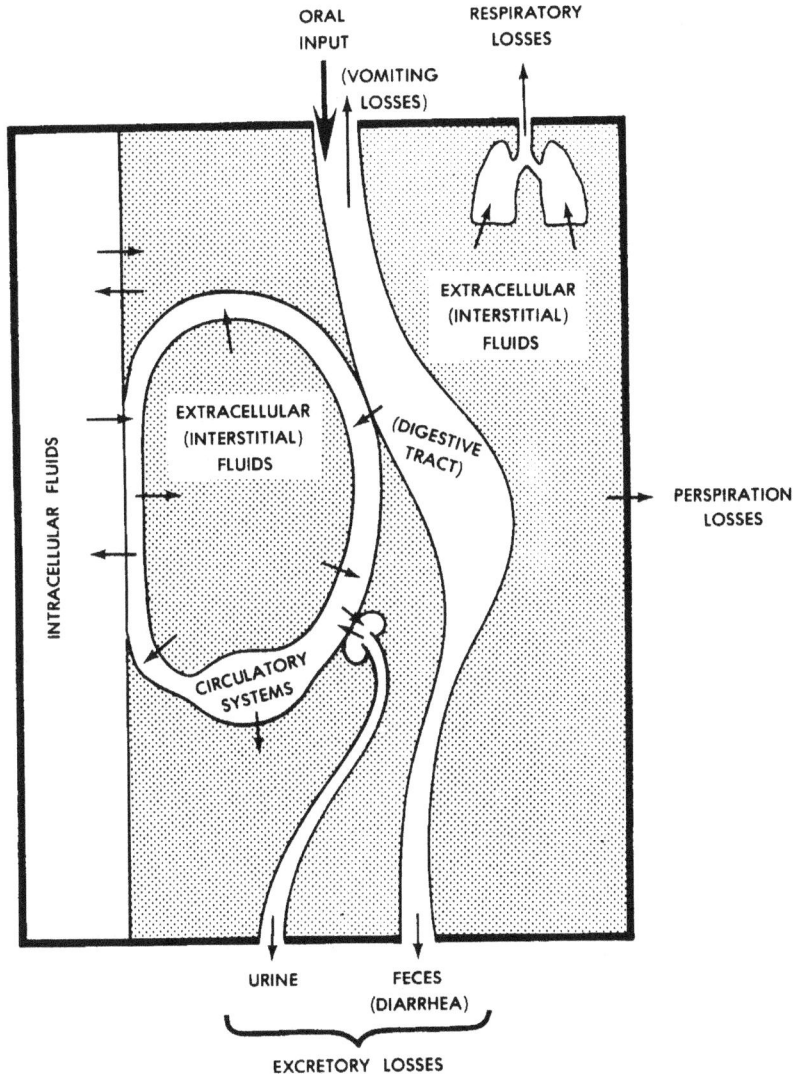

Figure 2-2. Scheme of the body fluids and fluid compartments.

a. Within the cell, we have seen that the major constituent is water. This fluid is called intracellular fluid ("within the cell").

b. Therefore, all other fluids are _extracellular_. The extracellular fluids are found in two different compartments.

(1) The tissue fluid is located among but not within the cells of the body. It is therefore called _interstitial_ or _intercellular_ fluid.

(2) In some systems, fluids serve as a vehicle to carry items around the body. These systems are called _circulatory systems_. The circulating fluid is called the plasma--the non-cellular component of blood.

2-6. ELECTROLYTES

Within the fluids of the body, there are certain chemicals known as electrolytes. Electrolytes are chemicals that dissociate ("break up") into ions ("charged particles") when they are dissolved. To maintain life and good health, electrolytes must be in balance. That is, they must be present in certain proportions and concentrations in each fluid compartment.

2-7. WATER

As we have mentioned, water is the main constituent of the human body.

a. **Some Physical Characteristics.** Water has several important physical characteristics that make it extremely useful to the body.

(1) First, it is a _fluid_. Therefore, it has the capacity to flow.

(2) Secondly, it is often called the "_universal solvent_." This refers to its ability to dissolve so many substances within itself. Thus, water is an excellent vehicle for the circulatory systems.

(3) Water is very useful in the temperature control mechanisms of the body. This is because of its _heat-carrying capacity_ and its tendency to remove large numbers of calories during evaporation.

b. **Sources**. Water thirst and water satiation is controlled by special centers in the hypothalamus of the brain. The human body obtains water in two primary ways:

(1) Most items that humans drink or eat consist largely of water.

(2) A second source of water is metabolic oxidation. This water is referred to as metabolic water. As various food substances are oxidized within the individual cell, water is one of the main by-products.

c. **Losses**.

(1) Perspiration. Water is continuously lost from the body in the form of perspiration or sweat. With high surrounding temperatures and/or vigorous exercise, the sweat is obvious. This is called sensible perspiration. Otherwise, the sweat is usually not obvious, and there is a low level of water loss. This is called insensible perspiration.

(2) Respiration. The surfaces of the lungs must be moist to ensure the passage of gases to and from the blood. Air is moistened within the respiratory passages and the alveoli of the lungs. Thus, moisture passes out of the body along with the exhaled breath.

(3) Urination. Water is also lost from the body in the form of urine. Urine carries nitrogenous wastes of protein metabolism, dissolved in the water.

(4) Vomiting and diarrhea. During vomiting and diarrhea, the body loses large quantities of water and dissolved electrolytes. In infants and the elderly, this loss of water and electrolytes can be very dangerous. Sometimes, even death may result.

2-8. DISSOLVED SUBSTANCES

As mentioned before, one of the characteristics of water that makes it so desirable is its capacity to dissolve almost anything ("universal solvent").

a. **Gases.** Oxygen and carbon dioxide are exchanged between air in the lungs and the blood. They are also exchanged between the blood and the individual cells of the body. At least in part, these gases are carried as dissolved substances in the water of the blood.

b. **Nutrients**. By nutrients, we mean the end products of digestion, and vitamins and minerals from the digestive system. By being dissolved in the water of the blood, these nutrients are distributed to the individual cells of the body.

c. **Wastes**. Wastes result from the metabolic processes of the body. Wastes are picked up from the individual cells and delivered dissolved in the water to the excretory organs of the body, such as the kidneys.

d. **Hormones**. Hormones are carried from the endocrine glands to specific target organs while dissolved in the water of the blood.

2-9. TISSUE FLUID CYCLE

That portion of the extracellular fluid found among the cells is called the tissue fluid, or interstitial fluid. Tissue fluid originates primarily with a fluid portion of the blood that escapes into the tissues from the capillaries. Part of this escaped fluid enters the beginning of the venous vessels. However, a large percentage of the tissue fluid is picked up by another circulatory system, the lymphatic system. Thus, there is a continuous flow of the fluids throughout the body. In addition, the intracellular fluid and the immediate extracellular fluid are continually being exchanged.

Section III. HOMEOSTASIS

2-10. INTRODUCTION

a. The body fluids play an important role in homeostasis. Homeostasis is the body's tendency to maintain a steady state. The tissue fluid forms the immediate environment of the living cell. In order to maintain the life processes of the individual cells, there must be appropriate concentrations of oxygen, carbon dioxide, nutrients, electrolytes, and other substances within the tissue fluid.

b. One of the chief functions of any organ system is to help to maintain this steady state. For example, the digestive system helps to maintain a steady concentration of nutrients. The respiratory system helps to maintain steady concentrations of oxygen and the removal of carbon dioxide.

c. All organ systems are at least partially controlled by a feedback mechanism. A feedback mechanism resembles the household thermostat. When the concentration of a substance is too low, the feedback mechanism stimulates an increased production and/or distribution. Once the level returns to normal, the feedback mechanism signals a decrease in production. There is a similar feedback mechanism for body temperature.

2-11. WATER BALANCE

The body has a natural requirement for a certain amount of water to continue its processes properly. Lack of fluid in the circulatory system can result in heart failure. Excessive amounts of fluid in the tissue spaces cause swelling of the body, known as edema. There are feedback mechanisms to maintain water balance.

2-12. ELECTROLYTE BALANCE

The electrolytes must also be in balance. Electrolyte balance is an important consideration when fluids are administered to a patient. See Figure 2-3 for an explanation of tonicity.

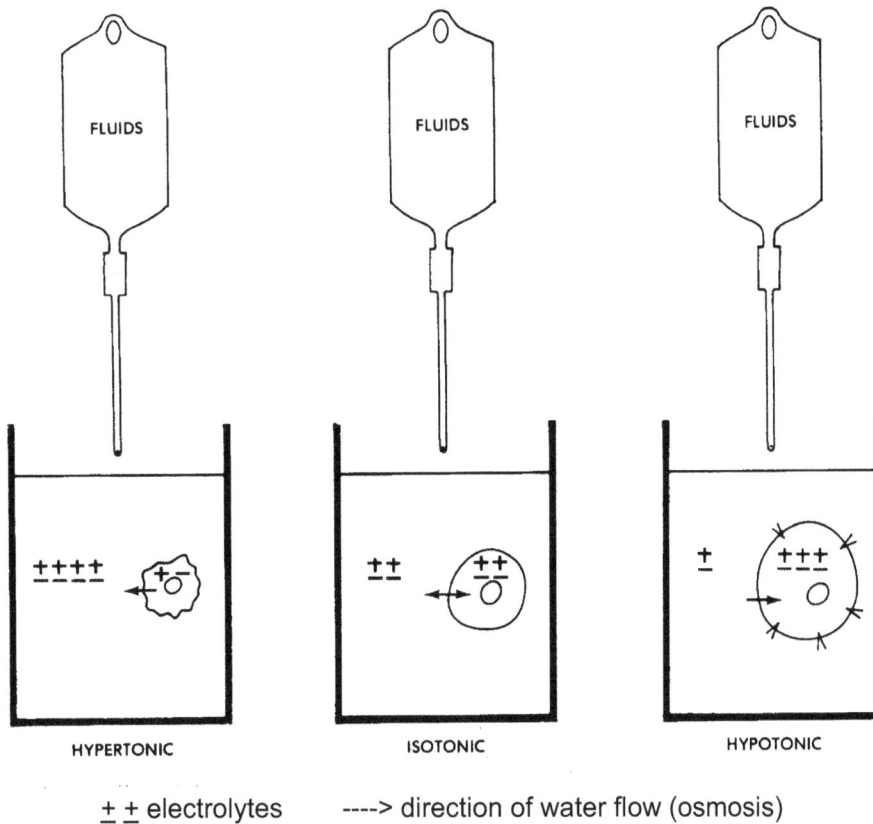

Figure 2-3. Tonicity (cell with semipermeable membrane, nonpermeable to electrolytes present).

$\pm$ $\pm$ electrolytes   ----> direction of water flow (osmosis)

a. **Hypertonicity.** If the overall concentration of electrolytes is greater in the tissue fluid surrounding a cell than it is in the intracellular fluid within the cell, the tissue fluid is hypertonic (noun: hypertonicity). The cell tends to be destroyed by loss of its fluid to the hypertonic environment.

b. **Hypotonicity.** If the overall concentration of electrolytes as less in the tissue fluid than it is in the intracellular fluid within the cell, the tissue fluid is hypotonic (noun: **hypotonicity**). In a hypotonic environment, fluid will enter a cell and cause it to swell and burst.

c. **Isotonicity.** If the concentrations of electrolytes are the same in the tissue fluid and the intracellular fluid, the situation is balanced (homeostatic). That is, the fluids are **isotonic**.

2-13. MOVEMENT OF MATERIALS INTO AND OUT OF THE CELL

We noted earlier that all substances that enter or leave the cell must pass through the cell membrane in some way.

a. **Semipermeability**. The permeability of a membrane is its capacity to allow materials to move through it. Since the cell membrane of animal cells is selective and does not allow all materials to pass through it, we say that it is semipermeable (noun: semipermeability).

b. **Diffusion**. Some materials readily pass through the membrane from an area of higher concentration to an area of lower concentration. This process is called diffusion. When materials require help to pass through the cell membrane, the process is referred to as facilitated diffusion.

c. **Active Transport**. In certain situations, materials pass through the cell membrane against the concentration gradient. In this case, an expenditure of energy is required. The process is called active transport. An example is the sodium/potassium pump, in which the sodium ions are forced out of the cytoplasm of the cell and into the surrounding tissue fluid and potassium ions are pumped back into the cell cytoplasm.

d. **Osmosis**. Sometimes a substance is not able to pass through the cell membrane. When the concentration of this substance is greater on one side of the cell membrane than the other, water will tend to pass through the membrane to the area of greater concentration. This process is called osmosis. This process involves the concept of tonicity, discussed in paragraph 2-12.

e. **Pinocytosis and Phagocytosis**. Sometimes, the cell membrane will engulf a minute amount of tissue fluid and its contents. This process is called pinocytosis. During pinocytosis, the cell membrane produces a vacuole to contain the engulfed material. When the cell membrane engulfs larger particles, such as bacteria or other cells, the process is called phagocytosis. After either pinocytosis or phagocytosis, digestive fluids may pass from the cytoplasm into the vacuole. The end products of digestion are absorbed from the vacuole into the cell cytoplasm.

2-14. MEMBRANE POTENTIALS

In living cells, there is generally a higher concentration of positively charged ions on the outside of the cell and a higher concentration of negatively charged ions on the inside of the cell. Thus, there is a concentration gradient (an electrical potential or polarity) across the membrane that we call the membrane potential that creates an electrical gradient.

a. **Resting Potential.** When the cell is in a resting state, the membrane potential is maintained by the sodium/potassium pump. The sodium/potassium pump actively transports 3 positive sodium ions (Na^+) to the outside of the cell membrane and

2 potassium ions to the inside of the cell membrane. This results in a negative charge inside the cell and a positive charge outside the cell, producing a potential or polarity across the membrane.

b. **Action Potential**. The electrical activity that occurs in a stimulated neuron or muscle fiber is called the action potential. This involves depolarization and subsequent repolarization. First, sodium ions move into the cell by diffusion. This reverses the polarity (depolarization). Second, potassium moves out of the cell by diffusion that causes repolarization. The sodium/potassium pump then restores the ionic balance by actively (energy required) pumping sodium back out and potassium back into the cell. These various electrical potentials can be measured with appropriate instruments.

Section IV. CELL GROWTH AND MULTIPLICATION

2-15. CELL GROWTH

a. The individual cells have the capacity to grow. They do this by acquiring various substances from the blood and converting them into appropriate cellular elements.

b. Sometimes, a tissue such as muscle tissue will increase in mass without an increase in the number of units. This condition is called hypertrophy.

2-16. CELL MULTIPLICATION

a. On the other hand, if an increase in tissue mass results from a greater number of cells, we refer to this as hyperplasia.

b. Cell multiplication is accomplished through a process called mitosis. In mitosis, the genetic material of the cell is doubled. Then, the cell divides into halves. One-half of the genetic material goes into each of the two daughter cells. In this manner, the two new cells each have the same genetic composition as the original cell.

Section V. EPITHELIAL CELLS AND TISSUES

2-17. INTRODUCTION

Tissues are groups of like cells together performing a common function or functions. The epithelial tissues are specialized to cover surfaces and line cavities. They are also secretory.

2-18. EPITHELIAL CELL TYPES

By observing microscopic preparations of epithelial tissues, one can classify the cells of epithelial tissues into three general types: columnar, cuboidal, and flat (squamous).

2-19. EPITHELIAL TISSUE TYPES

If an epithelial tissue consists of a single layer of cells, it is called a simple epithelial tissue. When there are several layers of cells, it is called a stratified epithelial tissue. In both cases, the epithelial tissue is further identified by the type of epithelial cell that forms the outermost layer of the tissue. For example, the outer layer (epidermis) of the skin is a stratified squamous epithelium; squamous cells form the outermost of many layers.

2-20. LINING OF SEROUS CAVITIES

The many serous cavities of the body are lined with a simple squamous epithelium. This epithelial tissue also secretes a serous fluid to act as a lubricant, reducing frictional forces of organs moving against each other. An example is the outer surfaces of the lungs, which move on the inside of the chest wall (within the pleural cavity) during breathing.

2-21. OUTER SURFACE OF THE BODY

The outer layer of the skin is a stratified squamous epithelium. In it, there are many layers of cells. The outermost layers consist of squamous, or flat, cells.

2-22. SECRETORY PROCESSES

Secretory epithelial cells, such as those in various glands, have a well-developed Golgi complex. In one type of secretory cells, the secretions are passed through the cell membrane. In another type of secretory cells, those of the sebaceous glands, a portion of the cell containing the secretion is sloughed off from the cell.

Section VI. FIBROUS CONNECTIVE TISSUE

2-23. INTRODUCTION

Tissues that generally support the body parts in various ways are known as the connective tissues (CT).

a. All of these connective tissues are characterized by having the major substance outside of the cell but formed by the cell. This extra-cellular material is called the matrix.

b. One type of CT is called the fibrous connective tissue (FCT). In FCT, the cell known as the fibroblast forms a long narrow thread-like structure known as the fiber. During the life of the individual, the fibroblast actually moves up and down the fiber. During this movement, it keeps the fiber in repair and restructures it in response to the stresses applied to the body.

2-24. TYPES OF FIBROUS CONNECTIVE TISSUE FIBERS

Two types of fibers are formed--the collagen or white fibers and the elastic or yellow fibers. The collagen fibers are limited in stretchability, particularly when compared to the elastic fibers.

2-25. FIBROUS CONNECTIVE TISSUES

The fibers of the FCT are variously organized to perform particular functions.

a. **Loose Areolar Fibrous Connective Tissue.** In some locations, the fibers are loosely arranged with spaces between them. This tissue serves as filler material in the spaces between the organs. This loose areolar FCT is also found between the skin and the underlying structures of the body. Thus, the skin is able to move more or less freely over the surface of these structures.

b. **Dense Fibrous Connective Tissue.** The fibers of dense FCT are closely packed and more or less parallel. As membranes, dense FCT envelops areas or structures of the body (as in capsules around organs). Other examples of dense FCT are ligaments and tendons. A ligament is a band of dense FCT that holds the bones together at a joint. A tendon attaches a muscle to a bone.

2-26. LENGTH AND TENSION

As a collagen fiber is increased in length, the tension (resistance to stretch) increases considerably. This can be shown by a length-tension (L-T) curve diagram, similar to the one in Figure 2-4.

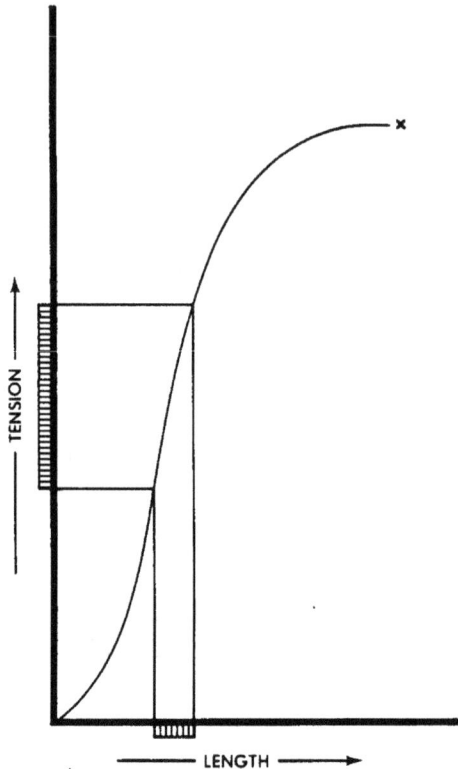

Figure 2-4. Length tension curve of an FCT fiber.

2-27. TEMPERATURE AND TENSION

a. The degree of elasticity (stretchability) of an FCT is more or less proportional to its temperature. The cooler it is, the less stretchable and the more subject to damage it is. On the other hand, as the fiber becomes warmer, its stretchability and resistance to damage increase.

b. This characteristic is the basis of warm-up exercises before participating in strenuous activities such as sports. By exercising to the point of sensible perspiration (para 2-7c), the body, temperature is raised to the desired level. At this level, the FCT are able to stretch and withstand the various forces applied to them.

Section VII. FATTY TISSUES

2-28. INTRODUCTION

Another supportive tissue of the body is fatty tissue (fat connective tissue). Here, the matrix is a lipid material, but found within the cell rather than outside of the cell.

2-29. LIPIDS

Lipids are fats, oils, and similar compounds such as fatty acids. Lipids are stored mostly in the form of neutral fat. <u>Neutral fat</u> consists of triglycerides, a type of molecule formed from glycerol (a type of alcohol) and three fatty acids. According to the length of each fatty acid, the triglyceride may be a liquid (oil) or a solid (fat). The triglycerides are kept in a liquid form, and even in cold weather, their lengths are adjusted in order to maintain a liquid state.

2-30. BROWN FAT AND YELLOW FAT

There are two types of fat within the body---brown fat and yellow fat. Both are excellent means of energy storage. When metabolized, they both yield large amounts of energy, especially when compared to carbohydrates. Brown fat is more common in infants and children, whereas adults tend to have mostly yellow fat.

2-31. TURNOVER OF FATS

Fats are essentially a temporary storage phenomenon. There is a continuous turnover of the triglycerides. There is a complete turnover within a 3-week period.

2-32. SOURCES

The diet is the major source of fat in the human body. Fats may be taken in as fats or converted from other substances, such as carbohydrates.

2-33. OBESITY

Obesity occurs when excessive amounts of fats and/or carbohydrates are taken into the body. When the energy contained in these compounds is not used in bodily activities, the surplus is generally stored as the triglycerides in fatty tissues of the body.

2-34. STORAGE OF FAT-SOLUBLE SUBSTANCES

a. A number of fat-soluble substances may be stored in the fat of the body. Vitamins A and D are fat-soluble.

b. In addition, organophosphoric compounds of modern pesticides are often stored in human fat. Although these compounds may have been required in food production, they may also be ingested along with the food.

c. The storage of such substances becomes particularly important when an individual goes on a crash diet. As fat is lost during such a diet, these fat-soluble substances are released into the general system. They may reach dangerous levels. In addition, the organs supported by the fat may become loose within the body and subject to injury.

2-35. CHOLESTEROL

Cholesterol is a special lipid-type substance. It is very important for the proper functioning of several structures and processes of the body, particularly in the liver. However, there are some indications that, in some individuals, excessive cholesterol may be damaging to the cardiovascular system of the body.

Continue with Exercises

EXERCISES, LESSON 2

REQUIREMENT. The following exercises are to be answered by completing the incomplete statement.

After you have completed all the exercises, turn to "Solutions to Exercises" at the end of the lesson, and check your answers.

1. All substances that enter or leave a cell must in pass through the cell _____. Resembling a circulatory system for the individual cell is the e_____ r_____. Granular particles concerned with protein synthesis are the r_____s. Spaces or cavities which serve functions at the cellular level such as digestion, respiration, excretion, and storage are the v_____s. A portion of the endoplasmic reticulum that aids in the final preparation of certain proteins and mucus-like substances is the _____ complex. The "powerhouses" of the cell are the _____a. Playing a major role in cell division are the two c_____s.

Each chromosome has a set of specific _____s. These determine the p_____ical and c_____ical characteristics of the body.

2. Adenosine triphosphate (ATP) provides _____y for cellular processes such as ac_____e tr_____t of substances across _____s, synthesis of chemical c_____s for the body, mechanical _____k (such as muscle _____n). When an ATP molecule provides _____y for such a process, it loses a _____e radical and becomes _____. Then, the cycle begins again as ADP is converted into _____ within the _____a.

3. The major component of living substances is _____. The fluid within the cell is called _____ fluid. Located among the cells is the _____l fluid. In the circulatory systems, fluids serve as a v_____e. Together, the interstitial and circulating fluids are called e_____ fluid.

4. Certain chemicals dissociate into ions when they are dissolved. These chemicals are called _____s. For good health, these chemicals must be in b_____. In other words, each fluid compartment must have a certain c_____n of a given electrolyte.

5.   Water has several important physical characteristics: First, it is a f_____;
therefore, it has the capacity of f____. Second, it is able to d_____ many substances
within itself; thus, it is an excellent v_____. Because of its h____-carrying capacity
and its ability to remove large numbers of _____s during evaporation, water is very
useful in controlling the body's _____ e.

6.   The human body obtains water in two primary ways: First, water is the major
component of items we d____k or ____. Second, as food substances are o_____ d
within individual cells, water is one of the main b_____s.

7.   Water is lost from the body during p_____n, r_____n, u_____n,
v_____g, and d_____a.

8.   Substances dissolved in the water of the body include g_____, n_____,
w_____, and h_____.

9.   Interstitial fluid originates primarily as the _____d's fluid portion which
escapes into the tissues from the _____s. Part of this fluid enters the b_____g
of the v_____s vessels. A large portion is picked up by the l_____system.

10.   The body's tendency to maintain a steady state is called h_____. As a part of
this, the body maintains appropriate concentrations of o_____, c_____d_____,
n_____s, e_____s, and other substances within the tissue fluid. A system
that helps to maintain the appropriate concentration of o_____ and c_____d_____
is the r_____y system. A system which helps to maintain the appropriate
concentration of n_____s is the d_____ system. Such organ systems are at
least partially controlled by f_____k mechanisms. These mechanisms resemble the
household t_____t.

11.   The body needs a certain amount of w_____ to function properly. Lack of fluid
may result in h_____ failure. Too much fluid tends to result in swelling, known as e_____.
To maintain water balance, there are f_____ mechanisms.

12.   If the concentration of electrolytes is greater in the tissue fluid than in the
intracellular fluid, the tissue fluid is _____tonic. If the concentration of electrolytes is
less in the tissue fluid than in the intracellular fluid, the tissue fluid is _____tonic.
If the concentration of electrolytes are equal in the tissue fluid and intracellular fluid, the
fluids are ____tonic.

13.   Assume that a substance is more concentrated on one side of a membrane than the other but that it cannot pass through the membrane. The process in which water passes to the side of greater concentration is called _____.

   If, however, the substance can easily pass through the membrane, the process in which the substance passes through the membrane to the area where it is less concentrated is called _____. If the substance needs assistance to pass through the membrane, we call the process f_____ d_____ n.

   Since the cell membrane allows only some types of substances to pass through it, the cell membrane is _____ble.

   When energy is used to move a substance across a membrane to an area of higher concentration, the process is called _____ e _____t.

   When a minute amount of tissue fluids is engulfed by the cell membrane, the process is _____ cytosis. When larger particles are engulfed, the process is _____ cytosis.

14.   When the cell is in a resting state, the membrane potential is maintained by the s_____ /p_____pump. This membrane potential is called the _____ing potential. The s_____ /p_____ pump actively transports 3 (positive)(negative) sodium ions to the outside of the cell membrane and 2 potassium ions to the inside of the cell membrane. This results in a _____tive charge inside the cell and a _____tive charge outside the cell.

   When a neuron or muscle fiber is stimulated, the resulting activity is called the _____ potential. This involves _____tion and subsequent _____tion. First, sodium ions move into the cell by _____n. This reverses the _____y. Second, potassium moves out of the cell by diffusion which causes _____tion.

15.   A condition in which tissue mass increases without an increase in the number of cells is called hyper_____. When tissue mass increases due to an increase in the number of cells, it is hyper_____. Another word for cell multiplication is m_____ .

16.   The epithelial tissue lining a serous cavity secretes a _____s fluid to act as a _____t. The secretion of sebaceous glands is formed as portions of the cells are _____ghed off.

17.   In FCT, the fibroblast moves up and down the ____. During this movement, it keeps the fiber in r_____r and restructures it in response to the s_____es applied to the body. The collagen fibers are limited in _____y, particularly when compared to the e_____c fibers. As a collagen fiber lengthens, the t_____n increases considerably. As an FCT becomes warmer, it becomes more _____able and more resistant to d_____ ; this is the basis of w_____-u__ exercises before more strenuous activities.

18.   Fats, oils, and fatty acids are types of _____ds. Such substances are stored mostly as n_____l fat, which consists of tri_____s. A molecule of tri_____ is formed from a glycerol and three fatty ____s. Within the body, triglycerides are kept in a (liquid) (solid) state by adjusting the length of each f_____a____. Within a 3-week period, there is a complete t_____r of the triglycerides. Fats may be taken in as ___s or converted from other substances, such as c_____s. When the diet contains more fats and carbohydrates than necessary for body activities, the result may be _____y.

Check Your Answers on Next Page

SOLUTIONS TO EXERCISES, LESSON 2

1.   All substances that enter or leave a cell must in some way pass through the cell membrane. Resembling a circulatory system for the individual cell is the endoplasmic reticulum. Granular particles concerned with protein synthesis are the ribosomes. Spaces or cavities that serve functions at the cellular level such as digestion, respiration, excretion, and storage are the vacuoles. A portion of the endoplasmic reticulum that aids in the final preparation of certain proteins and mucus-like substances is the Golgi complex. The "powerhouses" of the cell are the mitochondria. Playing a major role in cell division are the two centrioles.

Each chromosome has a set of specific genes. These determine the physical and chemical characteristics of the body. (para 2-2)

2.   Adenosine triphosphate (ATP) provides energy for cellular processes such as active transport of substances across membranes, synthesis of chemical compounds for the body, mechanical work (such as muscle contraction). When an ATP molecule provides energy for such a process, it loses a phosphate radical and becomes ADP. Then, the cycle begins again as ADP is converted into ATP within the mitochondria. (para 2-3b)

3.   The major component of living substances is water. The fluid within the cell is called intracellular fluid. Located among the cells is the interstitial fluid. In the circulatory systems, fluids serve as a vehicle. Together, the interstitial and circulating fluids are called extracellular fluid. (paras 2-4 and 2-5)

4.   Certain chemicals dissociate into ions when they are dissolved. These chemicals are called electrolytes. For good health, these chemicals must be in balance. In other words, each fluid compartment must have a certain concentration of a given electrolyte. (para 2-6)

5.   Water has several important physical characteristics: First, it is a fluid; therefore, it has the capacity of flow. Second, it is able to dissolve many substances within itself; thus, it is an excellent vehicle. Because of its heat-carrying capacity and its ability to remove large numbers of calories during evaporation, water is very useful in controlling the body's temperature. (para 2-7a)

6.   The human body obtains water in two primary ways: First, water is the major component of items we drink or eat. Second, as food substances are oxidized within individual cells, water is one of the main by-products. (para 2-7b)

7.   Water is lost from the body during perspiration, respiration, urination, vomiting, and diarrhea. (para 2-7c)

8.   Substances dissolved in the water of the body include gases, nutrients, wastes, and hormones. (para 2-8)

9.   Interstitial fluid originates primarily as the blood's fluid portion that escapes into the tissues from the capillaries. Part of this fluid enters the beginning of the venous vessels. A large portion is picked up by the lymphatic system. (para 2-9)

10.   The body's tendency to maintain a steady state is called homeostasis. As a part of this, the body maintains appropriate concentrations of oxygen, carbon dioxide, nutrients, electrolytes, and other substances within the tissue fluid. A system that helps to maintain the appropriate concentrations of oxygen and carbon dioxide is the respiratory system. A system that helps to maintain the appropriate concentration of nutrients is the digestive system. Such organ systems are at least partially controlled by feedback mechanisms. These mechanisms resemble the household thermostat. (para 2-10)

11.   The body needs a certain amount of water to function properly. Lack of fluid may result in heart failure. Too much fluid tends to result in swelling, known as edema. To maintain water balance, there are feedback mechanisms. (para 2-11)

12.   If the concentration of electrolytes is greater in the tissue fluid than in the intracellular fluid, the tissue fluid is hypertonic. If the concentrations of electrolytes is less in the tissue fluid than in the intracellular fluid, the tissue fluid is hypotonic. If the concentration of electrolytes are equal in the tissue fluid and intracellular fluid, the fluids are isotonic. (para 2-12)

13.   Assume that a substance is more concentrated on one side of a membrane than the other but that it cannot pass through the membrane. The process in which water passes to the side of greater concentration is called osmosis.

    If, however, the substance can easily pass through the membrane, the process in which the substance passes through the membrane to the area where it is less concentrated is called diffusion. If the substance needs assistance to pass through the membrane, we call the process facilitated diffusion.

    Since the cell membrane allows only some types of substances to pass through it, the cell membrane is semipermeable.

    When energy is used to move a substance across a membrane to an area of higher concentration, the process is called active transport.

    When a minute amount of tissue fluids is engulfed by the cell membrane, the process is pinocytosis. When larger particles are engulfed, the process is phagocytosis. (para 2-13)

14.   When the cell is in a resting state, the membrane potential is maintained by the sodium/potassium pump. This membrane potential is called the resting potential. The sodium/potassium pump actively transports three positive sodium ions to the outside of the cell membrane and two potassium ions to the inside of the cell membrane. This results in a negative charge inside the cell and a positive charge outside the cell.

When a neuron or muscle fiber is stimulated, the resulting activity is called the action potential. This involves depolarization and subsequent repolarization. First, sodium ions move into the cell by diffusion. This reverses the polarity. Second, potassium moves out of the cell by diffusion that causes repolarization. (para 2-14)

15.   A condition in which tissue mass increases without an increase in the number of cells is called hypertrophy. When tissue mass increases due to an increase in the number of cells, it is hyperplasia. Another word for cell multiplication is mitosis. (paras 2-15 and 2-16)

16.   The epithelial tissue lining a serous cavity secretes a serous fluid to act as a lubricant. The secretion of sebaceous glands is formed as portions of the cells are sloughed off. (paras 2-20, 2-22)

17.   In FCT, the fibroblast moves up and down the fiber. During this movement, it keeps the fiber in repair and restructures it in response to the stresses applied to the body. The collagen fibers are limited in stretchability, particularly when compared to the elastic fibers. As a collagen fiber lengthens, the tension increases considerably. As an FCT becomes warmer, it becomes more stretchable and more resistant to damage; this is the basis of warm-up exercises before more strenuous activities. (paras 2-23 thru 2-27)

18.   Fats, oils, and fatty acids are types of lipids. Such substances are stored mostly as neutral fat, which consists of triglycerides. A molecule of triglyceride is formed from a glycerol and three fatty acids. Within the body, triglycerides are kept in a liquid state by adjusting the length of each fatty acid. Within a 3-week period, there is a complete turnover of the triglycerides. Fats may be taken in as fats or converted from other substances, such as carbohydrates. When the diet contains more fats and carbohydrates than necessary for body activities, the result may be obesity. (paras 2-29 thru 2-33)

End of Lesson 2

LESSON ASSIGNMENT

LESSON 3   Envelopes of the Body.

LESSON ASSIGNMENT Paragraphs 3-1 through 3-42.

LESSON OBJECTIVES After completing this lesson, you should be able to
identify the functions of the envelopes of the body.

SUGGESTION   After completing the assignment, complete the
exercises at the end of this lesson. These exercises
will help you to achieve the lesson objectives.

LESSON 3

ENVELOPES OF THE BODY

Section I. INTRODUCTION

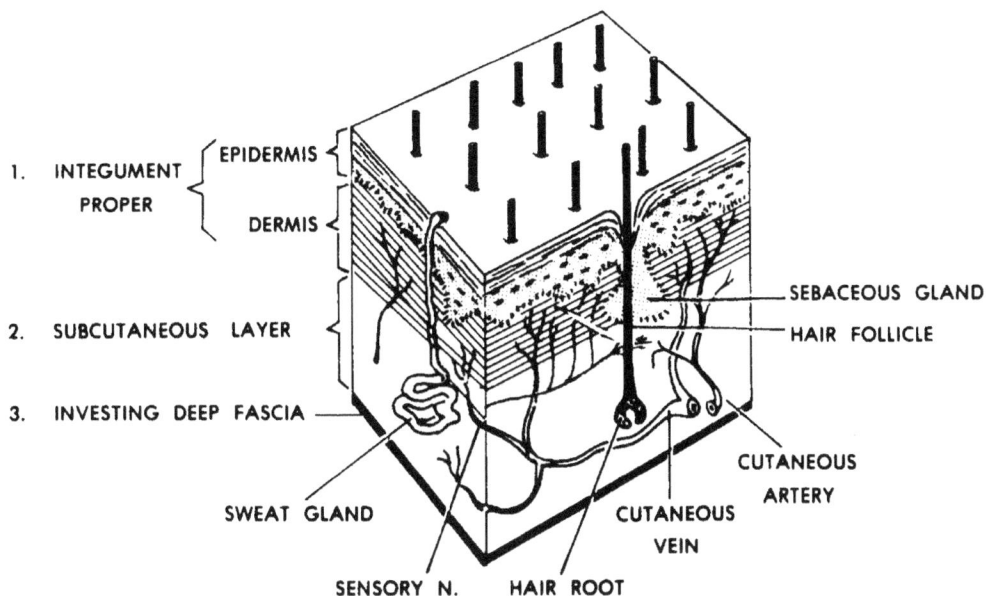

Figure 3-1. The integument and related structures.

3-1. INTRODUCTION

The envelopes of the body serve to protect the living structures within the body in a number of ways. The envelopes are like an air conditioner; they help to remove heat. The envelopes are like a blanket; they help to retain heat when the surrounding air is cold. One of the envelopes, the skin, is like a chemical factory; it manufactures vitamin D in the presence of sunlight. The skin is like an umbrella; it helps to protect us from the sun and the rain. The skin also protects the body from dehydration and friction.

3-2. ENVELOPES OF THE BODY

a. The human body has three concentric coverings (Figure 3-1), one inside of the other. The outermost layer is the integument proper (skin). Immediately beneath the skin is the subcutaneous layer. Beneath this layer is the investing deep fascia, a membrane which completely covers the remaining structures of the body.

b. These three concentric layers form complete envelopes around the body, except for the various openings.

3-3. THE INTEGUMENTARY SYSTEM

An organ system is a group of organs performing a common overall function. The outermost covering of the body is the integument proper, the largest single organ of the body. A number of structures are formed or derived from the various layers of the integument proper. These structures are known as the integumentary derivatives, sometimes referred to as "appendages." Together, the integument proper and the integumentary derivatives make up the integumentary system.

Section II. INTEGUMENT PROPER

3-4. INTRODUCTION

The integument proper has two major parts--the dermis and the epidermis. The dermis (or corium) is made up of rather dense FCT, forming a continuous layer around the body. On top of the dermis is the epidermis. The epidermis and dermis are interlocked by extensions of the dermis up into the epidermis. These extensions are known as papillae.

3-5. LAYERS OF EPIDERMIS

The epidermis is a stratified squamous epithelial tissue. This means that it has several layers of epithelial cells and that its outermost layer is made up of squamous (flat) epithelial cells.

a. **Mitotic Activity.** The layer adjacent to the dermis is known as the basal layer. The basal layer is made up of columnar epithelial cells. Since all of the mitotic (cell-multiplying) activity of the epidermis occurs in the basal layer, the basal layer is often called the germinative layer. This mitotic activity involves about 4 percent of the cells in the basal layer at any given time. It occurs primarily between midnight and 0400 hours.

b. **Migration of Cells to the Surface.** Over a period of weeks, new cells gradually migrate from the basal layer to the surface. During this migration to the surface, the cells change in shape from the original columnar to cuboidal and then finally to squamous. As the cells become squamous in form, they also become hardened, or cornified, through the development of a special type of protein. As they approach the surface, they die. Thus, the outermost layers of the epidermis are dead, horny scales.

3-6. SPLIT LINES

There are specific lines of tension or stress that varies from one area of the body to the next. The dense FCT of the dermis tends to be oriented along these lines. If a blunt probe is inserted into the dermis, the FCT fibers will separate to form a split. The lines of splits, or split lines, follow the lines of tension in the local area.

3-7. DERMATOGLYPHICS

The surfaces of the palms, soles, and digital pads of the hands and feet are thrown up into ridges and grooves. The patterns formed by these ridges and grooves are called dermatoglyphics. These dermatoglyphics are used as a means of identification, both by law enforcement agencies and by hospitals for newborns. We often refer to such procedures as fingerprinting or foot-printing.

3-8. CREASES

The body is jointed to allow motion. To facilitate motion of the joints, the skin develops natural creases. These creases are in relationship to the joints, but not exactly opposite to the joints.

3-9. THICKNESS

As the continuous covering of the body, the integument proper, or skin, is everywhere. However, the actual thickness of the dermis and/or epidermis varies considerably from very thin to very thick. For example, the thickest skin is located across the back between the shoulders.

3-10. PIGMENTATION

The integument proper of humans has some type of coloration (pigmentation). This coloration is because the presence of special chemicals called pigments. Black, red, and yellow are the most common colors of these pigments.

a. **Development**. Special cells are located in the dermis, just below the basal layer of the epidermis. These special cells provide the precursors of the pigments to the basal cells. As these basal cells migrate to the surface, the precursor materials are gradually converted into the actual pigments or colors.

b. **Genetic Control**. Genes control the type of color for each individual. There are various genes (sometimes multiple genes) for each color.

(1) When these genes are absent, the individual is an albino. There is a pink glow to the skin and eyes that is produced by the red color of the blood shining through the clear layers of the skin. There is also a whiteness of the skin produced by the refraction of light rays.

(2) Sometimes, the skin color varies for reasons other than genetic.

(3) Not only is the color of the integument determined by genes, the pattern of distribution of the color is determined by other genes.

Section III. INTEGUMENTARY DERIVATIVES

3-11. INTRODUCTION

A number of structures are derived from the layers of the integument proper. These structures are referred to as the integumentary derivatives or "appendages."

3-12. HAIRS

More or less covering the body are derivatives called hairs. The hairs of the body vary in construction from area to area. An individual's genes determine the specific construction, growth, and pattern of hairs for that individual. Sex hormones more or less control the distribution of hairs (sexual dimorphism). Also, in different cultures of human beings, different patterns of hair growth have arisen because of cultural selection.

3-13. NAILS

Another integumentary derivative is the nails. A nail covers the dorsal aspect of the end of each digit (fingers and toes).

3-14. GLANDS

The various glands are another kind of integumentary derivative.

a. **Sweat Glands**. There are at least two types of sweat (sudoriferous) glands:

(1) The general type throughout the body. This type produces a sensible and insensible perspiration. (See paragraph 2-7c(1).)

(2) A second type found in special areas. This type is found especially in the palms of the hands. Such sweat glands respond to emotional stresses to produce the "clammy" hands of the frightened individual.

b. **Sebaceous Glands**. Oil-producing (sebaceous) glands are usually found in relationship to the hair follicles. The oily product of these glands keeps the following structures flexible:

(1) The outer layers of the skin.

(2) The shafts of the hairs.

c. **True Scent Glands.** A third type of gland associated with the integument is the true scent gland. At least in older days, the product of these glands was supposed to be attractive to the opposite sex. (Here, we are not referring to the body odor known as BO. BO is a metabolic by-product produced by microorganisms located on the skin. These microorganisms act upon residue from perspiration, left after the water has evaporated.)

Section IV. FUNCTIONS OF THE INTEGUMENTARY SYSTEM

3-15. INTRODUCTION

The integumentary system forms the outermost covering of the human body. Thus, it is the boundary between the organism and the ambient (surrounding) environment. Because of this relationship, the integumentary system has a number of functions related to the environment and the individual's reactions to the environment.

3-16. REDUCTION OF FRICTION AND ITS EFFECTS

Over time, the body is likely to rub against many varied objects. The resulting frictional forces would be expected to damage the body surface. For comparison, consider the outer surfaces of older automobiles and other man-made objects.

a. **Hairs**. Hairs minimize friction by allowing surfaces to slip or slide over each other.

b. **Outer Dead Cells**. Where there is no hair (glabrous condition), the outer dead squamous cells rub off to reduce frictional forces. Within a couple of weeks after they arrive at the surface, the outer dead cells are removed during the activities of daily life.

c. **Thickening of the Integument**. The dermis and epidermis tend to become thicker whenever they are subjected to forces of pressures greater than average. Callouses are an extreme example of this.

3-17. WATERPROOFING

The outer layers of dead horny cells are kept flexible by oil from the sebaceous glands. Thus, these layers form an essentially waterproof covering for the body. This is very important in preventing general dehydration of the body. Dehydration (water loss) is a very important problem in burn patients who have lost a full thickness of the integument.

3-18. PROTECTION FROM SOLAR RADIATION

The integument also protects the body from excessive penetration of solar radiation. Solar radiation is blocked by pigments (para 3-10) and by the layers of dead **horny cells.**

3-19. GENERAL SENSIBILITY

Not the least of the functions of the integument is its general sensibility. As the interface between the organism and the immediate environment, the integument is subjected to many stimuli. A number of general sensory receptor organs are located in the integument and the underlying subcutaneous layer. These receptor organs continuously inform the brain of the conditions immediately surrounding the body. These conditions include pain, temperature, light and heavy pressures, touch, and so forth.

Section V. SUBCUTANEOUS LAYER

3-20. INTRODUCTION

Between the integument proper and the investing deep fascia is the middle layer called the subcutaneous layer.

SUB = under

CUTANEOUS = skin

In general, the subcutaneous layer is made up primarily of loose areolar FCT and fat. The fat tends to be localized in special areas that are different in the two sexes. (In affluent societies, there may be general obesity rather than localized fat.)

3-21. CUTANEOUS NAVL

Also found in the subcutaneous layer are the cutaneous NAVL (nerves, arteries, veins, lymphatics). In addition, some of the sensory receptors of the nervous system actually extend from the subcutaneous layer up into the papillae of the dermis, immediately below the epidermis.

a. **Cutaneous Capillaries**. The cutaneous capillaries of the subcutaneous layer tend to be localized at two levels. First, there is a superficial layer near the underside of the dermis. Second, there is a deeper layer near the investing deep fascia. These two layers of capillaries are more or less separated by the fatty tissue in the subcutaneous layer.

b. **Sensory Innervations**. If one looks at a zebra or a tiger, one can immediately see that the fur of these animals has a belt-like color pattern. There is also a belt-like pattern in the integument of humans. It is not a pattern of colors, as with zebras and tigers. It is a pattern of sensory innervations. A "belt" is innervated by a specific spinal nerve, left and right. This belt-like area is called a <u>dermatome</u>. We refer to the nerves supplying these areas as <u>segmental nerves</u> because they "segment" the integument into dermatomes. Except for the three dermatomes of the face, there is an overlap of adjacent dermatomes.

3-22. INTEGUMENTARY MUSCLES

Also associated with the subcutaneous layer are a number of integumentary muscles.

a. **Facial Muscles**. As the term implies, facial muscles are associated with the face. Facial muscles are mainly involved with the various openings of the face. They are able to open and close these openings. Because they are also used in visual communication, they are sometimes called <u>mimetic muscles</u> ("muscles of expression").

b. **Arrector Pili Muscles**. Another group of integumentary muscles is known as the arrector pili muscles. Ordinarily, the hairs and the hair follicles are at an angle to the skin rather than perpendicular (straight up or down). At times of emotional stress, the arrector pili muscles contract. In hairy areas, the contraction of these muscles, attached to the follicles, causes the hairs to stand "straight up." In glabrous areas, their contraction produces "goose bumps."

Section VI. INVESTING DEEP FASCIA

3-23. INTRODUCTION

The innermost of these three concentric layers is the investing deep fascia. The investing deep fascia is essentially a membrane of dense FCT completely surrounding the body. It overlies all of the remaining structures of the body.

3-24. VARIATIONS IN THICKNESS

a. The investing deep fascia varies in thickness in various parts of the body. This membrane is generally thicker the further inferior we go. In many areas, it is thick enough to be specifically named. For example, the investing deep fascia of the lower member is called the <u>fascia lata</u>.

b. The majority of the tissues of the body are made up primarily of water. Moreover, the interstitial spaces are filled with water. Therefore, the body within the investing deep fascia can be thought of as a hydrostatic column. As such, hydrostatic pressures become greater as one goes inferiorly in the body. Accordingly, the fascia becomes thicker to withstand the increasing pressures.

3-25. INTERMUSCULAR SEPTA

a. In the limbs of the upper and lower members, dense FCT membranes extend from the underside of the investing deep fascia to the bones. The membranes are known as the intermuscular septa. They divide the space within the investing deep fascia into discrete muscular compartments.

b. Each muscular compartment is a hydrostatic chamber. In a normal healthy human being, each compartment is full. Therefore, as arterial blood flows into a compartment, hydrostatic pressures are created which assist the flow of blood in the venous vessels back to the heart.

Section VII. BODY TEMPERATURE CONTROL

3-26. INTRODUCTION

In order to function properly, the human body must be maintained within a relatively narrow range of temperature.

3-27. SOURCES OF BODY HEAT

Body heat is derived from several sources.

a. **Muscle Contractions**. Muscle contractions produce a significant amount of heat. If muscles were very efficient, they would produce energy in the form of contractions and very little heat. Since muscles are inefficient, they produce much heat as they contract. For example, during strenuous physical exercise, the body temperature tends to rise by several degrees.

b. **Metabolic Activity.** Another source of heat in the body is certain organs such as the brain, liver, and so forth. These organs produce heat during their metabolic activity.

c. **Solar Radiation**. Another source of body heat is solar radiation. When received in excess, solar radiation can cause sunstroke.

3-28. TYPES OF BODY TEMPERATURE

a. **Core Temperature**. The core temperature is the temperature within the body proper. Normally, the core temperature is maintained within narrow limits. The core temperature of the blood is continuously monitored by special temperature detectors. These detectors are located in the hypothalamus of the brain.

b. **Peripheral Body Temperature.** The temperature of the body surface and the upper and lower members is called the peripheral body temperature. Peripheral body temperature can vary widely. Temperature receptors in the body periphery monitor the peripheral body temperature.

3-29. COUNTERCURRENT MECHANISM

In the limbs of the upper and lower members, the venous blood often has a low temperature. The return of this non-warmed blood to the core of the body might be dangerous. However, within the upper and lower members, the deep veins are generally located adjacent to the major arteries. As the venous blood flows toward the center of the body, it is gradually warmed by the arterial blood coming from the body. This condition is called the countercurrent mechanism.

3-30. REMOVAL OF HEAT

By selecting shady or cool surroundings, an individual can avoid becoming overheated. In other cases, however, the body heat may become excessive. In such cases, if the body is to remain healthy, the surplus body heat must be removed.

a. **Sweating.** Sweat (perspiration) is made up primarily of water, with various substances dissolved in it. As one of its physical characteristics, water has a relatively high heat-carrying capacity. In addition, it evaporates from the surface of the body. Another physical characteristic of water is that it removes large numbers of calories during evaporation.

b. **Radiation.** In addition, heat can be radiated directly from the surfaces of the body. This is particularly true of the surfaces of the axillae (armpit areas), the inside of the elbow areas, and the groin. These are areas where the skin tends to be thinner than average.

3-31. CONSERVATION OF HEAT

When the ambient (surrounding) temperature is cool or cold, the body must conserve heat rather than remove it.

a. **Less Sweating.** An immediate means of conserving heat is to stop sweating. This prevents heat loss by evaporation.

b. **Less Radiation.**

(1) In cool surroundings, the superficial capillaries are shut down. Thus, circulation is limited to the deep cutaneous capillaries. Because of the insulating fatty

tissues of the subcutaneous layer, these deep cutaneous capillaries radiate much less heat to the surface.

(2) If the exposed surface area is reduced, there will be less loss of body heat. This can even serve as a lifesaving measure. For example, if an individual has been in cold water (as in a shipwreck or other accident), his body can be folded to reduce exposure.

c. **Shivering**. During shivering, muscles contract without synchronization. Although this produces minimal motion, it produces considerable heat.

d. **Proper Clothing**. Obviously, proper clothing is a measure for conserving body heat.

e. **External Heat Sources**. External heat sources are commonly used by humans to conserve body heat.

Section VIII. VITAMIN D PRODUCTION

3-32. INTRODUCTION

Vitamin D is a fat-soluble vitamin. It is required by the body in relation to calcium metabolism.

3-33. MECHANISM OF PRODUCTION

The human body produces vitamin D in the integument. An organic compound known as ergosterol is converted into vitamin D by ultraviolet solar radiation.

3-34. CONTROL OF PRODUCTION

Excessive production of vitamin D can become lethal to a human being. The main purpose of skin pigmentation seems to be the limitation of vitamin D production. In their "original" distribution, the peoples of the equatorial (sunny) areas tended to be dark skinned. The peoples of subarctic (unsunny) areas tended to be light skinned.

Section IX. SUPERFICIAL WOUND HEALING

3-35. INTRODUCTION

A wound of the integument creates an opening. This opening is an avenue for infection and water loss.

3-36. RELATIONSHIP WITH SPLIT LINES

A wound crossing the split lines of the dermis tends to gape open. A wound parallel to the split lines closes easily. For this reason, when a surgeon can choose an incision, he tends to follow the split lines.

3-37. HEALING

A wound is healed by the reuniting of the margins. This is accomplished by the growth and multiplication of the cells at the margins of the wound.

3-38. SCARRING

Scars result from the healing process. In some human groups (for example, Orientals), scars can become quite large and are called keloids. For all groups, the scar (cicatrix) is much less prominent for wounds that parallel the split lines.

Section X. GENERAL ADAPTATIONS FOR GRASPING/HOLDING

3-39. INTRODUCTION

The hands grasp or hold onto things. The soles of the feet provide a nonslipping contact with the ground. For these reasons, frictional forces are maximized in the palms of the hands and the soles of the feet. This is accomplished by several adaptations of the coverings of the body in these areas.

3-40. ADAPTATIONS

These adaptations are described below:

a. The epidermis and dermis are quite thickened in these areas.

b. These two areas are hairless (glabrous).

c. The dermal papillae holding the dermis and epidermis together are increased in number and size.

d. The surface of the skin has many ridges and grooves. These, in effect, form miniature suction cups.

e. Deep in the palm and sole, there is a very dense FCT, referred to as the palmar aponeurosis and plantar aponeurosis. A thickened subcutaneous layer firmly attaches the modified integument to the underlying aponeurosis.

Section XI. VARIATIONS IN PENETRATION

3-41. VARIATIONS IN INFANTS AND THE ELDERLY

In infants and the elderly, substances more readily penetrate the skin than with other age groups. One such substance is hexachlorophene. Hexachlorophene is an ingredient in some soaps and detergents used to maintain a germ-free environment in the hospital. If the skin of the infant or elderly person is not thoroughly rinsed after the use of such soaps or detergents, the skin of these individuals will readily absorb the residual hexachlorophene. This may produce neurological damage.

3-42. VARIATIONS ACCORDING TO BODY AREA

This condition may also exist in other age groups in those areas where the skin is thinnest. These areas include the inner surfaces of the flexing joints, axillae, and groin and particularly the areas between the fingers and toes.

Continue with Exercises

EXERCISES, LESSON 3

REQUIREMENT. The following exercises are to be answered by completing the incomplete statements.

After you have completed all the exercises, turn to "Solutions to Exercises," at the end of the lesson and check your answers.

1.   The envelopes of the body are like an air conditioner; they help to remove _____. The envelopes are like a blanket; they help to retain _____ when the surrounding air is _____ d. The skin is like a chemical factory; it manufactures v_____ __ in the presence of sunlight. The skin is like an umbrella; it helps to protect us from the s___ and the r____.

2.   The mitotic activity of the epidermis occurs in the ____l layer.   At any given time, about __ percent of the cells in this layer are involved in m_____s. As cells migrate to the surface, they change shape from _____r to _____l and finally to _____s. As the cells become squamous, they also become h_____d, or c_____d.

3.   The color of the skin is due to special chemicals called _____s. Special cells located in the dermis provide the p_____s of pigments to the basal cells. As basal cells migrate to the surface, the precursors are gradually converted to the actual p_____s. The type of color for each individual is controlled by_____s.

4.   The integumentary system is the boundary between the organism and the surrounding e_____t. For this reason, the integumentary system has a number of functions related to the _____t.

Friction against the integument is reduced by _____s and outer dead ____s. When subjected to friction, the integument tends to become _____er.

The outer layers of cells are kept flexible by ___l from the sebaceous glands. This forms an essentially w_____f covering for the body. This is important in preventing general d_____n of the body.

Because of pigments and outer layers of dead cells, the integument helps to protect the body from excessive _____r radiation.

Receptor organs in the integument and the subcutaneous layer continuously inform the _____n of conditions immediately surrounding the body.

5. Sources of body heat include m_____ contractions, m_____c activity, and _____r radiation.

The core temperature is the temperature within the b____ p____r. The core temperature is continuously monitored by detectors in the h_____s of the brain. The temperature of the body surface and the upper and lower members is called the p_____l body temperature.

Blood within the deep veins of the upper and lower members is warmed by the adjacent major _____s. This situation is called the c_____t mechanism.

Heat is removed from the body by s_____g and ra____n.

Means of conserving heat are decreased s_____g, shutting down of the superficial _____s, reduction of the exposed s_____ a____, and external h__t s_____s.

6. The main purpose of skin pigmentation seems to be the limitation of the production of _____ ___.

7. The opening of a wound is an avenue for i_____n and w____ loss. In healing, the cells at the margins of the wound ___w and _____y to reunite the margins.

Check Your Answers on Next Page

SOLUTIONS TO EXERCISES, LESSON 3

1.   The envelopes of the body are like an air conditioner; they help to remove heat. The envelopes are like a blanket; they help to retain heat when the surrounding air is cold. The skin is like a chemical factory; it manufactures vitamin D in the presence of sunlight. The skin is like an umbrella; it helps to protect us from the sun and the rain. (para 3-1)

2.   The mitotic activity of the epidermis occurs in the basal layer. At any given time, about 4 percent of the cells in this layer are involved in mitosis. As cells migrate to the surface, they change shape from columnar to cuboidal and finally to squamous. As the cells become squamous, they also become hardened, or cornified. (para 3-5)

3.   The color of the skin is because of special chemicals called pigments. Special cells located in the dermis provide the precursors of pigments to the basal cells. As basal cells migrate to the surface, the precursors are gradually converted to the actual pigments. The type of color for each individual is controlled by genes. (para 3-10)

4.   The integumentary system is the boundary between the organism and the surrounding environment. For this reason, the integumentary system has a number of functions related to the environment.

Friction against the integument is reduced by hairs and outer dead cells. When subjected to friction, the integument tends to become thicker.

The outer layers of cells are kept flexible by oil from the sebaceous glands. This forms an essentially waterproof covering for the body. This is important in preventing general dehydration of the body.

Because of pigments and outer layers of dead cells, the integument helps to protect the body from excessive solar radiation.

Receptor organs in the integument and the subcutaneous layer continuously inform the brain of conditions immediately surrounding the body. (paras 3-15 thru 3-19)

5.   Sources of body heat include muscular contractions, metabolic activity, and solar radiation.

The core temperature is the temperature within the body proper. The core temperature is continuously monitored by detectors in the hypothalamus of the brain. The temperature of the body surface and the upper and lower members is called the peripheral body temperature.

Blood within the deep veins of the upper and lower members is warmed by the adjacent major arteries. This situation is called the countercurrent mechanism.

Heat is removed from the body by sweating and radiation.

Means of conserving heat are decreased sweating, shutting down of the superficial capillaries, reduction of the exposed surface area, and external heat sources. (paras 3-27 thru 3-31)

6.   The main purpose of skin pigmentation seems to be the limitation of the production of vitamin D. (para 3-34)

7.   The opening of a wound is an avenue for infection and water loss. In healing, the cells at the margins of the wound grow and multiply to reunite the margins. (paras 3-35, 3-37)

End of Lesson 3

LESSON ASSIGNMENT

LESSON 4   The Skeletal System.

LESSON ASSIGNMENT   Paragraphs 4-1 through 4-40.

LESSON OBJECTIVES   After completing this lesson, you should be able to:

> 4-1.   Identify and describe functions of major skeletal components.

> 4-2.   Match important skeletal elements with their functions.

SUGGESTION   After completing the assignment, complete the exercises at the end of this lesson. These exercises will help you to achieve the lesson objectives.

LESSON 4

THE SKELETAL SYSTEM

Section I. GENERAL

4-1. INTRODUCTION

The skeleton forms the framework for the human body. It is composed of individual bones. These bones meet (are articulated with) each other at joints.

4-2. GENERAL FUNCTIONS

a. **Support.** In general, the skeleton supports the body.

b. **Motion and Locomotion.** Because of the joints and the attached skeletal muscles, the parts of the body can move with respect to each other (motion). Also, because of such linkages in the lower members, the entire body can be moved from place to place (locomotion).

c. **Protection.** Certain parts of the skeleton are structured to protect vital organs.

d. **Hematopoiesis.** The skeleton is also involved in formation of blood (hematopoiesis) cells.

e. **Storage.** Moreover, the skeleton stores various minerals.

Section II. TISSUES AND TISSUE PROCESSES OF SKELETAL ELEMENTS

4-3. CONNECTIVE TISSUES

The skeletal elements are made up of several types of connective tissues. In general, connective tissues tend to connect and/or support. These tissues are characterized by an extracellular material referred to as the matrix.

a. In the formation of the individual organs known as the bones, bone tissues make up the main portion of each bone, on an FCT framework.

b. Certain bone surfaces are covered with cartilage connective tissue.

4-4. PIEZOELECTRIC EFFECT

a. Each bone is built around an FCT framework on which the apatite crystals are deposited in a regular order. Apatite is a mineral, a form of calcium phosphate. (Another mineral found in bones is calcium carbonate.)

b. When compressed, the apatite crystals produce a local electric current. This phenomenon is known as the piezoelectric effect.

c. Presumably, this piezoelectric effect is produced in the bones of the lower limb during walking. We know that tissues respond to local electric current. When walking casts are used, fractured lower members tend to heal much more rapidly than when the patient is bedridden. Bones tend to lose mass when they are not subjected to forces as great as ordinary.

4-5. BUILDING UP, TEARING DOWN, AND REBUILDING OF BONE TISSUE

a. The living cells of the bones are osteocytes. When these cells are building up bone tissue, they are called osteoblasts. When they are tearing down bone tissue, they are called osteoclasts.

b. This building up, tearing down, and rebuilding are continuous processes throughout the life of the individual human being. The building and rebuilding respond specifically to the directions of force applied to the body at that particular time. Therefore, throughout the life of the individual, the skeleton can be remodeled and changed continuously in reaction to applied forces.

Section III. DEFINITION AND TYPES OF BONES

4-6. DEFINITION

Bones are those individual organs that are elements of the skeletal system.

4-7. TYPES

The individual bones of the skeleton can be categorized into three major groups according to their general shapes:

a. Long.

b. Flat.

c. Irregular.

Section IV. A "TYPICAL" LONG BONE

4-8. GENERAL STRUCTURE

A "typical" <u>long bone</u>, as the name implies, has more length than width. (See Figure 4-1.)

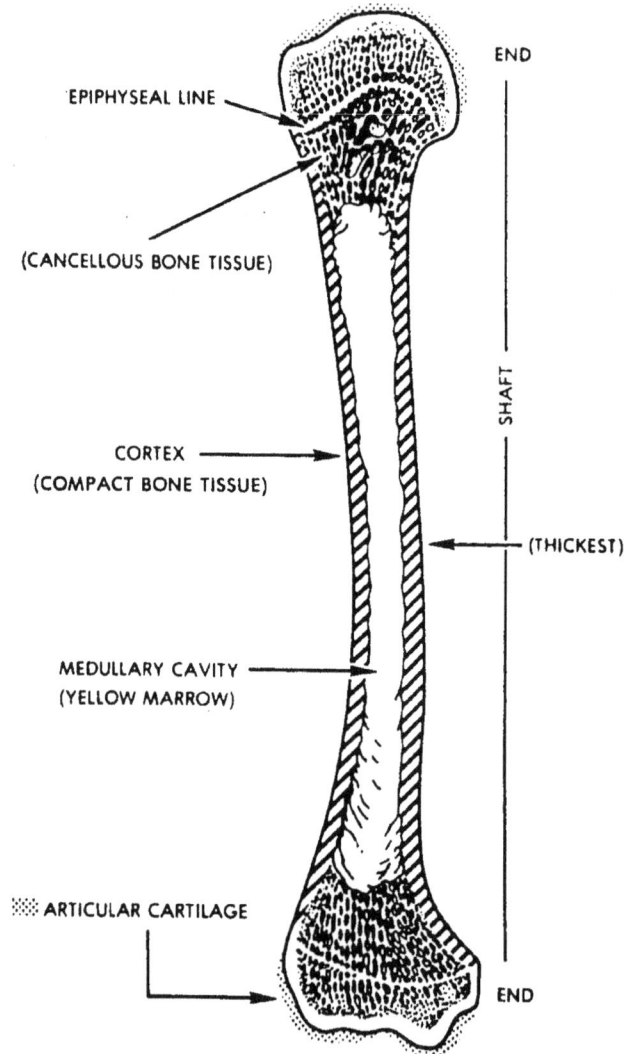

EPIPHYSEAL LINE

END

(CANCELLOUS BONE TISSUE)

CORTEX
(COMPACT BONE TISSUE)

SHAFT

(THICKEST)

MEDULLARY CAVITY
(YELLOW MARROW)

ARTICULAR CARTILAGE

END

Figure 4-1. "Typical" long bone section.

a. **Shaft (Diaphysis).** In effect, the long bone has a shaft, with proximal and distal ends. The shaft tends to be cylindrical in form.

(1) It has a cortex (outer portion) of dense bony tissue called compact bone tissue. The cortex is usually thickest at the middle of the shaft.

(2) The inside of the shaft is usually hollow, except that it is filled with yellow marrow (in adults, but red marrow in small children and infants).

b. **Ends (Epiphyses).** At the ends of the long bone, the cortex is much thinner. Each end is filled with a lattice-or sponge-like network of bony tissue, called cancellous bony tissue. The strands of bone forming this lattice are called trabeculae. The trabeculae are aligned with the lines of applied forces, particularly tension and compression. The spaces within the cancellous bony tissue are filled with red marrow.

c. **Some Special Parts.** The skeletal muscles pull and create tensions at their attachments to the bone. These tensions will often cause the bone to react and form spines, tubercles, ridges, and the like.

d. **Articular Cartilages.** The surface of each end of the bone is covered by an articular cartilage. This cartilage is located where the bone contacts another bone at a joint. The cartilage is made up of hyaline-type cartilage tissue. The articular cartilage makes the movement between the bones smoother.

e. **Periosteum.** The periosteum surrounds the bone, except where the articular cartilages are located. The periosteum is an envelope of the bone and consists mainly of dense FCT. In fact, the periosteum may be considered the outermost portion of the bone.

(1) However, the periosteum has a special layer of cells immediately adjacent to the surface of the bone. Since this layer is able to produce bone material, it is called the osteogenic layer of the periosteum.

(2) When a long bone is fractured or a portion of the bone is lost without losing the periosteum, the fracture is healed by the combined action of the osteogenic layer of the periosteum and the osteoblasts of the bone itself.

f. **NAVL.** Associated with the periosteum are the "service tissues." These are the NAVL (nerves, arteries, veins, and lymphatics), which nourish and stimulate the living tissues of the bone and periosteum.

(1) Neurovascular bundle. Branches from the main NAVL of the body go as a unit to the bone. This unit, the neurovascular bundle, consists of NAVL within a common fibrous connective sheath.

(2) <u>Branches of neurovascular bundle</u>. Portions of these NAVL spread out through the periosteum as periosteal branches over the outer surfaces of the bone. Other branches penetrate through the cortex of the bone to spread out through the medullary (or marrow) cavity. The holes through the cortex are known as the <u>nutrient canals</u>. The branches are known as the <u>nutrient branches</u>.

4-9. ORIGIN AND DEVELOPMENT

a. A long bone begins in the fetus as a hyaline cartilage model of the bone.

b. At the appropriate time, the cartilage model is invaded by a mass of material that begins to destroy the cartilage and replace it with bone tissue. This invading mass and the subsequently developed bone structure are called the <u>primary center of ossification</u>, or <u>diaphysis</u>.

c. At about the time of birth or thereafter, a <u>secondary center of ossification</u>, or <u>epiphysis</u>, develops at each end of the developing long bone.

d. A plate of cartilage, called the <u>epiphyseal plate</u>, remains between the diaphysis and each epiphysis. In the early years of life, the cartilage grows faster than the diaphysis can tear it down. This results in gradual lengthening of the long bone.

e. At the proper time, between puberty and adulthood, the bone development overtakes completely destroys the cartilage. After this, the diaphysis and the epiphysis are solidly fused to one another. The dense bony line of fusion between the diaphysis and epiphysis is called the <u>epiphyseal line</u>. The epiphyseal line is easily visible in the radiographs ("x-rays") of young adults.

f. While the bone has been growing in length, it also grows in width. The osteogenic layer of the periosteum gradually adds bony tissue to the outside surface of the bone. At the same time, osteoclastic activity removes bone material from the wall of the marrow cavity.

g. Many factors are involved in the process of bone growth. One of the primary factors is a hormone of the anterior pituitary gland known as <u>somatotropin</u>. Overproduction of somatotropin in a young person (before fusion of the ossification centers) results in <u>gigantism</u>. Overproduction of somatotropin in adults (after fusion of the ossification centers) results in a condition called <u>acromegaly</u>. Acromegaly involves excessive growth of the jaw, hands, and feet.

h. Throughout the entire life of the individual, the continuous tearing down (osteoclastic activity) and rebuilding (osteoblastic activity) remodel the bony substance. These processes occur in response to the forces or stresses applied to the body.

Section V. A "TYPICAL" FLAT BONE

4-10. GENERAL STRUCTURE

Another category of bones consists of the flat bones. (See Figure 4-2.)

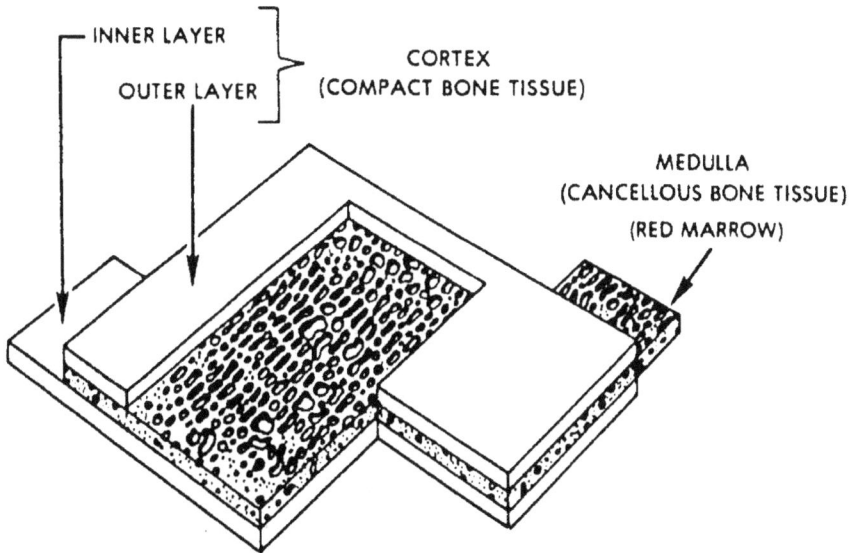

Figure 4-2. "Typical" flat bone section.

    a. The flat bones have two layers of dense bony tissue, called <u>tables</u>. Thus, there is an <u>inner table</u> and an <u>outer table</u>.

    b. Generally, between the two tables is a layer of cancellous bony tissue.

    (1) The spaces of this cancellous bony tissue are filled with red marrow. In adults, the red marrow of the flat bones is the primary blood-cell forming area of the body.

    (2) As with the cancellous tissue of the long bone, the cancellous tissue of the flat bone is organized into <u>trabeculae</u>. The trabeculae are oriented in the same directions as the lines of applied forces, much like the struts of a building.

    (3) Adjacent to the nasal cavities, many flat bones are hollowed to form the paranasal sinuses. These hollow spaces take the place of cancellous bony tissue. The development of the mastoid bone is likewise formed by the extension of the air-filled cavity of the middle ear into the mastoid bone.

c. The outer surface of the outer table and the under surface of the inner table are covered with periosteum. The periosteum is similar to that described for the "typical" long bone.

d. At their margins, flat bones are articulated with other flat bones and held together by FCT. These fibrous connections are usually called sutures.

4-11. ORIGIN AND DEVELOPMENT

Flat bones generally begin as membranous, FCT models within the fetus. Again, an invasion of material forms an ossification center. This center tears down and replaces the FCT with bone tissue. The ossification center continues to grow outward. In time, a full plate of bone has been formed. Then, the flat bone grows at its margins until adulthood.

4-12. SPECIAL CONDITIONS OF THE FLAT BONES OF THE CRANIUM

The flat bones of the skull are somewhat special.

a. **Curved Shape.** They are generally curved. Together, they form a sphere which surrounds and protects the brain.

b. **Healing of Fractures.** When the growth of the cranial flat bones is complete, the osteogenic layer of the periosteum disappears.

(1) Cracks and/or line fractures of cranial flat bones will usually heal by the activity of the osteoblasts within the bone.

(2) However, when bone substance is lost and a spatial defect ("hole") remains, the missing portions of the table(s) will not be replaced. Osteoblastic activity will repair only the margins of the spatial defect ("hole").

c. **Variations in Brain Injury.**

(1) In a young individual, the flat bones of the skull are not yet fully developed. The cranium as a whole is relatively flexible. An injury to the brain, resulting from a force applied to the cranium, will usually be located immediately below the location of the applied force.

(2) In an older adult, the flat bones of the skull have fully developed and are more or less fused to each other. The cranium is a relatively solid sphere. An injury to the brain, resulting from a force applied to the cranium, will usually be found on the opposite side from the applied force. Often, the applied force will be diverted around the sphere to the base of the cranium. There, the diverted force may cause fractures of the cranium at the apertures (openings) in its base.

Section VI. SESAMOID BONES

4-13. GENERAL

The sesamoid bones are another kind of bone. Sesamoid bones develop in place within tendons of skeletal muscles where the tendons sustain excessive pressures. Since the sesamoid bone absorbs these pressures, it protects the tendon from wear and tear.

4-14. EXAMPLE-PATELLA

The primary example of sesamoid bones is the patella (kneecap). In the form of a simple pulley mechanism, the tendon of the quadriceps femoris muscle passes over the distal end of the femur. Located at this point within the tendon is the patella.

Section VII. DEFINITION AND TYPES OF JOINTS

4-15. INTRODUCTION

a. Where two bones meet each other, this junction is referred to as a joint or articulation.

b. The joints of the human skeleton may be characterized, in general, in three different ways.

4-16. MATERIAL HOLDING JOINT TOGETHER

First, they are characterized by the type of material that holds the bones together at the joint.

a. If the bones are fused together with bony tissue, the articulation is called a synosteosis.

b. Thus, in a synchondrosis, the bones are held together by cartilage tissue.

c. In a syndesmosis, the bones are held together by FCT.

NOTE: A synovial articulation is somewhat different and will be described in detail in the next section.

4-17. RELATIVE MOBILITY

A second way of categorizing joints of the human skeleton is according to relative mobility.

a. The junctions of some bones are nonmobile, such as a synosteosis.

b. Others are semimobile, as seen with some syndesmoses.

c. Being structured to facilitate motion, synovial articulations (see the next section) are mobile to various degrees.

4-18. DEGREES OF FREEDOM

The term degrees of freedom refers to the number of planes in which movement is permitted. This also equals the number of axes around which motion can take place at a particular joint.

a. **One Degree of Freedom.** One degree of freedom means that the joint is uniaxial. Motion can take place in a single plane around one axis only. An example is a "hinge" joint.

b. **Two Degrees of Freedom.** Two degrees of freedom mean that the joint is biaxial. Motion can take place around two different axes.

c. **Three Degrees of Freedom.** With three degrees of freedom, we say that the joint is multiaxial. Motion can take place around the three axes in all three planes. An example is "ball and socket" type joints.

Section VIII. A "TYPICAL" SYNOVIAL JOINT

4-19. INTRODUCTION

A synovial joint is structured to facilitate freedom of motion in one or more of the three planes around the three axes of any given joint. The "typical" synovial joint (Figure 4-3) is a schematic representation rather than an actual synovial joint, but it contains the structural features common to all synovial joints.

4-20. BONES

The synovial articulation is formed between two bones. These bones are parts of the skeleton. They are levers of motion. To them are attached skeletal muscles, which provide the forces for motion.

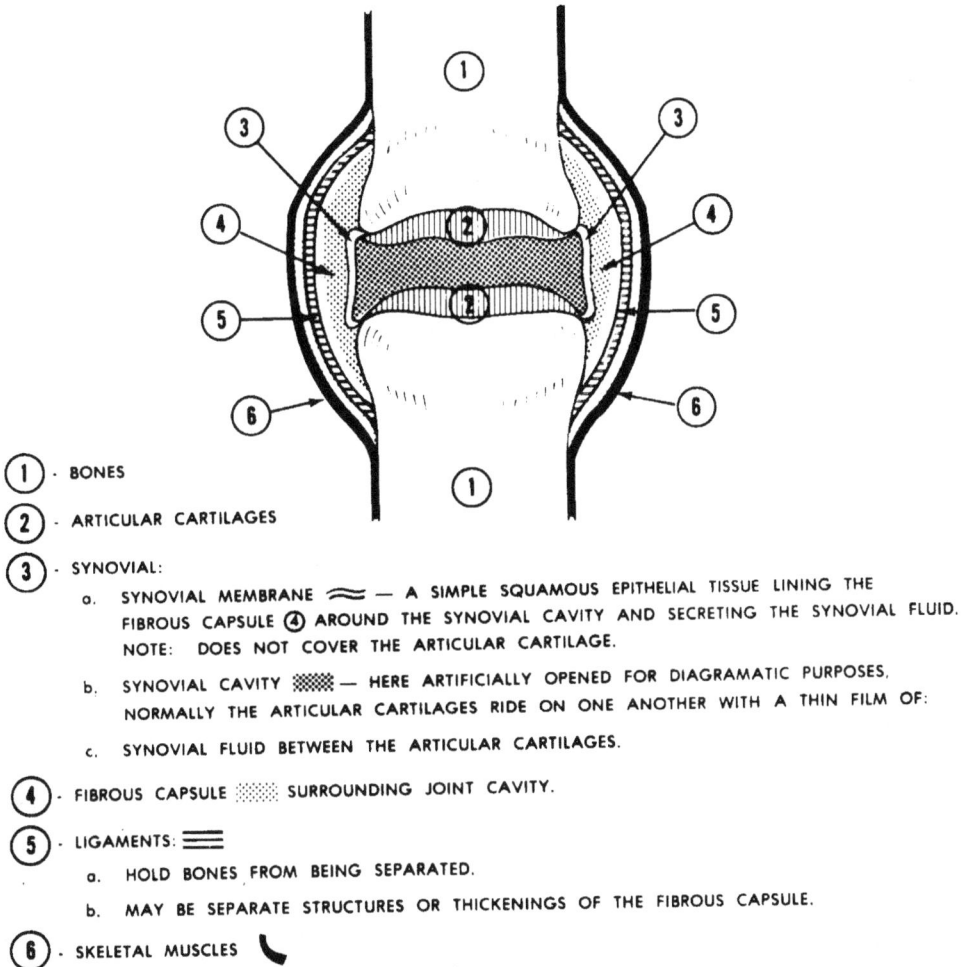

Figure 4-3. A "typical" synovial joint--diagrammatic.

Legend for Figure 4-3:

(1) - BONES

(2) - ARTICULAR CARTILAGES

(3) - SYNOVIAL:

  a. SYNOVIAL MEMBRANE ≈ — A SIMPLE SQUAMOUS EPITHELIAL TISSUE LINING THE FIBROUS CAPSULE (4) AROUND THE SYNOVIAL CAVITY AND SECRETING THE SYNOVIAL FLUID. NOTE: DOES NOT COVER THE ARTICULAR CARTILAGE.

  b. SYNOVIAL CAVITY ▓▓ — HERE ARTIFICIALLY OPENED FOR DIAGRAMATIC PURPOSES, NORMALLY THE ARTICULAR CARTILAGES RIDE ON ONE ANOTHER WITH A THIN FILM OF:

  c. SYNOVIAL FLUID BETWEEN THE ARTICULAR CARTILAGES.

(4) - FIBROUS CAPSULE ▒▒ SURROUNDING JOINT CAVITY.

(5) - LIGAMENTS: ≡

  a. HOLD BONES FROM BEING SEPARATED.

  b. MAY BE SEPARATE STRUCTURES OR THICKENINGS OF THE FIBROUS CAPSULE.

(6) - SKELETAL MUSCLES ↰

4-21. ARTICULAR CARTILAGES

Covering a portion of each bone is an articular cartilage. The portions covered are the ends that would otherwise be in contact during the motions of the joint. Each articular cartilage has a relatively smooth surface and some ability to act as a shock absorber.

4-22. JOINT CAPSULE

The joint area is surrounded by a dense FCT capsule that encloses the joint area.

4-23. SYNOVIAL MEMBRANE, FLUID, AND CAVITY

The inner surface of this fibrous capsule is lined with a synovial membrane. The synovial membrane secretes a synovial fluid into the synovial cavity, or joint space. The synovial fluid is a very good lubricant. Thus, it minimizes the frictional forces between the moving bones.

4-24. LIGAMENTS

The bones of the synovial joint are held together by ligaments. Ligaments are very dense FCT structures that keep the bones from being pulled apart. These ligaments may occur as either discrete, individual structures or as thickenings of the fibrous capsule.

4-25. SKELETAL MUSCLES

The skeletal muscles cross the synovial joint from one bone to the other. They are attached to the bones. The tonic (continuous) contraction of these skeletal muscles holds the opposing surfaces of the bones tightly together. When properly stimulated, these muscles contract and cause motion of the bones around the joint.

4-26. TYPES OF SYNOVIAL JOINTS

Synovial joints are often referred to by their geometric or mechanical structure.

a. **Ball-and-Socket Joint.** The ball-and-socket synovial joint has one bone with a rounded head, a "ball." The other bone has a corresponding cavity, the "socket." The ball-and-socket joint is usually multiaxial.

b. **Hinge Joint.** In the hinge joint, the geometry of the bony surfaces and the disposition of the ligaments are such as to allow the parts to fold on each other, around a single axis only.

c. **Others.** There are other special arrangements of the synovial joints to produce specific motions. An example: Rotation of the head at the pivot-type joint of atlas and axis (the upper two vertebrae).

Section IX. THE AXIAL SKELETON

4-27. INTRODUCTION TO THE HUMAN SKELETON

As a whole, the human skeleton (Figure 4-4) is the supporting framework of the body. The skeleton is composed of the individual bones and the articulations between them. The human skeleton is generally considered in two major subdivisions: the axial skeleton and the appendicular skeleton.

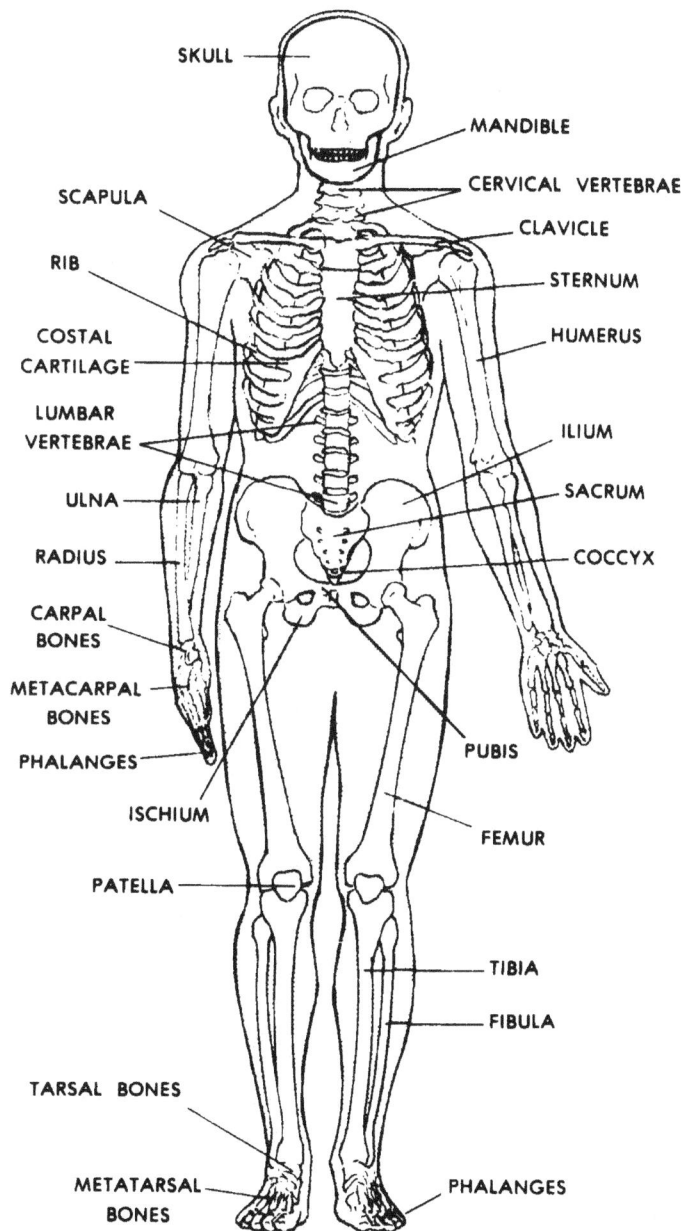

Figure 4-4. Anterior view of the human skeleton.

4-28. INTRODUCTION TO THE AXIAL SKELETON

The axial skeleton (Figure 4-5) is the central supporting framework of the body. Its major components are the vertebral column (spine), the thoracic cage, and the skull.

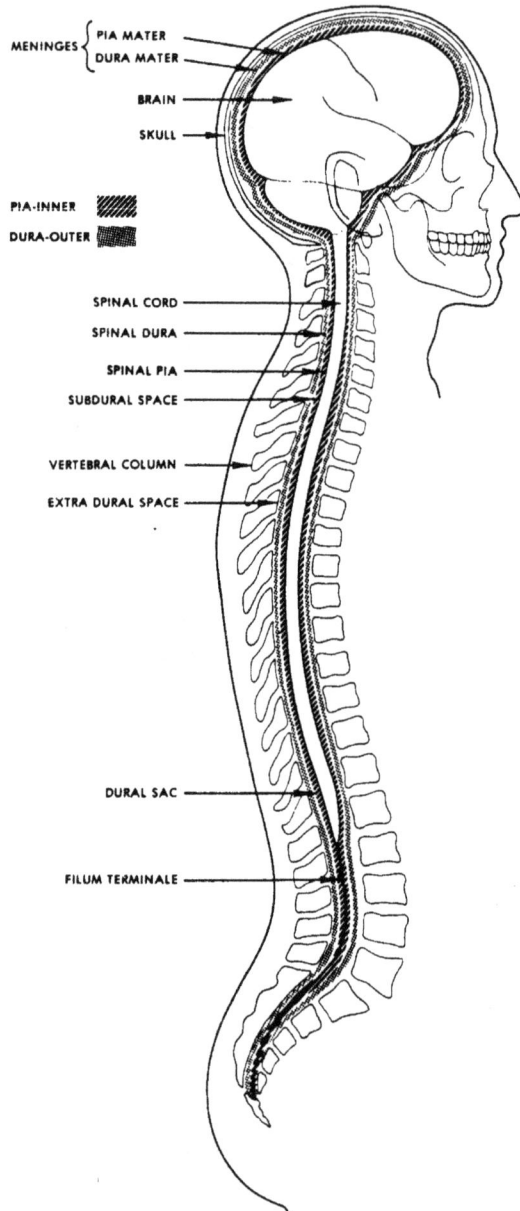

Figure 4-5. Midsagittal section of skull and vertebral column with CNS and meninges in place.

4-29. SKULL

The skull is the skeleton of the head region. It is located on the top of the vertical vertebral column. It has two major functional subdivisions: the cranium and the facial (visceral) skeleton.

a. **Cranium.** The cranium is a spherical container that protects the brain. At the base of the cranium is a series of openings. Blood vessels and nerves enter and leave the cranial cavity through these openings.

b. **Facial Skeleton.** The facial skeleton is also referred to as the visceral skull. It is attached to the anterior and inferior surfaces of the cranium. It is the skeleton of the entrances of the respiratory and digestive systems and the orbits containing the eyes.

4-30. NOTE ABOUT THE VERTEBRAL COLUMN

The vertebral column is a series of individual segments, the vertebrae, and one on top of the other.

4-31. MOTIONS OF THE HEAD

The upper part of the vertebral column, the neck region, and associated muscles provide the head with its various motions. The upper two vertebrae are specifically constructed for head motions.

a. The articulation between the occipital base of the skull and the atlas (the first cervical vertebra) is specially constructed for anterior-posterior motions of the head ("nodding").

b. Between the atlas (the first cervical vertebra) and the axis (the second cervical vertebra) is a special pivotal-type joint. This joint facilitates rotary (turning) motions of the head.

4-32. WEIGHT BEARING

a. The vertebral bodies and the associated intervertebral discs are the primary mechanism for supporting the body weight.

b. In the lumbar and lumbosacral regions, the articular processes of the vertebrae is also weight bearing. (A bony projection extends upward and another extends downward from each right and left side of the neural arch of each of these vertebrae.) These projections are the articular processes. Through them, as well as through the vertebral bodies and discs, adjacent vertebrae are articulated with each other.

c. The specially constructed sacrum, at the lower end of the vertebral column, receives the body weight from above and transfers it to the pelvic bones of the lower members.

4-33. PROTECTION OF THE SPINAL CORD AND ITS MEMBRANES

Whereas the cranium protects the brain, the neural arches protect the spinal cord and its membranes (meninges). The neural arches of the individual vertebrae arch over the spinal cord and its membranes. The continuous series of neural arches forms a continuous spinal canal.

4-34. MOTION OF THE VERTEBRAL COLUMN

Together, the vertebrae, the intervertebral discs, and the associated ligaments form a semiflexible rod. This allows a certain amount of motion to the vertebral column in addition to its supporting role.

a. **Role of Processes.** The spinous and transverse processes of the neural arches serve as attachments for skeletal muscles. By acting as levers, these processes enable the skeletal muscles to move the vertebrae.

b. **Role of Intervertebral Discs.** The intervertebral discs between adjacent vertebrae serve several functions.

(1) First, they allow motion to occur between adjacent vertebrae. The relative thickness of the individual intervertebral disc determines the amount of motion possible between the adjacent vertebrae. The total movement of the vertebral column (spine) is the sum of the motions of the individual intervertebral discs.

(2) Secondly, the intervertebral disc acts as a shock absorber. As such, it minimizes the shocks that are transmitted to the vertebral column by the contact of the heels with the floor during walking, jumping, etc.

(3) During the course of a day standing and sitting, the individual becomes about an inch shorter than he was at the beginning of the day. This is less true of older individuals. After a good night's rest in a horizontal position, these discs regain their original thickness. As an astronaut works at zero gravity, he retains his full height.

(4) With age, individuals tend to lose height. This is because the intervertebral discs shrink somewhat over the years. Since these discs also become less flexible, there is less compression from morning until night. Thus, the height in the evening is closer to the morning height than with a younger person.

c. **Role of Curvatures of Vertebral Column.** As a whole, the vertebral column has four curvatures. Two of these are concave to the front; two are concave to the rear. As do the intervertebral discs, these curvatures function as shock absorbers for the body.

4-35. FUNCTIONS OF THE RIB CAGE

The thoracic cage consists of the ribs, the sternum, and thoracic vertebrae. The 12 pairs of ribs are attached posteriorly to the thoracic vertebrae. Anteriorly, the upper 10 pairs of ribs attach directly or indirectly (via costal cartilages) to the sternum.

a. **Motion.** Because of the segmentation of the thoracic cage into vertebrae and ribs, motion can occur in the thoracic region of the body.

b. **Costal Breathing.** The special construction of the ribs and their costal cartilages allows costal breathing to take place.

c. **Protection.** In addition, the rib cage encloses such vital structures as the lungs, the heart, and the liver and gives them protection.

Section X. THE APPENDICULAR SKELETON

4-36. INTRODUCTION

The appendicular skeleton consists of the bones of the upper and lower members.

4-37. THE GIRDLES

Each member is attached ("appended") to the axial skeleton by a skeletal element called a girdle.

a. **Pelvic Girdles.** The girdle of each lower member is called the pelvic girdle. Each pelvic girdle is attached firmly to the corresponding side of the sacrum. With their ligaments, the two pelvic girdles and sacrum together form a solid bony circle known as the bony pelvis.

b. **Pectoral Girdles.** The girdle of each upper member is called the pectoral girdle. Unlike the pelvic girdles, each pectoral girdle is very loosely attached to the axial skeleton. The sole attachment is by the sternoclavicular joint, which in turn is constructed to increase the degrees of motion.

4-38. GENERAL STRUCTURE OF THE LIMBS

Both the upper and lower members have limbs arranged in three segments. The proximal segment has one bone. The middle segment has two bones. The distal segment has many bones arranged in a five-rayed (pentadactyl) pattern.

4-39. FUNCTIONS OF THE LOWER MEMBER

a. **Body Support.** The skeleton of the lower member is strongly constructed in a columnar fashion for body support. The foot at the lower end of the lower limb extends at a 90° angle. Therefore, the foot forms a base for the body during the erect, standing posture.

b. **Locomotion.** At the same time, the lower limb has a series of linkages that enable the body to move from place to place.

4-40. FUNCTIONS OF THE UPPER MEMBER

The grasping hand is the distal segment of the upper member. The flexible construction of the pectoral girdle and the bones of the upper limb serve to place the grasping hand into as many positions as possible. This is particularly helpful in grasping food and placing it into the mouth. The grasping hand also serves as a tool-holding device. (When we study the nervous system, we shall see that a significant portion of the brain and special pathways are present in order to control the movements of this grasping hand.)

Continue with Exercises

EXERCISES, LESSON 4

REQUIREMENT. The following exercises are to be answered by completing the incomplete statements. After you have completed all the exercises, turn to "Solutions to Exercises" at the end of the lesson, and check your answers.

1.   The skeleton _____s (holds up) the body.

    Joints and attached skeletal muscles enable the parts of the body to move with respect to each other; this is called _____n. Such linkages in the lower members make l_____n possible.

    The skeleton helps to p_____t vital organs.

    The skeleton is involved in the formation of _____d (h_____s) cells.

    The skeleton also stores various _____s.

2.   Each bone is built upon a framework of _____ . Upon this framework, _____e crystals are deposited in regular order. When compressed, these crystals produce a local _____c c_____t. This phenomenon is called the _____electric effect. Bones tend to lose mass when they are not subjected to at least ordinary _____s.

3.   The living cells of the bones are osteo_____. When these cells are building up bone tissue, they are called osteo_____. When they are tearing down bone tissue, they are called osteo_____. The building and rebuilding respond directly to the directions of _____ applied to the body.

4.   The envelope surrounding the "typical" long bone is the p_____m. Adjacent to the surface of the bone, there is a special layer of bone-forming cells called the osteo_____c layer. When a long bone is fractured without loss of the periosteum, the fracture is healed by the combined action of the _____c layer of the periosteum and the osteo_____s of the bone itself.

5.   In the early years of life, near each end of the long bones, there is a plate of cartilage called the epi_____ plate. Between puberty and adulthood, this cartilage is replaced by _____ development. The dense bony line remaining is called the _____l line.

Meanwhile, the bone also grows in w_____h. As bony tissue is added to the outside of the bone by the _____c layer, o_____c activity removes bone material from the wall of the marrow cavity.

6.   When the growth of the cranial flat bones is complete, the osteogenic layer of the _____m disappears. Osteoblastic activity repairs only the margins of a spatial defect. Thus, the missing portions of the tables (will) (will not) be replaced.

7.   a.   In a young individual, if the brain is injured by a force applied to the cranium, where will the injury usually be located? _____.

      b.   In an older adult, the injury will usually be located _____ _____ or it may be diverted to the _____.

8.   Enclosing the joint area of a "typical" synovial joint is the joint _____. Lubricating the joint is the _____ fluid. Holding the bones together at the joint are the _____ts and skeletal _____s. Producing motion when properly stimulated are the skeletal _____s.

9.   The upper part of the vertebral column, the neck region, and associated muscles provide the head with its various _____s. The upper two vertebrae are specifically constructed for motions of the_____.

10.   The vertebral bodies, the intervertebral discs, and the articular processes of the vertebrae serve to s_____t the body w_____t. The sacrum receives the b____ w_____ from above and transfers it to the pelvic bones.

11.   A semiflexible rod is formed by the _____e, the inter-vertebral _____s, and the associated _____ts. The spinous and transverse processes of the neural arches serve as _____ts for skeletal muscles and act as _____s.

       The intervertebral discs allow motion to occur between adjacent _____e. Second, they act as _____k_____s.

       The curvatures of the vertebral column also function as _____k_____s for the body.

12.   The construction of the upper member serves to place the grasping _____ into as many _____s as possible. This is particularly helpful in _____ing _____ and placing it into the _____.

Check Your Answers on Next Page

SOLUTIONS TO EXERCISES, LESSON 4

1.   The skeleton <u>supports</u> (holds up) the body.

    Joints and attached skeletal muscles enable the parts of the body to move with respect to each other; this is called <u>motion</u>. Such linkages in the lower members make <u>locomotion</u> possible.

    The skeleton helps to <u>protect</u> vital organs.

    The skeleton is involved in the formation of <u>blood</u> (<u>hematopoiesis</u>) cells.

    The skeleton also stores various <u>minerals</u>. (para 4-2)

2.   Each bone is built upon a framework of <u>FCT</u>. Upon this framework, <u>apatite</u> crystals are deposited in regular order. When compressed, these crystals produce a local <u>electric</u> <u>current</u>. This phenomenon is called the <u>piezoelectric</u> effect. Bones tend to lose mass when they are not subjected to at least ordinary <u>forces</u>. (para 4-4)

3.   The living cells of the bones are <u>osteocytes</u>. When these cells are building up bone tissue, they are called <u>osteoblasts</u>. When they are tearing down bone tissue, they are called <u>osteoclasts</u>. The building and rebuilding respond direly to the directions of <u>force</u> applied to the body. (para 4-5)

4.   The envelope surrounding the "typical" long bone is the <u>periosteum</u>. Adjacent to the surface of the bone, there is a special layer of bone-forming cells called the <u>osteogenic</u> layer. When a long bone is fractured without loss of the periosteum, the fracture is healed by the combined action of the <u>osteogenic</u> layer of the periosteum and the <u>osteoblasts</u> of the bone itself. (para 4-8e)

5.   In the early years of life, near each end of the long bones, there is a plate of cartilage called the <u>epiphyseal</u> plate. Between puberty and adulthood, this cartilage is replaced by <u>bone</u> development. The dense bony line remaining is called the <u>epiphyseal</u> line.

    Meanwhile, the bone also grows in <u>width</u>. As bony tissue is added to the outside of the bone by the <u>osteogenic</u> layer, <u>osteoclastic</u> activity removes bone material from the wall of the marrow cavity. (para 4-9d-f)

6.   When the growth of the cranial flat bones is complete, the osteogenic layer of the <u>periosteum</u> disappears. Osteoblastic activity repairs only the margins of a spatial defect. Thus, the missing portions of the tables <u>will not</u> be replaced. (para 4-12b)

7.   a. In a young individual, if the brain is injured by a force applied to the cranium, where will the injury usually be located? <u>Immediately below the location of the applied force</u>.

   b. In an older adult, the injury will usually be located <u>on the opposite side from the applied force</u> or it may be diverted to the <u>base of the cranium</u>. (para 4-12c)

8.   Enclosing the joint area of a "typical" synovial joint is the joint <u>capsule</u>. Lubricating the joint is the <u>synovial</u> fluid. Holding the bones together at the joint are the <u>ligaments</u> and skeletal <u>muscles</u>. Producing motion when properly stimulated are the skeletal <u>muscles</u>. (paras 4-22 thru 4-25)

9.   The upper part of the vertebral column, the neck region, and associated muscles provide the head with its various <u>motions</u>. The upper two vertebrae are specifically constructed for motions of the <u>head</u>. (para 4-31)

10.   The vertebral bodies, the intervertebral discs, and the articular processes of the vertebrae serve to <u>support</u> the body <u>weight</u>. The sacrum receives the <u>body</u> <u>weight</u> from above and transfers it to the pelvic bones. (para 4-32)

11.   A semiflexible rod is formed by the <u>vertebrae</u>, the intervertebral <u>discs</u>, and the associated <u>ligaments</u>. The spinous and transverse processes of the neural arches serve as <u>attachments</u> for skeletal muscles and act as <u>levers</u>.

   The intervertebral discs allow motion to occur between adjacent <u>vertebrae</u>. Second, they act as <u>shock</u> <u>absorbers</u>.

   The curvatures of the vertebral column also function as <u>shock</u> <u>absorbers</u> for the body. (para 4-34)

12.   The construction of the upper member serves to place the grasping <u>hand</u> into as many <u>positions</u> as possible. This is particularly helpful in <u>grasping</u> <u>food</u> and placing it into the <u>mouth</u>. (para 4-40)

End of Lesson 4

LESSON ASSIGNMENT

LESSON 5   Physiology and Actions of Muscles.

LESSON ASSIGNMENT   Paragraphs 5-1 through 5-24.

LESSON OBJECTIVES   After completing this lesson, you should be able to:

5-1.   Match elements of muscle function with their descriptions.

5-2.   Given a list of statements about muscle function, select the false statement.

5-3.   Given incomplete statements about muscle function, complete the statements.

SUGGESTION   After completing the assignment, complete the exercises at the end of this lesson. These exercises will help you to achieve the lesson objectives.

LESSON 5

PHYSIOLOGY AND ACTIONS OF MUSCLES

Section I. MUSCLE TISSUES

5-1. INTRODUCTION

The term <u>muscle</u> (like the term <u>bone</u>) is used with two distinctly different meanings. In one case, the term is used to designate tissues. In the other case, the term refers to individual, discrete organs of the body. However, the structure and actions of <u>tissues</u> are often quite different in detail from the structure and actions of <u>organs</u>.

5-2. ACTIONS OF MUSCLE TISSUES

a. Tissues of the body are collections of like cells performing a common function. Muscle tissues are specialized to produce tension by contraction. In fact, they function solely by contraction.

b. As a by-product, muscle tissues also produce heat. (<u>Shivering</u> is a state in which the muscles of the body are primarily concerned with producing heat. Shivering involves contractions that are not synchronized and therefore do not produce motion.)

c. As used in muscle physiology, the term <u>contraction</u> is not necessarily synonymous with the term <u>shortening</u>. Rather, <u>contraction</u> means the production of tension through the interaction of the muscle tissues.

5-3. TYPES OF MUSCLE TISSUES

There are three types of muscle tissue:

a. **Smooth**. Smooth muscle tissue consists of elongated cellular elements. It is found mainly in the walls of visceral organs and blood vessels.

b. **Striated.** Striated muscle tissue is composed of fibers. These fibers represent the fusion of many cells into a single functioning fiber (syncytium). Under the microscope, these fibers appear to have a transverse pattern of light and dark banding.

c. **Cardiac.** Cardiac muscle tissue is also composed of banded fibers. However, its fibers have a branched character. Cardiac muscle tissue is found only in the wall of the heart.

5-4. MICROSCOPIC ANATOMY OF THE STRIATED MUSCLE TISSUE

The striated muscle fiber is a syncytium (para 5-3b).

a. The fiber, as a whole, is surrounded by a membrane known as the sarcolemma. The sarcolemma has specialized invaginations that enter the interior of the fiber at right angles to the sarcolemma. These are called transverse tubules (T-tubules). The T-tubules connect with the extracellular space and allow interstitial fluid to flow in and through the striated muscle fiber.

b. The fiber is filled with a type of intracellular fluid called sarcoplasm.

SARCO = flesh

c. Within the sarcoplasm is a tubular system called the sarcoplasmic reticulum that stores calcium, which is necessary for the muscle activation and contraction.

d. Myofilaments are found in the sarcoplasm.

MYO = muscle

FIL = thread

Myofilaments are long complexes of protein molecules, either actin or myosin. Thus, there are two main types of myofilaments: actin and myosin. The myosin filaments are thicker and have appendages known as myosin "bridges." The myosin filaments are surrounded by the thinner actin filaments.

e. Great numbers of well-developed mitochondria (the "powerhouse" elements of cells) are found in striated muscle fibers.

5-5. CONTRACTION OF A STRIATED MUSCLE FIBER

a. **"Sliding Filament" Theory**. The current consensus of opinion of how a striated muscle fiber contracts is known as the "sliding filament" theory (Figure 5-1). This theory emphasizes the role of the myosin bridges. Energy is provided by the mitochondria in the form of ATP. With this energy, the myosin bridges swing and draw the actin filaments over the myosin filaments. The length of the striated muscle fiber is thus shortened.

b. **"All-or-None" Phenomenon**. When stimulated to contract by a nervous impulse, a striated muscle fiber contracts totally or not at all. This is the "all-or-none" phenomenon. The striated muscle fiber has a threshold of stimulation. Below this threshold, the fiber will not act. When stimulated at or above this threshold, the fiber will contract totally every time.

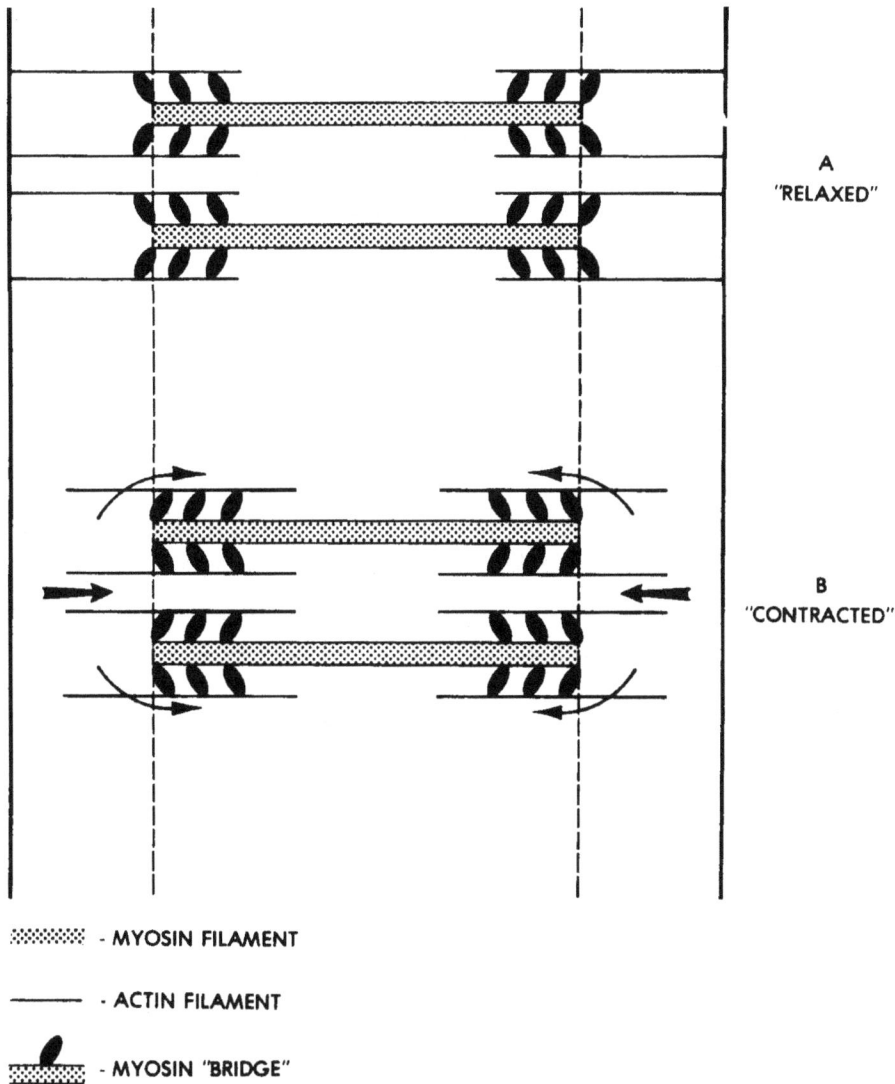

A
"RELAXED"

B
"CONTRACTED"

▒▒▒ - MYOSIN FILAMENT

——— - ACTIN FILAMENT

▬▬ - MYOSIN "BRIDGE"

Figure 5-1. Schematic diagram of the "sliding filament" theory.

c. **Length-Tension Curve**. The contraction of a striated muscle fiber produces tension (force). The amount of this tension varies with the length of the fiber at each moment of contraction. This tension is greatest when the fiber is at its resting length. The tension is proportionately less when the fiber is shorter or longer than its resting length. These variations in tension according to differences in fiber length may be plotted. The resulting curve is called the length-tension curve of the striated muscle fiber.

Section II. SKELETAL MUSCLES

5-6. INTRODUCTION

An <u>organ</u> is a collection of tissues that together perform a particular function. The individual muscles of the body are individual organs. Their overall function is to produce effects by the production of tensions. An individual muscle of the body is made up of muscle tissues, fibrous connective tissues (FCT), and the muscular NAVL.

5-7. KINDS OF MUSCLES WITH STRIATED MUSCLE FIBERS

Several kinds of muscles have striated muscle fibers as their muscle tissue. These include the:

a. **Skeletal Muscles**. The skeletal muscles are attached to the bones of the skeleton. Since they cross joints, they produce motion at these joints.

b. **Branchiomeric Muscles**. The branchiomeric muscles are those associated with the jaws, pharynx, palate, and larynx.

c. **Extraocular Muscles**. The extraocular muscles are within the orbit. They are attached to and move the eyeball.

d. **Integumentary Muscles**. The integumentary muscles are developed in association with the deep surface of the skin (integument proper). A prime example of the integumentary muscles consists of the facial (mimetic) muscles.

5-8. MAKEUP OF AN INDIVIDUAL SKELETAL MUSCLE

The individual skeletal muscle is composed primarily of striated muscle fibers and FCT fibers.

a. **Striated Muscle Fibers**. There are two types of striated muscle fibers--fast (white) and slow (red).

(1) <u>Fast (white)</u>. The fast striated muscle fibers can contract rapidly and strongly but only for a short time.

(2) <u>Slow (red)</u>. The slow striated muscle fibers tend to contract more slowly but for a sustained duration. The red color of slow striated muscle fibers is because of <u>myoglobin protein</u>. This protein has the capacity to store oxygen within the sarcoplasm. Thus, oxygen is available for the production of energy during the contraction.

b. **FCT Fibers**.

(1) Endomysium. The endomysium is a meshwork of FCT that surrounds each striated muscle fiber individually.

(2) Perimysium. A group of these striated muscle fibers is bound together in a bundle (fascicle) by an FCT envelope known as the perimysium.

(3) Epimysium. The entire muscle is bound within an FCT sheath called the epimysium.

5-9. EFFECTS OF TEMPERATURE ON FCT FIBERS

When the FCT fibers are relatively cold, they are stiffer and more liable to break. As the FCT fibers become warmer, they also become more elastic. Thus, warm-up exercises are always strongly suggested before engaging in vigorous activity.

5-10. GENERAL STRUCTURE OF A SKELETAL MUSCLE

A skeletal muscle generally has two major subdivisions.

a. **Fleshy Belly**. The main portion is the fleshy belly, where muscle tissue is located.

b. **FCT Attachments**. At the ends of the belly, the FCT continue and form some sort of attachment to the bones.

(1) In the case of many skeletal muscles, this attachment is a discrete cord of dense FCT known as a tendon.

(2) If the tendon is broad and flat rather than cord-like, we call it an aponeurosis.

(3) Often, we cannot see the tendon-like structure of attachment. Rather, the fleshy belly seems to be attached directly to the surface of the bone. Such an attachment is called a fleshy attachment. However, in reality, the FCT still forms the actual attachment to the bone.

(4) Muscle soreness is often the result of the tearing of the FCT attachment to a bone.

5-11. TYPES OF SKELETAL MUSCLES ACCORDING TO FIBER PATTERN

Skeletal muscles are categorized according to the manner in which the muscle fibers are oriented to the tendons of attachment.

a. In some muscles, the fibers are quite long and parallel and extend the length of the muscle (from attachment to attachment). This type of skeletal muscle is referred to as a ribbon or strap muscle.

b. In other muscles, the striated muscle fibers are oriented obliquely between the two tendons of attachments. Such muscles are said to have a quadrilateral structure.

c. If the striated muscle fibers appear to be attached to one tendon in a feather-like arrangement, the muscle structure is known as pennate.

(1) If all of the fibers are on one side of the tendon, the muscle structure is unipennate.

(2) If the fibers are on two sides, the muscle structure is bipennate.

(3) If the feather-like arrangement is branched, the muscle structure is multipennate.

5-12. EFFECTS OF FIBER PATTERNS

Thus, ribbon muscles have long fibers. On the other hand, pennate (especially multipennate) muscles have great numbers of short fibers. These different structures of skeletal muscles affect both a muscle's relative strength and its distance of contraction.

a. **Relative Strength**. The strength of a skeletal muscle is proportional to the cross-sectional area of its fibers. Therefore, a multipennate muscle is generally much stronger than a ribbon muscle.

b. **Distance of Contraction**. On the other hand, the longer the fibers of a muscle, the greater will be its distance of contraction. As a very loose rule of thumb, a skeletal muscle can contract to three-fifths of its resting length. The ribbon muscles (such as the rectus abdominis M., which flexes the trunk) have long distances of contraction. The multipennate muscles have the least distance of contraction (but are very strong and stable).

5-13. SOME BASIC PHYSIOLOGY OF THE SKELETAL MUSCLES

a. **Length-Tension Curve**. In paragraph 5-5c, we described the length-tension curve for a striated muscle fiber. A length-tension curve can also be constructed for a whole skeletal muscle. However, the FCT fibers of the skeletal muscle provide an additional component to the tension produced by the muscle fibers. As the muscle is extended beyond its resting length, the tension produced by the FCT fibers becomes greater and greater. Thus, the tension produced by a whole skeletal muscle increases greatly with increased length.

b. **Fatigue**. Oxygen is used by the mitochondria of the muscle to produce energy in the form of ATP.

(1) As a muscle is used, its oxygen supply becomes depleted. Naturally, this depletion occurs more quickly in white striated muscle fibers than it does in red striated muscle fibers. With continued exercise, however, the oxygen becomes depleted in both types of fibers.

(2) However, ATP can still be formed, but much less efficiently, in a sequence which is anaerobic (without oxygen). In this anaerobic sequence, the glucose is only partially decomposed. The ultimate product of the anaerobic sequence is lactic acid.

(3) Lactic acid accumulates in the sarcoplasm of the muscle fibers. As this occurs, the muscle becomes stiffer and is no longer able to function well. This condition is called fatigue. An oxygen debt has been built up during the anaerobic production of ATP. This debt must be paid (the muscle must become replenished with oxygen) before the muscle will be able to function properly again.

c. **Tonus**. Tonus is a state of semicontraction of the musculature of the body. The degree of tonus varies considerably with the state of health and exercise of the individual. Tonus serves to remove the slack from the skeletal muscles so they can act immediately when called upon. Also, at the joints, tonus serves to keep the opposing surfaces of the bones close together. This helps to prevent injury to the articular cartilages during muscular contractions.

5-14. WOUND HEALING IN SKELETAL MUSCLES

After a skeletal muscle is injured, the wound area undergoes a specific series of changes.

a. Special body cells collect in the area and remove dead and dying tissue. At the margins of the wound, the healthy striated muscle fibers dedifferentiate (lose their special character and become more simple in structure).

b. If damaged tissue and foreign materials have been properly removed (debridement) and if the edges of the live muscle tissue are closely fitted to each other, the regenerating muscle fibers will actually join and produce a whole muscle again.

c. If a great amount of muscle tissue is missing, a defect will remain in the muscle. Some physicians have developed the "minced muscle" technique, used to replace these defects.

Section III. SOME SKELETOMUSCULAR MECHANICS

5-15. INTRODUCTION

The skeletal and muscular systems of the body work together to produce motions and locomotion of the body. All of these actions are mechanical in nature. They utilize the various mechanics as studied in physics.

a. **Vectors**. The various forces produced by contracting muscles have specific direction and magnitude. As such, these vectors or forces when plotted are represented by arrows whose length corresponds to the magnitude of the force and whose direction corresponds to the direction of the force.

b. **Lever Systems**. The majority of the motions are of the rotary type and occur around an axis or fulcrum. These motions follow the physics of lever systems. The third class of lever (Figure 5-2) is the most common.

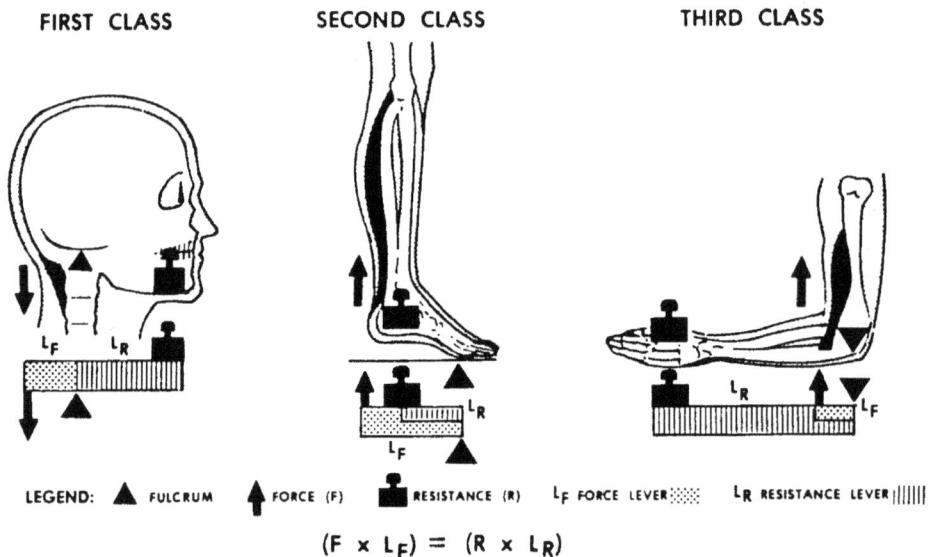

FIRST CLASS   SECOND CLASS   THIRD CLASS

LEGEND: ▲ FULCRUM ↑ FORCE (F) ■ RESISTANCE (R) L_F FORCE LEVER L_R RESISTANCE LEVER

$$(F \times L_F) = (R \times L_R)$$

Figure 5-2. Types of lever systems.

c. **Simple Pulley Systems**. Another common mechanism of the human body is the simple pulley system. Here, the direction of force can be at an angle to the muscle. This is achieved by having the muscle's tendon go around a bony eminence in the same way as a rope goes around a single pulley.

d. **Pendulums**. During locomotion, the body uses several pendulums in the swinging of the upper and lower limbs.

5-16. THE SKELETOMUSCULAR UNIT

The skeletomuscular unit (Figure 5-3) is a working concept of muscle and skeleton producing motion. The components of an S-M unit are: bones, a joint, and skeletal muscle(s).

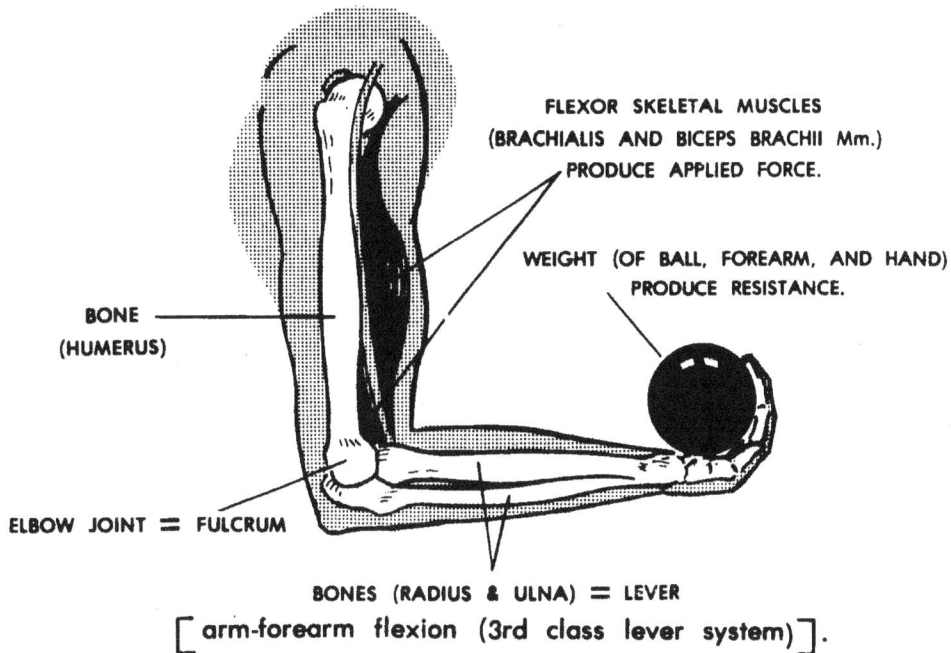

FLEXOR SKELETAL MUSCLES
(BRACHIALIS AND BICEPS BRACHII Mm.)
PRODUCE APPLIED FORCE.

WEIGHT (OF BALL, FOREARM, AND HAND)
PRODUCE RESISTANCE.

BONE
(HUMERUS)

ELBOW JOINT = FULCRUM

BONES (RADIUS & ULNA) = LEVER
[arm-forearm flexion (3rd class lever system)].

Figure 5-3. The skeletomuscular unit.

a. **Bones**. Bones act as levers and as attachment sites for skeletal muscles.

b. **Joint (Articulation).** The joint is the center, fulcrum, point, or axis of motion.

c. **Skeletal Muscle(s).** Skeletal muscles apply the forces for motion. Any given motion utilizes a group of muscles working together.

5-17. POTENTIAL ROLES OF A SKELETAL MUSCLE

During a given rotary motion, a skeletal muscle may have one of several different roles to play. During the motion, a muscle may change from one role to another.

a. **Prime Mover**. Of a group of muscles acting upon a moving part, the one producing the strongest and most direct force is in the prime mover role. Its force is in the direction of the motion being produced.

b. **Synergist**. When another skeletal muscle produces an added force in the same general direction as the prime mover, it is referred to as a synergist.

c. **Neutralizer**. The muscles moving a part are often arranged so that they tend to move the part at a small angle from the intended direction. In such cases, an additional muscle, the neutralizer, is present to counteract and correct the direction of pull.

d. **Antagonist**. Muscles whose lines of pull are opposite to the direction of motion are referred to as antagonists. Antagonists are extremely important for making a smooth, coordinated motion. They tend to adjust the actual direction, speed, and distance of the motion. Without proper antagonists, the motions of the body parts become uncontrolled and flailing. When the motion is completed, the antagonist contracts and returns the part moved to its original position.

e. **Stabilizer**. A stabilizer is a skeletal muscle that ensures that the joint being moved is properly maintained.

f. **Fixator**. When one joint is moved, the other joints of the body must be kept immobile so that the desired motion can take place normally. The skeletal muscles that hold these other joints immobile are called fixators.

5-18. SECONDARY ROLES OF SKELETAL MUSCLES

Most skeletal muscles are not directly aligned with the desired motions of the joints. This means that they are potentially able to produce secondary motions at these joints. This potential secondary role of a muscle is very important to medical personnel for two reasons:

a. First, during evaluation of a patient's muscular system, a muscle may only appear to be working properly. In fact, it may not be functioning. Its action may have been taken over by another muscle acting in its secondary role.

b. Next, one may know that a muscle is no longer functioning properly. In such a case, it may be possible to design exercises to develop the secondary role of another muscle so that it will perform the action of the first muscle as a part of a rehabilitation program.

5-19. OTHER FUNCTIONS OF SKELETAL MUSCLES

Besides moving the body parts around joints, skeletal muscles also perform other purposes in the human body.

a. Some muscles are specially designed to maintain the erect posture of the human body.

b. <u>Breathing</u> is the process by which air is moved into and out of the lungs. The skeletal muscles of the rib cage and the abdominal cavity produce the various muscular actions of breathing.

c. The <u>interior pressures</u> of the trunk must be increased by the muscles of the trunk wall for two purposes:

(1) Evacuation of substances from the body.

(2) Stabilization so that the trunk can act as a base for work of the upper members.

d. Skeletal muscles can also produce a more or less continuous contraction to immobilize an area of the body. This occurs around painful areas, such as inflamed joints or fractures. This muscular response is called <u>splinting</u>.

5-20. EFFECTS OF EXERCISE OR THE LACK OF IT

a. **Atrophy**. Whether by choice or as a result of injury or illness, a skeletal muscle may not be used. Without use, the striated muscle tissue tends to be lost. The general process in which muscle or another type of tissue decreases is called <u>atrophy</u>. Where the muscle tissue has been, there is an invasion of FCT and fat.

A = without

TROPHY = growth

b. **Hypertrophy**. When a muscle is exercised to capacity, the muscle responds by increasing in mass. The increased mass results from an increase in the diameter of the individual muscle fibers. The number of muscle fibers does not increase. This general process is called <u>hypertrophy</u>.

c. **Types of Exercises**.

(1) <u>Isometric</u>. An activity in which a muscle produces tension without a change in length is called an <u>isometric exercise</u>.

ISO = same

METRIC = measurement

For example, if you clasp your hands together and pull without actually moving them, you are participating in an isometric exercise. It has been shown that isometric exercises build muscle strength rapidly. On the other hand, the skeletomuscular system may still lack range of motion.

(2) <u>Isotonic</u>. In isotonic exercises, the active muscles change in length. As the prime mover decreases in length, the antagonistic muscle increases in length. However, both muscles are producing tension.

Section IV. NERVOUS CONTROL OF SKELETAL MUSCLES

5-21. INTRODUCTION

Generally, skeletal muscle tissue contracts in response to a signal from the nervous system. The skeletal muscles of one side of the body are controlled by the opposite side of the brain. Thus, injury to the left side of the brain tends to result in paralysis of the right side of the body.

5-22. NEUROVASCULAR BUNDLE AND MOTOR POINT

The nerves of the body extend from the CNS to the individual muscles. Going to the individual skeletal muscle is the <u>neurovascular bundle</u>. This contains the NAVL for that muscle within a common FCT sheath. The point where this bundle enters the muscle is called the <u>motor point</u>. In a clinic or laboratory, this is the last point where a stimulus can be applied to make the whole muscle contract.

5-23. SENSORY INPUT TO THE CNS FROM THE SKELETAL MUSCLE

The central nervous system (CNS) receives information from the individual skeletal muscle. It also sends commands for action to the muscle.

a. **General Sensations**. The usual general sensations of pain, temperature, pressure, etc., are included in the input from the skeletal muscle.

b. **Stretch Receptors**. Associated with the individual skeletal muscle are two sense organs which analyze the degree of tension or stretch of the muscle as a whole.

(1) <u>The stretch reflex</u>. The <u>muscle spindle</u> is located within the substance of the fleshy belly of the muscle. The muscle spindle is very sensitive to the length of the muscle. It continuously sends information about the specific length of the muscle.

(2) <u>The Golgi tendon organ reflex</u>. Another stretch receptor is the <u>Golgi tendon organ</u>. As its name implies, it is located in the tendon of the muscle. When it informs the CNS that the stretch is excessive, the CNS commands the muscle to relax.

5-24. MOTOR COMMANDS FROM THE CNS TO THE SKELETAL MUSCLE

a. **Motor Homunculus**. The various parts of the body are represented in the substance of the brain. If one plots the sequence and the amount of tissue devoted to each part of the body, one comes up with a caricature of the human being. This caricature (distorted image) is referred to as the motor homunculus.

b. **Pyramidal/Extrapyramidal Motor Systems**. Various collections of neurons and their processes carry commands for actions to the individual skeletal muscles. Originating in the brain, these neurons and processes pass through the brain stem into the spinal cord. In general, they are grouped into the pyramidal motor system and extra pyramidal motor system.

(1) Since the pyramidal motor system is subject to volitional control, it can be used for testing during medical examinations.

(2) The extra pyramidal motor system is more automatic. For the most part, control in this system is non-volitional.

c. **Modulation of Commands**. Several areas of the brain act as coordinators and modulators of the muscle activity of the body. These areas include the cerebellum and the basal ganglia. The sequential patterns of action to produce an overall motion appear to be programmed in the brain, particularly the cerebellum.

d. **Motor Neurons**. The individual motor neuron has its cell body in the brainstem or spinal cord. The axon of the motor neuron passes out of the CNS to become a part of the nerves going to the individual skeletal muscles.

e. **Motor Units**. In the skeletal muscle, the individual motor neuron (axon) has a terminal branching so that it contacts several striated muscle fibers. The actual number of striated muscle fibers contacted (innervated) by a single motor neuron are together known as a motor unit.

(1) When its motor units are small (involving fewer muscle fibers), a muscle can produce very fine actions. The extra ocular muscles are an example of this.

(2) With larger motor units, the muscle action is coarse.

(3) A variable number of motor units may be called into action at a given moment. The number recruited is the number needed for the required action.

f. **Neuromuscular Junctions**. At the end of each branch of the terminal branching of the motor neuron, is an enlargement known as the bouton.

(1) The bouton has a specific relationship with the sarcolemma of the striated muscle fiber. There is no actual physical contact. Instead, there is a little space known as the synaptic cleft.

(2) Across this space to the striated muscle fiber, the command message is carried in the form of a special chemical <u>acetylcholine</u> (ACh). Once the message has been transferred, the ACh is degraded to no longer function.

(3) Nerve gases and organic phosphate insecticides produce their effects by interfering with the transmission or reception of messages across the synaptic cleft.

g. **Axial Versus Appendicular Muscular Control**. The musculature of the body can be thought of in two categories: axial and appendicular.

(1) <u>The axial musculature</u> includes the skeletal muscles of the trunk and the upper and lower girdle regions.

(2) The <u>appendicular musculature</u> includes the skeletal muscles of the upper and lower limbs beyond the girdles.

(3) These two categories are important because they are controlled by the nervous system in different ways. Also, they react quite differently to various physiological and nervous situations.

(4) The muscles that operate the hands tend to be very specifically and highly controlled by the nervous system.

Continue with Exercises

EXERCISES, LESSON 5

REQUIREMENT. The following exercises are to be answered by completing the incomplete statements.

After you have completed all the exercises, turn to "Solutions to Exercises" at the end of the lesson, and check your answers.

1. Muscle tissues are specialized to produce t_____ by contraction. In fact, they function solely by _____n. As a by-product, muscle tissues also produce _____t. The term "contraction" means the production of _____n through the interaction of the muscle tissues.

2. Myofilaments are long complexes of p_____n molecules. There are two main types of myofilaments: _____in and _____in. The myosin filaments are th_____er and have appendages known as myosin _____s. The myosin filaments are surrounded by thinner _____n filaments. Great numbers of well-developed _____a are found in striated muscle fibers.

3. A popular theory explaining the contraction of striated muscle fibers is the "_____ing _____t" theory. This theory emphasized the role of the _____n _____s, which swing and draw the _____n filaments over the _____n filaments.

What is the "all-or-none" phenomenon concerning the contraction of striated muscle fibers?

The tension produced by a striated muscle fiber is potentially greatest when the fiber is at its _____ing _____h.

4. Striated muscle fibers are found in _____l muscles, _____iomeric muscles, extra_____r muscles, and _____y muscles.

5. The individual skeletal muscle is composed primarily of _____d muscle fibers and ____ fibers. White striated muscle fibers are (fast) (slow). Red striated muscle fibers are (fast) (slow).

The fast striated muscle fibers can contract rapidly and strongly but for a _____ time. The slow striated muscle fibers can contract for a _____ time.

6. Muscle soreness is often the result of the tearing of the _____ attachment to the bone.

7. A multipennate muscle is generally much (weaker) (stronger) than a ribbon muscle. The ribbon muscles have a (longer) (shorter) distance of contraction than that of the multipennate muscles.

8. As a muscle extends beyond its resting length, the tension produced by FCT fibers becomes _____er and _____er. Thus, as a whole skeletal muscle lengthens, the tension produced (increases) (decreases) greatly.

9. In the anaerobic sequence for the production of ATP, the ultimate product is _____ acid. As this occurs, the muscle becomes _____er and unable to function well. Before the muscle can function well again, the muscle must be replenished with _____.

10. At the margins of a wound to a skeletal muscle, the healthy striated muscle fibers ded_____te. The regenerating muscle fibers will actually join and produce a whole muscle again if there has been proper removal of _____d tissue and _____n materials (deb_____t) and if the edges of the live muscle tissue are c_____ly _____ed to each other.

11. The potential secondary role of a skeletal muscle is important. First, it may mask the fact that another muscle is not _____ing _____ly. Second, when a muscle is known to work improperly, another muscle's secondary role can be developed through _____s so that it will perform the action of the first muscle.

12. Some muscles are specially designed to maintain the erect _____e of the human body.

The skeletal muscles of the rib cage and the abdominal cavity produce the various muscular actions of _____ing.

The muscles of the trunk wall increase the interior pressures of the trunk to assist in ev_____n of substances from the body and stabilize the trunk to act as a base for work of the _____r_____s.

There is also a muscular response used to immobilize an area of the body. This is called _____ing.

13. The general process in which muscle or another type of tissue decreases is called
_____y. A muscle increases in mass through a process called _____y.

An activity in which a muscle produces tension without a change in length is called
an _____ic exercise. In isotonic exercises, the active muscles change in _____h.

14. The skeletal muscles of one side of the body are controlled by the
(opposite) (same) side of the brain. Thus, injury to the left side of the brain tends to
result in paralysis of the (left) (right) side of the body.

15. The last point where a stimulus can be applied to make a whole muscle contract is
the _____ point. This is the point where the n_____r bundle enters the
muscle. This bundle contains the _____ for that muscle within a common FCT sheath.

16. The Golgi tendon organ is located in the _____n of the muscle. The muscle
spindle is located within the _____y _____y of the muscle. These two organs are both
_____h receptors.

17. A muscle with small motor units can produce very _____e actions. With larger motor
units, the muscle action is _____.

Check Your Answers on Next Page

SOLUTIONS TO EXERCISES, LESSON 5

1. Muscle tissues are specialized to produce tension by contraction. In fact, they function solely by contraction. As a by-product, muscle tissues also produce heat. The term "contraction" means the production of tension through the interaction of the muscle tissues. (para 5-2)

2. Myofilaments are long complexes of protein molecules. There are two main types of myofilaments: actin and myosin. The myosin filaments are thicker and have appendages known as myosin bridges. The myosin filaments are surrounded by thinner actin filaments. Great numbers of well-developed mitochondria are found in striated muscle fibers. (para 5-4d, e)

3. A popular theory explaining the contraction of striated muscle fibers is the "sliding filament" theory. This theory emphasized the role of the myosin bridges, which swing and draw the actin filaments over the myosin filaments.

    What is the "all-or-none" phenomenon concerning the contraction of striated muscle fibers? When stimulated to contract by a nervous impulse, a striated muscle fiber contracts totally or not at all.

    The tension produced by a striated muscle fiber is potentially greatest when the fiber is at its resting length. (para 5-5)

4. Striated muscle fibers are found in skeletal muscles, branchiomeric muscles, extraocular muscles, and integumentary muscles. (para 5-7)

5. The individual skeletal muscle is composed primarily of striated muscle fibers and FCT fibers. White striated muscle fibers are fast. Red striated muscle fibers are slow.

    The fast striated muscle fibers can contract rapidly and strongly but for a short time. The slow striated muscle fibers can contract for a long time. (para 5-8)

6. Muscle soreness is often the result of the tearing of the FCT attachment to the bone. (para 5-10b (4))

7. A multipennate muscle is generally much stronger than a ribbon muscle. The ribbon muscles have a longer distance of contraction than that of the multipennate muscles. (para 5-12)

8. As a muscle extends beyond its resting length, the tension produced by FCT fibers becomes greater and greater. Thus, as a whole skeletal muscle lengthens, the tension produced increases greatly. (para 5-13a)

9.   In the anaerobic sequence for the production of ATP, the ultimate product is <u>lactic</u> acid. As this occurs, the muscle becomes <u>stiffer</u> and unable to function well. Before the muscle can function well again, the muscle must be replenished with <u>oxygen</u>. (para 5-13b)

10.   At the margins of a wound to a skeletal muscle, the healthy striated muscle fibers <u>dedifferentiate</u>. The regenerating muscle fibers will actually join and produce a whole muscle again, if there has been proper removal of <u>damaged</u> tissue and <u>foreign</u> materials (<u>debridement</u>) and if the edges of the live muscle tissue are <u>closely fitted</u> to each other. (para 5-14)

11.   The potential secondary role of a skeletal muscle is important. First, it may mask the fact that another muscle is not <u>working properly</u>. Second, when a muscle is known to work improperly, another muscle's secondary role can be developed through <u>exercises</u> so that it will perform the action of the first muscle. (para 5-18)

12.   Some muscles are specially designed to maintain the erect <u>posture</u> of the human body.

The skeletal muscles of the rib cage and the abdominal cavity produce the various muscular actions of <u>breathing</u>.

The muscles of the trunk wall increase the interior pressures of the trunk to assist in <u>evacuation</u> of substances from the body and stabilize the trunk to act as a base for work of the <u>upper members</u>.

There is also a muscular response used to immobilize an area of the body. This is called <u>splinting</u>. (para 5-19)

13.   The general process in which muscle or another type of tissue decreases is called <u>atrophy</u>. A muscle increases in mass through a process called <u>hypertrophy</u>.

An activity in which a muscle produces tension without a change in length is called an <u>isometric</u> exercise. In isotonic exercises, the active muscles change in <u>length</u>. (para 5-20)

14.   The skeletal muscles of one side of the body are controlled by the <u>opposite</u> side of the brain. Thus, injury to the left side of the brain tends to result in paralysis of the <u>right</u> side of the body. (para 5-21)

15.   The last point where a stimulus can be applied to make a whole muscle contract is the <u>motor</u> point. This is the point where the <u>neurovascular</u> bundle enters the muscle. This bundle contains the <u>NAVL</u> for that muscle within a common FCT sheath. (para 5-22)

16. The Golgi tendon organ is located in the <u>tendon</u> of the muscle. The muscle spindle is located within the <u>fleshy belly</u> of the muscle. These two organs are both <u>stretch</u> receptors. (para 5-23)

17. A muscle with small motor units can produce very <u>fine</u> actions. With larger motor units, the muscle action is <u>coarse</u>. (para 5-24e)

End of Lesson 5

LESSON ASSIGNMENT

LESSON 6   The Human Digestive System.

LESSON ASSIGNMENT   Paragraphs 6-1 through 6-37.

LESSON OBJECTIVES   After completing this lesson, you should be able to:

        6-1.   Identify the overall function of and processes involved in the human digestive system.

        6-2.   Identify two key facts about digestion.

        6-3.   Match features or structures of the digestive system with their functions.

        6-4.   Given a list of statements about the physiology of the digestive system, select the false statement.

SUGGESTION   After completing the assignment, complete the exercises at the end of this lesson. These exercises will help you to achieve the lesson objectives.

LESSON 6

THE HUMAN DIGESTIVE SYSTEM

Section I. INTRODUCTION

6-1. GENERAL FUNCTION

       The overall function of the human digestive system (Figure 6-1) is to provide materials to be used by the individual cells of the body. These materials are used by the cells:

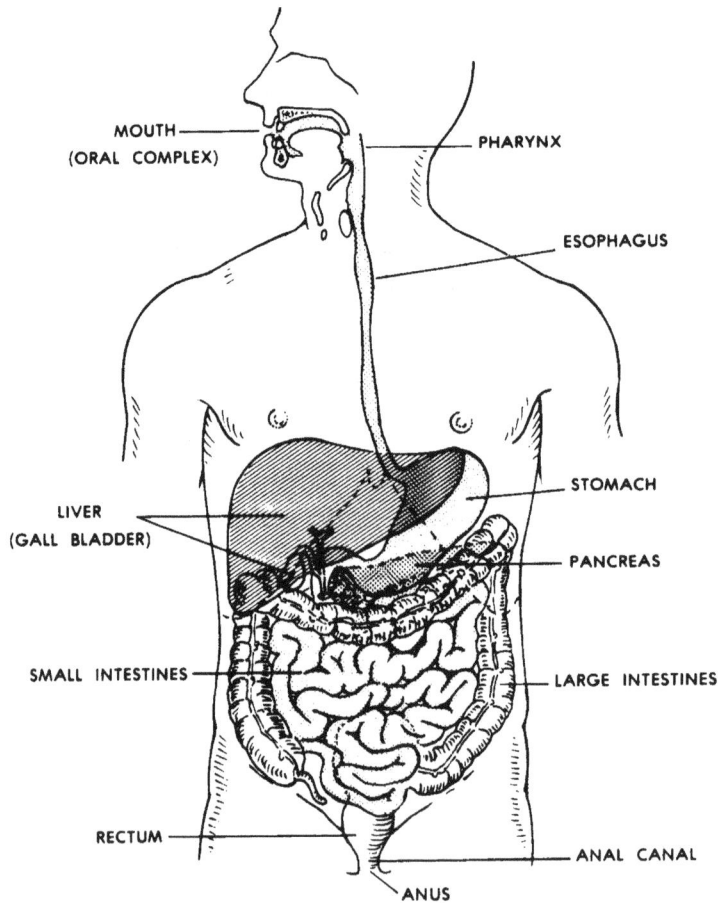

Figure 6-1. The human digestive system.

a. As energy for life processes.

b. For growth and repair of body tissues.

6-2. THE ENERGY CYCLE

The body requires that all of its energy be brought into it from external sources.

a. **Solar Radiation**. The ultimate source of all energy for living things on Earth is the Sun. This energy reaches the Earth in the form of solar radiation.

b. **Photosynthesis**. This radiant energy is stored by plants as the chemical bonds of glucose molecules. The process for doing this is called <u>photosynthesis</u>.

PHOTO = light

SYNTHESIS = put together

This takes place in the presence of the green substance called chlorophyll.

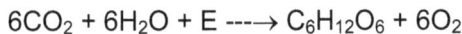

$$6CO_2 + 6H_2O + E ---\rightarrow C_6H_{12}O_6 + 6O_2$$

Carbon Dioxide + Water + Energy YIELDS Glucose + Oxygen

c. **Food Consumption**. The green plants are then utilized as food by various animals. Ultimately, either the green plants or the animals that ate the green plants are consumed by humans.

d. **Digestion and Metabolic Oxidation**. Through the processes of digestion, the glucose is released. It is then delivered to the cells of the body by the circulatory system. Within the cells of the body, the energy is released from the glucose by the chemical process known as metabolic oxidation:

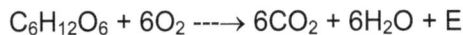

$$C_6H_{12}O_6 + 6O_2 ---\rightarrow 6CO_2 + 6H_2O + E$$

Glucose + Oxygen YIELDS Carbon Dioxide + Water + Energy

e. **Production and Use of ATP**. The released energy is then used to produce the compound known as ATP (adenosine triphosphate). This metabolic oxidation and the production of ATP occur in the mitochondria. For this reason, the mitochondria are known as the "powerhouses" of the cell. When energy is required for carrying on any of the life processes, it is obtained from the ATP.

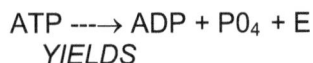

$$ATP ---\rightarrow ADP + PO_4 + E$$
$$YIELDS$$

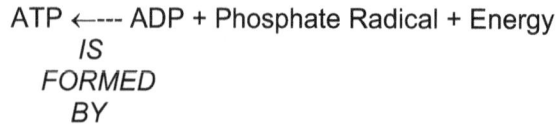

ATP $\longleftarrow$ ADP + Phosphate Radical + Energy
        IS
    FORMED
        BY

6-3. FOODS

A food is any substance utilized by a living thing for energy (or for growth and repair).

a. There are both plant and animal sources for foods. One can eat grains in the form of bread, and one can eat the meat of an animal that ate such grains.

b. Making up foods are specific substances known as <u>foodstuffs</u>. In general, foodstuffs are in three categories:

(1) Carbohydrates (starches and sugars).

(2) Lipids (fats and oils).

(3) Proteins.

c. In addition, other necessary items are also parts of foods. These include water, minerals, vitamins, and so forth.

d. In the human digestive system, the following processes are involved:

(1) Ingestion (taking in) of foods.

(2) Initial processing.

(3) Storage.

(4) Digestion.

(5) Absorption.

(6) Elimination of unused materials.

Section II. INGESTION AND INITIAL PROCESSING OF FOODS

6-4. INGESTION

a. **Hunger.** When an individual needs foods, he experiences a sensation known as hunger. The hypothalamus area of the brain controls the degree of hunger or satiation (feeling of being well fed). To do this, the hypothalamus receives various types of information from throughout the body.

b. **Food Selection.** When food is presented, an individual goes through a process of food selection. He or she has a greater appetite for some foods than others. This process is related both to previous learning and to current, internal chemical requirements.

c. **Biting.** Together, the upper and lower incisors (anterior teeth) create two cutting surfaces like a pair of scissors. As food items are placed in the opening of the oral cavity, bite-size chunks of food are cut off. These chunks are usually just the right size for the mouth to handle.

6-5. TWO KEY FACTS ABOUT DIGESTION

In general terms, there are two key facts to understand about digestion:

a. First, digestion is a chemical process. Through a process called hydrolysis, food is broken down into its constituent parts.

b. Second, this chemical process takes place only at wet surfaces of the food.

6-6. MASTICATION

During the process known as mastication (chewing), the food particles are gradually broken down into smaller and smaller pieces. At the same time, the total surface area of the food increases greatly.

a. This grinding and crushing of the food particles are accomplished by the posterior teeth, the premolar and molar teeth. For this purpose, these teeth have broad, opposing surfaces.

b. Together, the tongue and cheeks act to keep the food particles between the surfaces of the grinding teeth. This is accomplished as the lower jaw moves up and down.

6-7. SALIVA

a. Secreting fluids into the oral cavity are such glandular structures as the salivary glands and the buccal glands. (The buccal glands are serous and mucous glands on the inner surfaces of the cheeks.) These fluids are collectively known as the saliva.

b. Saliva serves to wet the surface areas of the food particles produced by mastication. In addition, saliva also dissolves some of the molecules of the food items.

c. Taste buds sample these dissolved molecules and test the quality of the food being eaten. Taste buds are located on the tongue and the back of the oral cavity.

d. Another component of the saliva is mucus. The mucus tends to hold the food particles together as a bolus. Since the mucus also makes this bolus somewhat slippery, the bolus can slide readily through the initial portion of the digestive tract.

Section III. SWALLOWING (DEGLUTITION)

6-8. INTRODUCTION

When the food has been adequately broken down (increased surface area), wetted thoroughly, and tested (tasted), it is ready to be swallowed.

a. The bolus is moved posteriorly out of the mouth (oral cavity) into the pharynx and then down through the esophagus to the stomach.

b. The pharynx is common to both the digestive and respiratory systems. Therefore, as the bolus passes through the pharynx, both the upper and lower air passageways must be protected. Otherwise, food particles might enter the passageways.

6-9. MOVEMENT OUT OF THE ORAL CAVITY

a. **Initial Movement of the Bolus.** There are intrinsic muscles in the tongue. Through their action, the tongue arches upward and presses against the hard palate, the roof of the mouth. This initiates the posterior movement of the bolus.

b. **Action of the Hyoid Complex.** The muscles of the hyoid bone pull the hyoid bone upward and force the tongue upward into the oral cavity. This closes up the front part of the oral cavity and forces the bolus further to the rear.

c. **Action of the Soft Palate.** As the bolus approaches the pharynx, the soft palate is raised. Thus, the soft palate serves as a trap door to close the upper air passageway. By tensing to resist the pressure from the bolus of food, the soft palate ensures the continued backward movement of the bolus into the pharynx.

6-10. MOVEMENT THROUGH THE PHARYNX

a. **Pharyngeal Constrictor Muscles.** The wall of the pharynx contains three pharyngeal constrictor muscles. By wavelike contractions, these muscles force the bolus down into the beginning of the esophagus.

b. **Action of the Epiglottis.** As the hyoid bone's muscles raise the tongue up into the oral cavity, they also raise the larynx. The larynx is raised because it is attached to the inferior margin of the hyoid bone. As the larynx is raised, its epiglottis automatically turns down over the opening of the larynx. Thus, food is prevented from entering the lower-air passage-way.

6-11. MOVEMENT THROUGH THE ESOPHAGUS

The esophagus is a tube with muscular walls. It extends from the pharynx above, through the neck and thorax, to the stomach in the abdomen. Wavelike contractions (peristalsis) move the bolus through the esophagus to the stomach.

Section IV. TEMPORARY STORAGE

6-12. INTRODUCTION

a. The stomach is a saclike enlargement of the digestive tract. By way of the esophagus, the stomach receives the food that has been processed in the oral cavity.

b. The stomach's capacity is great enough to allow the individual to take in enough food material at one time to last for an extended period of time. This allows the individual to engage in activities other than eating.

c. In addition, certain digestive processes are initiated in the stomach.

d. The food is retained in the stomach for varying lengths of time, depending upon the types of food eaten, the condition of the individual, and many other factors.

6-13. ADAPTATIONS OF THE STOMACH FOR THE STORAGE FUNCTION

The stomach is adapted as a storage area in several ways.

a. Its wall is quite stretchable. The mucosal lining of the stomach is thrown up into longitudinal folds called rugae. These rugae flatten out as the stomach capacity increases.

b. At each end of the stomach, there is a structure to keep the contents from leaving the stomach.

(1) At the point where the esophagus enters the stomach, there is a "gastroesophageal valve." This valve appears to be functional, although it has not been demonstrated anatomically.

(2) At the other end of the stomach is the well-developed pyloric valve.

6-14. ADAPTATIONS OF THE STOMACH FOR ADDITIONAL FOOD PROCESSING

a. **Gastric Glands.** The mucosal lining of the stomach contains a number of gastric glands. These gastric glands produce gastric digestive juices for initiating digestion, particularly of proteins. Some of the gastric glands also produce hydrochloric acid. Thus, chyme, the mixture produced by the stomach, is quite acid.

b. **Additional Musculature.** A third inner, oblique layer of muscle has been added to the stomach wall. With the three layers of muscles, the contents of the stomach are thoroughly mixed.

Section V. DIGESTION AND ABSORPTION

6-15. INTRODUCTION

The small intestines are the primary area of the body for digestion of foodstuffs. Digestion occurs through the action of enzymes. The results of the digestion are the end-products. These end-products (molecules or particles) are of such size that they can be absorbed through the walls of the small intestines. The end-products are then distributed throughout the body by the body's circulatory systems.

6-16. DIGESTION AS A CHEMICAL PROCESS

a. Digestion is the chemical process that breaks foodstuffs down into their basic constituents. In general, chemical processes are expected to occur at a rate proportional to the temperature. However, in the human body, the temperature is not high enough for the chemical process of digestion to produce a sufficient quantity of the materials needed.

b. Therefore, digestive enzymes are present to maintain the appropriate rates of reaction. Digestive enzymes are catalysts. A catalyst is a substance that improves the rate of a reaction without being consumed itself. Because of digestive enzymes, digestion proceeds at a pace fast enough to provide the materials needed by the body.

c. The majority of digestion in humans takes place in the small intestines. The small intestines are located in the central part of the abdomen, immediately beneath the abdominal wall. In healthy individuals, a flap called the greater omentum is draped over the small intestines (between them and the anterior abdominal wall). The greater omentum has a great deal of fat for insulation. It is richly supplied with blood vessels for heat. Some might compare the greater omentum to an "electric blanket" for the small intestines.

FOODSTUFF	ENZYME CLASS	END PRODUCTS
Carbohydrates	Amylases	Simple Sugars
Lipids	Lipases	Fatty Acids and Glycerol
Proteins	Proteases	Amino Acids

Table 6-1. Foodstuffs, enzyme classes, and end-products of digestion.

6-17. DIGESTIVE ENZYMES

a. The digestive process begins in the oral cavity. The saliva contains enzymes which initiate the digestion of complex carbohydrates.

b. In the stomach, the gastric glands produce enzymes that initiate the digestion of proteins.

c. In the small intestines, there are digestive enzymes for all three classes of foodstuffs--carbohydrates, lipids, and proteins. Enzymes for completing the digestion of these three classes are found in the fluids produced by the pancreas and glands in the mucosa of the small intestines. Moreover, there is a fluid called bile that is produced by the liver and stored in the gallbladder for release into the small intestines. Bile helps in the digestion of lipids.

d. The presence or absence of certain enzymes is genetically determined. Therefore, some individuals may have difficulty digesting certain foods.

6-18. TIME AND LENGTH

The length of the small intestines appears to be just right. The time it takes for material to travel from beginning to end is just about right for the completion of digestion.

6-19. ABSORPTION

The end-products of digestion are absorbed primarily through the walls of the small intestines.

a. **Surface Area.** The amount of absorption is proportional to the surface area of the walls which contact the contents. Two anatomical specializations serve to increase this surface area:

    (1) There are permanent circular folds (plicae circulares) in the mucosal lining of the small intestines.

    (2) The entire inner surface of the mucosa is covered with villi. Villi are minute, fingerlike processes that extend into the lumen (cavity) of the small intestines.

b. **Capillaries.** The simple sugars and amino acids are absorbed into the blood capillaries. Most of the fatty acids and glycerol are absorbed into the lymphatic capillaries.

6-20. HEPATIC VENOUS PORTAL SYSTEM

All of the blood capillaries in the absorptive areas of the digestive tract join to form the hepatic portal venous system. A venous portal system is a system that begins in capillaries, which join to form veins, which in turn end in another group of capillaries. The hepatic portal vein carries the blood from the absorptive areas of the digestive system to the liver.

6-21. THE LIVER

In the liver, a number of actions are performed on the blood. Excess materials are removed and stored. For example, some glucose is stored as glycogen. Toxic materials are degraded, microorganisms are removed, and so forth. The "treated" blood is then routed from the liver to the heart and then throughout the body.

6-22. UTILIZATION OF THE LIPIDS

The lipid materials, such as fatty acids and glycerol, are carried to the venous system beyond the liver.

a. Lipid materials are a high-energy item. They are stored as fat throughout the body so that they will be available when needed for energy.

b. Body fat also serves as insulation in the subcutaneous tissues. It gives buoyancy to the body in water.

c. Cholesterol is a very important substance in the body. It participates in the functioning of the liver and in other activities of the body.

d. However, there are certain medical conditions in which physicians prescribe a low-cholesterol and/or low-fat diet.

Section VI. SOME PROTECTIVE MECHANISMS ASSOCIATED WITH THE HUMAN DIGESTIVE SYSTEM

6-23. CONTINUITY WITH SURROUNDING ENVIRONMENT

The human digestive system is essentially a continuous tube. It is open at both ends. Therefore, the lumen (cavity) connects directly with the surrounding environment.

a. Along with the ingested food, almost anything can pass through the mouth into the digestive system. Almost anything does enter the digestive system.

b. The digestive tract is open to the surrounding environment also at the other end, the anus.

6-24. COMMENT ABOUT THE RETICULOENDOTHELIAL SYSTEM

As indicated above, a variety of toxic materials and/or microorganisms may be included with the ingested foods. To protect against these undesired materials, special protective mechanisms are associated with the human digestive system. Such protective mechanisms are said to belong to the reticuloendothelial system. This term refers to the association of such mechanisms with a particular layer of epithelial cells.

6-25. COMMENT ABOUT LYMPHOID TISSUES

a. The lymphocyte is an important type of white blood cell that is also found in the interspaces of a tissue called lymphoid (or lymphatic) tissue. Lymphocytes signal other types of white blood cells to phagocytize (engulf) foreign materials found within the body. The lymphoid tissues are particularly important in individuals from birth until about 15 years of age. The mass of lymphoid tissue found in the body of a 12-year-old is about twice the mass found in a full-grown adult. (Between 6 and 15 years of age, the immune system of the blood becomes the primary protector of the body from disease.)

b. The lymphoid tissues are a primary component of the reticuloendothelial system.

6-26. TONSILS

Tonsils are aggregates of lymphoid tissue found at the beginning of the pharynx. There are three pairs of tonsils. Together, they form a ring of lymphoid tissue at the beginning of the pharynx. This ring, called Waldeyer's ring, completely surrounds the entrance to the pharynx from both the mouth (digestive entrance) and the nose and nasal chambers (respiratory entrance).

a. In the upper recess of the pharynx is the pair of pharyngeal tonsils (commonly known as the adenoids).

b. On either side, below the soft palate, are the <u>palatine tonsils</u>. These are the tonsils that one sees most frequently in small children.

c. On the back of the root of the tongue are the <u>lingual tonsils</u>.

6-27. "TONSILS" OF THE SMALL INTESTINES

Lymphoid aggregates of varying size are found in the walls of the small intestines. In the ileum portion, in particular, these aggregates are large enough to be easily observed and are called <u>Peyer's patches</u>. These might be considered "tonsils" of the small intestines.

6-28. "TONSILS" OF THE LARGE INTESTINE

At the beginning of the large intestine, at the inferior end of the cecum, is a structure known as the <u>vermiform appendix</u>. Since the vermiform appendix is actually a collection of lymphoid tissue, it should be considered the "tonsil" of the large intestine.

6-29. KUPFFER'S CELLS

As we have seen, blood from the absorptive areas of the gut tract is collected and delivered to the liver by the hepatic venous portal system. As this blood passes through the sinusoids (channels) of the liver, it is acted upon by cells called Kupffer's cells. These cells line the sinusoids. Since Kupffer's cells remove harmful substances from the blood, they are considered part of the reticuloendothelial system.

6-30. THE MAMMARY GLAND

a. When the newborn baby is nursed by its mother, the initial secretion of the mammary glands is called <u>colostrum</u>. Although this colostrum lacks nutrients, it is loaded with antibodies. These antibodies provide the infant with its primary protection for the first 6 months of life.

b. After a few days, the mammary gland produces the natural food for the human infant. As the infant suckles at the mother's breast, there is a certain amount of <u>reflux</u> (backward flow) into the milk ducts of the mammary gland. Should the infant develop an upper respiratory infection, the organisms causing the infection will be included in this reflux. Generally by the next time the infant suckles, the mammary gland will have produced the appropriate antibodies. These antibodies are delivered to the infant for its protection.

Section VII. VITAMINS

6-31. INTRODUCTION

a. There is a group of chemicals that are required in very small quantities from outside the body for the proper functioning of the body. These substances are called vitamins.

b. Vitamins are found in varying amounts in different foods. In fact, many processed foods contain artificial vitamin supplements.

c. Vitamins can be considered in two major categories--water-soluble vitamins and fat-soluble vitamins.

6-32. WATER-SOLUBLE VITAMINS

The water-soluble vitamins include vitamin C, B-complex vitamins, and others. There is a daily requirement for water-soluble vitamins. This is because they are excreted continuously with the urine.

a. **Vitamin B_1 (Thiamine Hydrochloride).** Vitamin B_1 is present in liver, bananas, lean pork, and whole grain cereals.

b. **Vitamin B_2 (Riboflavin).** Riboflavin is found in milk, milk products, leafy green vegetables, fruit, and liver.

c. **Vitamin B_6 (Pyridoxine Hydrochloride).** Vitamin B_6 is found in whole grain cereals, yeast, milk, fish, eggs, and liver.

d. **Nicotinic Acid (Niacin) and Nicotinamide (Niacinamide).** These are present in meat, liver, milk, peanuts, and whole grain cereals.

e. **Vitamin B_{12}.** Vitamin B_{12} is found in liver, milk, eggs, and cheese.

f. **Folic Acid.** Folic acid is found in leafy green vegetables and liver.

g. **Vitamin C (Ascorbic Acid).** Sources of vitamin C include citrus fruits, tomatoes, bell peppers, paprika, and all leafy green vegetables.

6-33. FAT-SOLUBLE VITAMINS

On the other hand, fat-soluble vitamins can be accumulated in the fat of the body:

a. **Vitamin A.** Vitamin A is mainly obtained from yellow-colored vegetables of all sorts (carrots, squash, and so forth.).

b. **Vitamin D.** Vitamin D is produced in the skin by the activity of solar radiation. It is also present in fish liver oils, butter, and egg yolk.

c. **Vitamin K.** Vitamin K is important in blood clotting. It is actually produced by microorganisms located in the large intestines. This source of vitamin K may be lost during the administration of antibiotics. Vitamin K also occurs in such foods as alfalfa, spinach, cabbage, and egg yolk.

d. **Vitamin E.** The function of vitamin E in humans is not known. Research indicates that vitamin E has important functions in various species, but the specific function varies from species to species.

Section VIII. ELIMINATION OF UNUSED MATERIALS

6-34. UNDIGESTED FOOD MATERIALS

a. **Nondigestible Food Materials.** A number of substances within food materials cannot be digested by the human digestive system. One important material in this group is called cellulose. Cellulose is a complex carbohydrate found in plants. Cellulose is commonly referred to as "bulk" or "fiber."

b. **Other Undigested Food Materials.** When individuals consume great quantities of foods, a portion of it will not be digested.

c. **Passage Out of the Small Intestines.** This undigested material will pass out of the small intestines with the non-digestible materials. The resulting fluid mass enters the large intestines through the ileocecal valve.

6-35. LARGE INTESTINES

a. **Consolidation of Contents.** In the large intestines, this fluid mass is gradually consolidated into a semisolid mass called feces. The major function of the large intestines then is salvage. Water is the primary salvage item. In addition to water, some previously unabsorbed endproducts of digestion can be absorbed here. At the same time certain excretions from the body can be deposited in the fecal mass.

b. **Mucus.** As the contents increase in solidity, mucus is added to facilitate their movement through the large intestines. (Previously, we have seen the addition of mucus to the bolus in the mouth to facilitate movement.) This mucus is produced by unicellular glands in the mucosal lining of the large intestines. (Because of their microscopic appearance, these unicellular glands are called goblet cells.)

c. **Organisms.** Many microorganisms are found within the lumen or cavity of the large intestines. Certain microorganisms are responsible for the production of vitamin K. Depending on the type of food present, some species of microorganisms produce various gases (flatulence). On occasion, pathogenic organisms may be present and cause problems for the individual.

6-36. STORAGE OF FECES

Toward the lower end of the large intestines, the contents (feces) have become relatively consolidated. This consolidated mass is retained (stored) mainly in the rectum and the lower portion of the sigmoid colon.

6-37. ELIMINATION

At the appropriate time, the feces is passed out of the body (defecation). The feces passes through the anal canal and anus. This is accomplished by the relaxation of the anal sphincter muscles.

Continue with Exercises

EXERCISES, LESSON 6

REQUIREMENT. The following exercises are to be answered by completing the incomplete statements.

      After you have completed all the exercises, turn to "Solutions to Exercises" at the end of the lesson, and check your answers.

1.   The overall function of the human digestive system is to provide _____s to be used by the individual _____s of the body.

2.   The radiant energy of the Sun is stored by plants as the chemical bonds of _____ molecules. The process for doing this is called_____.

      Ultimately, humans consume either the green _____s themselves or the _____s which ate the green plants.

      Through the processes of _____n, the glucose is released. It is then delivered to the cells of the body by the _____y system.

      Within the cells of the body, the energy is released from the glucose molecules by the process known as _____c_____n. The released energy is then used to produce the compound ____. Metabolic oxidation and the production of ATP occur within the _____a. The energy for any of the life processes is obtained directly from ____.

3.   The three categories of foodstuffs are c_____s, l_____s, and p_____s. Other necessary items include w_____, m_____s, and v_____s.

4.   The following processes are involved in the human digestive system:

      a. I_____n of foods.

      b. Initial _____g.

      c. _____ge.

      d. D_____n.

      e. A_____n.

      f. E_____n of unused materials.

5. When an individual needs food, he experiences the sensation of _____r. This is controlled by the h_____s area of the brain, which receives i_____n from various parts of the body for this purpose.

The process of food selection is related both to previous _____g and to internal _____l requirements.

As food enters the oral cavity, bite-size chunks of food are cut off by the upper and lower _____s. These chunks are about the right size for the _____ to handle.

6. There are two key facts about digestion:

a. First, digestion is a _____l process. Food is broken down into its constituent parts through the process of _____s.

b. Second, this chemical process takes place only at ___t surfaces of the food.

7. Food processes are broken down into smaller and smaller pieces through the process of _____n, or _____g. This greatly increases the total s_____ a____ of the food. The grinding and crushing are accomplished by the p_____r and _____r teeth. Keeping the food between the surfaces of the grinding teeth are the _____e and the _____s.

8. The fluids secreted into the oral cavity by the _____y glands and the _____l glands are collectively known as _____. These fluids serve to ____t the surface areas of the food particles. Saliva also d_____s some of the molecules of food items. These dissolved molecules are tested by the _____e ____s. Food particles are held together as a bolus by the m_____, which also makes the bolus somewhat slippery.

9. The bolus is moved posteriorly out of the _____h into the p_____ and then down through the _____s to the stomach. Both the upper and lower air passageways must be protected as the bolus passes through the _____.

10. The actions of the tongue are produced by its _____c muscles and the muscles of the _____ bone.

As the bolus approaches the pharynx, the upper air passageway is closed by the ____t_____e, which also t_____s to resist the pressure from the bolus.

11. Wavelike contractions of the three pharyngeal c_____r muscles force the bolus into the beginning of the _____s.

As the larynx is raised along with the tongue and the hyoid bone, its epi_____s turns down over the opening of the _____. Thus, food is prevented from entering the lower ____ passageway.

12. The esophagus is a tube with m_____r walls. It extends from the _____ above, through the neck and thorax, to the _____ in the abdomen. Wavelike contractions, called p_____s, move the bolus through the esophagus to the stomach.

13. Because of the stomach's capacity, the individual can engage in activities other than _____g. In addition, certain _____ve processes are initiated in the stomach.

14. One way the stomach is adapted as a storage area is that its wall is quite _____ble. Its lining has folds called ____ae.

Another adaptation is that, at each end, there is a _____e or similar structure to keep contents from leaving. The "gastroesophageal _____e" has not been demonstrated anatomically. At the other end of the stomach is the well-developed _____c valve.

15. The mucosal lining of the stomach contains a number of _____c glands. The mixture produced by the stomach, called _____e, is quite (acid) (basic).

The three layers of muscles help to ensure that the contents of the stomach are thoroughly ____d.

16. Digestion occurs through the actions of chemicals called _____s. The end products (molecules or particles) are small enough to be absorbed through the walls of the small _____s.

Digestive enzymes are present to maintain the appropriate r____s of reaction. A catalyst is a substance that improves the ____ of reaction without being _____d itself. Digestive enzymes are _____s. Without digestive enzymes, digestion would be too ____w to provide materials needed by the body.

17.   The majority of digestion in humans takes place in the _____ _____ s. Draped over these is a flap called the greater _____m. This flap has fat for _____n and many blood vessels for _____t. Thus, the greater omentum may be compared to an "_____c _____t" for the small intestines.

18.   The saliva contains enzymes which initiate the digestion of complex _____ s.

       In the stomach, the gastric glands produce enzymes which initiate the digestion of _____ s.

       In the small intestines, there are digestive enzymes for c_____ s l____s, and p_____s. These enzymes are found in the fluids produced by the p_____ and glands in the m_____a of the small intestines. Moreover, the liver produces a fluid called ____, which is stored in the g_____r for release into the small intestines; this fluid helps in the digestion of _____s.

19.   The absorptive area of the walls of the small intestines is increased by permanent circular _____s (plicae circulares) and by finger like processes called _____i.

20.   Simple sugars and amino acids are absorbed into the _____d capillaries. Most of the fatty acids and glycerol are absorbed into the _____c capillaries.

21.   The blood capillaries absorbing substances from the digestive tract join to form the h_____c p____l v___s system. A venous p____l system begins in _____s, which join to form ____s, which in turn end in another group of _____s. The hepatic portal vein carries blood from the absorptive area of the digestive system to the

_____.

22.   In the liver, excess materials are removed and _____d. For example, some glucose is stored as _____n. Toxic materials are degraded. Microorganisms are r_____d. The "treated" blood is then routed from the liver to the _____ and then throughout the body.

23.   Lipid materials are stored as ____ throughout the body so that they will be available when needed for _____y.

24.   The lumen of the digestive system connects directly with the s_____ing e_____t. For this reason, special _____ve mechanisms are associated with the human digestive system. Such mechanisms belong to the reticulo_____ system.

A primary component of the _____endothelial system are the _____d tissues. An important type of cell found within these tissues is the_____cyte. These cells signal other types of white blood cells to _____ze foreign materials. These tissues are more important in the (child) (adult).

The aggregate of lymphoid tissue at the beginning of the pharynx are called _____s.

Peyer's patches might be considered the "_____s" of the small intestines.

At the beginning of the large intestine, at the inferior end of the cecum, is the vermiform _____, which might be considered the"_____" of the large intestine.

Lining the sinusoids of the liver and removing harmful substances from the blood are _____'s cells. These cells are also considered to be part of the _____l system.

25.   During nursing, the initial secretion of the mammary glands is called c_____m. Although this secretion lacks nutrients, it is loaded with _____s. These provide the infant with its primary p_____n for the first 6 _____s of life.

Later, if the infant has an upper respiratory infection, the mammary gland will produce the appropriate _____s. This is because of a _____x of fluid into the milk ducts of the mammary gland as the infant sucks.

26.   Required in very small quantities from outside the body are substances called v_____s. These can be considered in two major categories-- _____-soluble and _____-_____.

Water-soluble vitamins include the ___-complex vitamins, vitamin ___, and others. There is a daily requirement for water-soluble vitamins because they are continuously excreted with the _____.

On the other hand, fat-soluble vitamins accumulate in the ____ of the body.

27.   An important nondigestible food material is _____ose, commonly referred to as "_____r" or "____k." Other undigested materials may be because of the consumption of _____t quantities of food. Undigested food materials enter the large intestines through the ile_____ valve.

28.   A major function of the large intestines is to salvage _____r. To facilitate movement, _____s is added to the contents of the large intestines. Microorganisms in the large intestines manufacture vitamin __. Some microorganisms can act upon certain foods to produce _____s. Feces is stored in the _____m and the lower portion of the s_____d colon. Defecation is accomplished by relaxation of the ___l _____r muscles.

Check Your Answers on Next Page

SOLUTIONS TO EXERCISES, LESSON 6

1.   The overall function of the human digestive system is to provide <u>materials</u> to be used by the individual <u>cells</u> of the body. (para 6-1)

2.   The radiant energy of the Sun is stored by plants as the chemical bonds of <u>glucose</u> molecules. The process for doing this is called <u>photosynthesis</u>.

       Ultimately, humans consume either the green <u>plants</u> themselves or the <u>animals</u> that ate the green plants.

       Through the processes of <u>digestion</u>, the glucose is released. It is then delivered to the cells of the body by the <u>circulatory</u> system.

       Within the cells of the body, the energy is released from the glucose molecules by the process known as <u>metabolic</u> <u>oxidation</u>. The released energy is then used to produce the compound <u>ATP</u>. Metabolic oxidation and the production of ATP occur within the <u>mitochondria</u>. The energy for any of the life processes is obtained directly from <u>ATP</u>. (para 6-2)

3.   The three categories of foodstuffs are <u>carbohydrates</u>, <u>lipids</u>, and <u>proteins</u>. Other necessary items include <u>water</u>, <u>minerals</u>, and <u>vitamins</u>. (para 6-3b, c)

4.   The following processes are involved in the human digestive system:

       a. <u>Ingestion</u> of foods.

       b. Initial <u>processing</u>.

       c. <u>Storage</u>.

       d. <u>Digestion</u>.

       e. <u>Absorption</u>.

       f. <u>Elimination</u> of unused materials. (para 6-3d)

5.   When an individual needs food, he experiences the sensation of hunger. This is controlled by the <u>hypothalamus</u> area of the brain, which receives <u>information</u> from various parts of the body for this purpose.

       The process of food selection is related both to previous <u>learning</u> and to internal <u>chemical</u> requirements.

As food enters the oral cavity, bite-size chunks of food are cut off by the upper and lower incisors. These chunks are about the right size for the mouth to handle. (para 6-4)

6.   There are two key facts about digestion:

    a. First, digestion is a chemical process. Food is broken down into its constituent parts through the process of hydrolysis.

        b. Second, this chemical process takes place only at wet surfaces of the food. (para 6-5)

7.   Food processes are broken down into smaller and smaller pieces through the process of mastication, or chewing. This greatly increases the total surface area of the food. The grinding and crushing are accomplished by the premolar and molar teeth. Keeping the food between the surfaces of the grinding teeth are the tongue and the cheeks. (para 6-6)

8.   The fluids secreted into the oral cavity by the salivary glands and the buccal glands are collectively known as saliva. These fluids serve to wet the surface areas of the food particles. Saliva also dissolves some of the molecules of food items. These dissolved molecules are tested by the taste buds. Food particles are held together as a bolus by the mucus, which also makes the bolus somewhat slippery. (para 6-7)

9.   The bolus is moved posteriorly out of the mouth into the pharynx and then down through the esophagus to the stomach. Both the upper and lower air passageway must be protected as the bolus passes through the pharynx. (para 6-8)

10.   The actions of the tongue are produced by its intrinsic muscles and the muscles of the hyoid bone.

        As the bolus approaches the pharynx, the upper air passageway is closed by the soft palate, which also tenses to resist the pressure from the bolus. (para 6-9)

11.   Wavelike contractions of the three pharyngeal constrictor muscles force the bolus into the beginning of the esophagus.

        As the larynx is raised along with the tongue and the hyoid bone, its epiglottis turns down over the opening of the larynx. Thus, food is prevented from entering the lower air passageway. (para 6-10)

12.   The esophagus is a tube with muscular walls. It extends from the pharynx above, through the neck and thorax, to the stomach in the abdomen. Wavelike contractions, called peristalsis, move the bolus through the esophagus to the stomach. (para 6-11)

13.   Because of the stomach's capacity, the individual can engage in activities other than eating. In addition, certain digestive processes are initiated in the stomach. (para 6-12)

14.   One way the stomach is adapted as a storage area is that its wall is quite stretchable. Its lining has folds called rugae.

Another adaptation is that, at each end, there is a valve or similar structure to keep contents from leaving. The "gastroesophageal valve" has not been demonstrated anatomically. At the other end of the stomach is the well-developed pyloric valve. (para 6-13)

15.   The mucosal lining of the stomach contains a number of gastric glands. The mixture produced by the stomach, called chyme, is quite acid.

The three layers of muscles help to ensure that the contents of the stomach are thoroughly mixed. (para 6-14)

16.   Digestion occurs through the actions of chemicals called enzymes. The end products (molecules or particles) are small enough to be absorbed through the walls of the small intestines. (para 6-15)

Digestive enzymes are present to maintain the appropriate rates of reaction. A catalyst is a substance that improves the rate of reaction without being consumed itself. Digestive enzymes are catalysts. Without digestive enzymes, digestion would be too slow to provide materials needed by the body. (para 6-16)

17.   The majority of digestion in humans takes place in the small intestines. Draped over these is a flap called the greater omentum. This flap has fat for insulation and many blood vessels for heat. Thus, the greater omentum may be compared to an "electric blanket" for the small intestines. (para 6-16c)

18.   The saliva contains enzymes that initiate the digestion of complex carbohydrates.

In the stomach, the gastric glands produce enzymes that initiate the digestion of proteins.

In the small intestines, there are digestive enzymes for carbohydrates, lipids, and proteins. These enzymes are found in the fluids produced by the pancreas and glands in the mucosa of the small intestines. Moreover, the liver produces a fluid called bile, which is stored in the gallbladder for release into the small intestines; this fluid helps in the digestion of lipids. (para 6-17)

19.   The absorptive area of the walls of the small intestines is increased by permanent circular folds (plicae circulares) and by fingerlike processes called villi. (para 6-19a)

20.   Simple sugars and amino acids are absorbed into the blood capillaries. Most of the fatty acids and glycerol are absorbed into the lymphatic capillaries. (para 6-19b)

21.   The blood capillaries absorbing substances from the digestive tract join to form the hepatic portal venous system. A venous portal system begins in capillaries, which join to form veins, which in turn end in another group of capillaries. The hepatic portal vein carries blood from the absorptive area of the digestive system to the liver. (para 6-20)

22.   In the liver, excess materials are removed and stored. For example, some glucose is stored as glycogen. Toxic materials are degraded. Microorganisms are removed. The "treated" blood is then routed from the liver to the heart and then throughout the body. (para 6-21)

23.   Lipid materials are stored as fat throughout the body so that they will be available when needed for energy. (para 6-22a)

24.   The lumen of the digestive system connects directly with the surrounding environment. For this reason, special protective mechanisms are associated with the human digestive system. Such mechanisms belong to the reticuloendothelial system.

        A primary component of the reticuloendothelial system are the lymphoid tissues. An important type of cell found within these tissues is the lymphocyte. These cells signal other types of white blood cells to phagocytize foreign materials. These tissues are more important in the child.

        The aggregate of lymphoid tissue at the beginning of the pharynx are called tonsils.

        Peyer's patches might be considered the "tonsils" of the small intestine.

        At the beginning of the large intestine, at the inferior end of the cecum, is the vermiform appendix, which might be considered the "tonsil" of the large intestines.

        Lining the sinusoids of the liver and removing harmful substances from the blood are Kupffer's cells. These cells are also considered to be part of the reticuloendothelial system. (paras 6-23 thru 6-29)

25.   During nursing, the initial secretion of the mammary glands is called colostrum. Although this secretion lacks nutrients, it is loaded with antibodies. These provide the infant with its primary protection for the first 6 months of life.

        Later, if the infant has an upper respiratory infection, the mammary gland will produce the appropriate antibodies. This is due to a reflux of fluid into the milk ducts of the mammary gland as the infant sucks. (para 6-30)

26.   Required in very small quantities from outside the body are substances called vitamins. These can be considered in two major categories--water-soluble and fat-soluble.

Water-soluble vitamins include the B-complex vitamins, vitamin C, and others. There is a daily requirement for water-soluble vitamins because they are continuously excreted with the urine.

On the other hand, fat-soluble vitamins accumulate in the fat of the body. (paras 6-31 thru 6-33)

27.   An important nondigestible food material is cellulose, commonly referred to as "fiber" or "bulk." Other undigested materials may be due to the consumption of great quantities of food. Undigested food materials enter the large intestines through the ileocecal valve. (para 6-34)

28.   A major function of the large intestines is to salvage water. To facilitate movement, mucus is added to the contents of the large intestines. Microorganisms in the large intestines manufacture vitamin K. Some microorganisms can act upon certain foods to produce gases. Feces is stored in the rectum and the lower portion of the sigmoid colon. Defecation is accomplished by relaxation of the anal sphincter muscles. (paras 6-35 thru 6-37)

End of Lesson 6

LESSON ASSIGNMENT

LESSON 7   The Human Respiratory System and Breathing.

LESSON ASSIGNMENT   Paragraphs 7-1 through 7-41.

LESSON OBJECTIVES   After completing this lesson, you should be able to:

                                  7-1. Match characteristics and processes of breathing and respiration with their descriptions.

                                  7-2. Given a list of sentences about respiration or breathing, select the false statement.

                                  7-3. Complete incomplete sentences about breathing or respiration.

SUGGESTION   After completing the assignment, complete the exercises at the end of this lesson. These exercises will help you to achieve the lesson objectives.

LESSON 7

THE HUMAN RESPIRATORY SYSTEM AND BREATHING

Section I. INTRODUCTION

7-1. PURPOSE OF RESPIRATION AND BREATHING

a. The processes of respiration and breathing serve to provide oxygen to the body cells. This oxygen is used in the process of metabolic oxidation. In metabolic oxidation, the energy trapped in glucose molecules is released for use in the body's activities.

b. Also, the carbon dioxide (CO_2) produced during metabolic oxidation and any other unwanted gases are removed from the body.

7-2. DEFINITIONS

a. **Respiration**. In general, respiration is the exchange of gases. In the human body, two kinds of respiration take place.

(1) <u>External respiration</u>. In external respiration, gases are exchanged between the blood and the surrounding air.

(2) <u>Internal respiration</u>. In internal respiration, gases are exchanged between the blood and the individual cells of the body.

b. **Breathing.** On the other hand, breathing is the process by which air is moved into and out of the lungs.

(1) <u>Types</u>. In humans, there are two types of breathing. In <u>costal breathing</u>, the rib cage is used. In <u>diaphragmatic breathing</u>, there is reciprocal interaction between the diaphragm and the abdominal wall.

(2) <u>Direction of air flow</u>. When the air flows inward, we call it <u>inhalation</u> (inspiration). When the air flows outward, we call it <u>exhalation</u> (expiration).

7-3. PHYSICAL PRINCIPLES

Both respiration and breathing are essentially physical processes. Air and/or various gases are moved from one place to another. Their movement is because of differences in their relative pressures from one space to another.

a. **Pressure Gradient.** Consider a situation in which there are two separate but connected spaces. If the concentration or pressure of that substance is greater in one space than the other, then there is a pressure gradient for that substance. As a result, the substance will move from the area of higher pressure to the area of lower pressure.

b. **Boyle's Law.** Assume that we have a container and we can change the volume of the container without allowing a gas to escape. Boyle's law tells us that if we increase the volume, the pressure inside will decrease. Likewise, if we decrease the volume, the pressure inside will increase.

c. **Pascal's Law.** If a closed container is filled with a fluid, a pressure applied to the fluid will produce an equal pressure at each and every point on the inner surface.

d. **Surface Area**. Most phenomena in breathing and respiration take place at one surface or another. As surface area increases, more gases can be exchanged or treated.

7-4. GENERAL ANATOMY AND CONSTRUCTION OF THE HUMAN TRUNK

The human trunk (Figure 7-1) can be considered a hollow cylinder. A muscular membrane, the thoracic diaphragm, extends across this hollow and divides the trunk into upper and lower cavities.

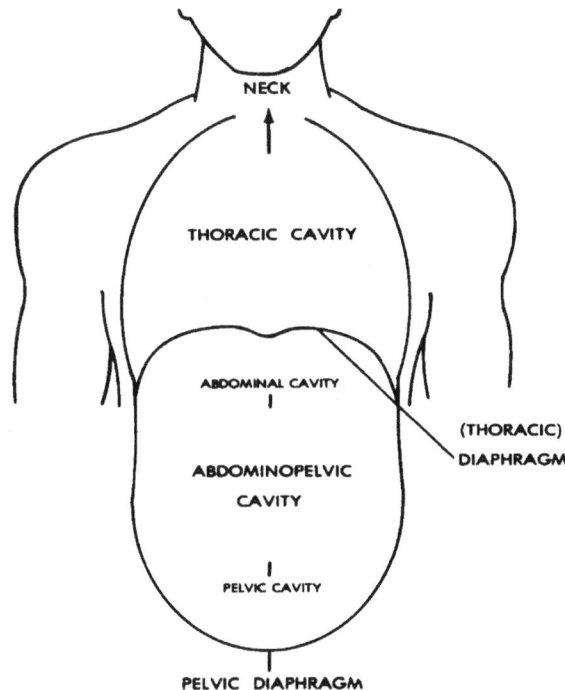

Figure 7-1. Schematic frontal section of the human trunk.

a. **Thoracic Cavity.** The thoracic cavity is the space of the trunk above the diaphragm. It is open to the outside by way of the neck and head. Since the wall of the thorax is reinforced by special muscles, bones, and cartilages, we can consider the thorax to be a "solid-walled container" filled with gas.

b. **Abdominopelvic Cavity.** The abdominopelvic cavity is the rest of the trunk cavity below the diaphragm. The abdominopelvic cavity is a closed system. Its walls are "elastic" since they are made up of musculature. The abdominopelvic cavity is filled with a fluid continuum. This fluid continuum consists primarily of water contained in the soft tissues of the abdomen and the pelvis.

Section II. INTRODUCTION TO HUMAN BREATHING

7-5. DEFINITION

Breathing is basically the process of moving air into and out of the lungs.

7-6. USE OF PRESSURE GRADIENTS

Breathing is accomplished by manipulating the pressure gradient between the surrounding atmosphere and the thoracic cavity. For all practical purposes, the pressure of the surrounding atmosphere can be considered a constant. Thus, the desired pressure gradients are achieved by changing the pressure within the thoracic cavity. The pressure in the thoracic cavity alternates so that it is less and then greater than the pressure of the surrounding atmosphere.

7-7. TYPES OF HUMAN BREATHING

The two types of human breathing are costal and diaphragmatic. They may be used individually and independently, or they may be used in combination.

7-8. LUNG CAPACITIES

a. **Total Lung Capacity.** From the instant of the "first breath," the lungs have a certain total volume called the total lung capacity. This is the entire volume of air in the lungs after one inhales as much as one can. Total lung capacity equals the sum of the residual volume and the vital capacity.

b. **Residual Volume.** After the "first breath," the lungs are never completely emptied. Thus, there is a certain portion of air that is always present in the lungs. After one exhales as much air as possible, the portion remaining in the lungs is called the residual volume. In actuality, this is not "dead air," because air circulation continually refreshes the air of the residual portion.

c. **Vital Capacity.** The vital capacity of the lung is the total amount of air that can be exchanged during total filling and emptying of the lung. For example, if one inhales as much air as one can and then exhales as much as possible, the volume exhaled would be the vital capacity.

7-9. BREATHING CYCLES

A breathing (respiratory) cycle is a sequence in which the lungs are filled and emptied to produce an exchange of the air in the lungs. The cycle includes an inhalation of air (filling of the lung with air), then a rapid exhalation (emptying), and then a short rest period. See Figure 7-2 for a representation of the "filling" of the lungs.

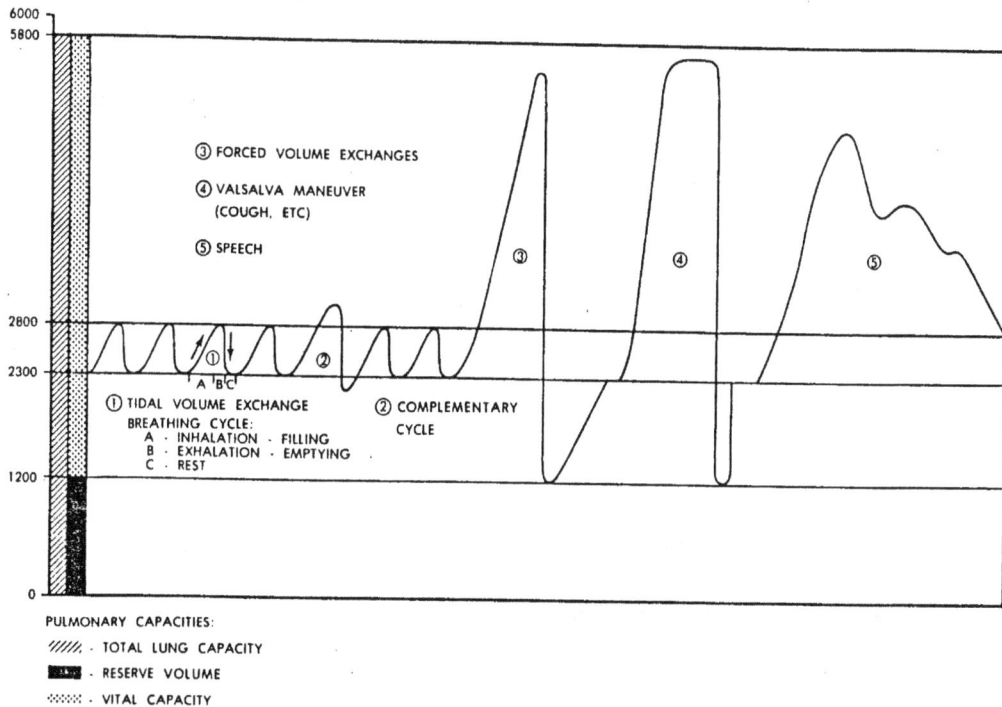

Figure 7-2. "Filling" of the lungs.

a. **Volume Exchanges During Breathing.** The amount of air exchanged in a given period depends upon the rate and depth (volume) of breathing. Rate and depth are adjusted according to physiological demand. The rate of respiration is the number of breathing cycles per minute.

b. **Some Types of Breathing Cycles.**

(1) Quiet ("tidal") breathing. As one takes part in ordinary, low-level activity, the breathing cycles are of the quiet type. This type involves only a minimal exchange of air.

(2) Complementary cycle. Over a period of time, quiet breathing may not totally satisfy the oxygen requirements of the body. Thus, we can observe a breathing cycle with a slightly greater volume exchange called the complementary cycle. It provides a little extra oxygen to make up the difference.

(3) Forced breathing. In forced breathing, the volumes of air exchanged are much greater than in quiet breathing. The actual volume exchanged depends upon the oxygen demand.

(4) Holding of breath. One can inhale a volume of air and hold it for a period. If one makes an exhalation effort but still holds the air inside the lungs, it is called Valsalva's maneuver (forced expiration against a closed glottis).

(5) Cough. If one suddenly releases the air, terminating Valsalva's maneuver, the result is a cough. If the musculature of a patient's abdominal wall is paralyzed, the patient cannot execute the Valsalva's maneuver and cannot produce a cough.

(6) Speech. During speech or vocalization, the breathing cycles overlap. That is, the subsequent cycle begins before the previous one is ended. The purpose of this is to maintain a continuous outflow of air.

Section III. COSTAL ("THORACIC") BREATHING

7-10. DEFINITION

Costal breathing is breathing accomplished by moving of the rib cage as a whole.

7-11. ANATOMY OF THE HUMAN RIB CAGE

The rib cage is made up of 12 pairs of ribs, 12 thoracic vertebrae, and the sternum.

a. **Ribs.**

(1) Structure of a "typical" rib. Each rib is a flat-type bone that is curved laterally. Along its inferior margin is a subcostal groove.

(2) Attachments.

(a) All 12 pairs of ribs are attached posteriorly to the thoracic vertebrae.

(b) Anteriorly, the upper 10 pairs of ribs are attached directly or indirectly to the sternum. The indirect attachments are made through costal cartilages to the ribs above.

(c) It is important to note that both the posterior and anterior articulations are located essentially in the midline of the body, back and front.

(3) <u>Costal cartilages</u>. The costal cartilages are bars of cartilage of varying lengths. Since costal cartilages are elastic, they can be twisted (deformed) and returned to their original shape.

b. **Sternum.** The sternum is located in the midline anteriorly, immediately beneath the skin. (Since the sternum is a flat bone with hematopoietic (blood-forming) red marrow and is so close to the surface of the body, it is a convenient location for taking a sample of hematopoietic tissue for clinical examination--the sternal punch.)

(1) The sternum is made up of three parts--the manubrium above, the body as the main portion, and the xiphoid process below.

(2) Where the manubrium articulates with the top of the body of the sternum is a sternal angle (Louis' angle). The sternal angle is important in costal breathing, since it allows for greater expansion of the rib cage. (In the clinic, the sternal angle is important as a landmark. It marks the site of the second rib and is used to identify locations on the chest wall.)

c. **Thoracic Vertebrae.** Posteriorly, there are 12 thoracic vertebrae, joined by intervertebral discs. Their curvature, the thoracic curvature, is concave anteriorly. During breathing, this curvature straightens and thus increases the expansion of the rib cage.

d. **Segmentation.** The segmentation of the thorax is produced by both the intervertebral discs and the intercostal spaces between adjacent ribs. Such segmentation of the rib cage allows motion to take place, especially bending to the right or left.

e. **Intercostal Muscles.** The intercostal spaces are filled by two layers of intercostal muscles. The intercostal muscles extend from the vertebrae behind to the sternum in front. A strengthening "plywood effect" is created by the arrangement of the two layers at a right angle to each other. Therefore, these muscles help to maintain the "solid-wall" condition of the thorax. For this reason, a pressure gradient can be maintained between the inside and outside of the thorax.

f. **Skeletal Muscles Attached to the Rib Cage.** Various skeletal muscles are attached to the rib cage. Some extend from above and draw the rib cage upward. Others extend from below and draw the cage downward.

7-12. COSTAL INHALATION

In costal inhalation, the lungs are expanded and inflated with air because of upward movement of the rib cage. The expansion of the rib cage is sufficient to allow the needed volume of air to enter the lungs. There are two different types of movements of the ribs that produce this expansion of the rib cage.

a. One type of movement involves the so-called "bucket handle" effect. As each rib swings upon its ends, like a bucket handle swinging up from the sides of the bucket, the rib moves upward and outward laterally. As this type of movement occurs on both sides of the rib cage, the transverse diameter of the rib cage increases from side to side.

b. The second type of movement is described as follows: The lowest points of the ribs are their front ends at the sternum. During inhalation, these front ends move upward and forward along with the sternum. This increases the diameter of the thoracic cavity from front to back (anterior-posterior (A-P) diameter).

c. The increases in the transverse and A-P diameters enlarge the volume of the thoracic cavity and thus decrease the pressure of the air inside (Boyle's law). Thus, there is a relatively higher atmospheric pressure outside. This pushes air into the respiratory passageways and into the alveoli of the lungs. The alveoli are inflated by this inflowing air.

7-13. COSTAL EXHALATION

a. The lungs empty during costal exhalation, a process that is essentially the reverse of costal inhalation. The rib cage moves downward as a whole.

(1) In small-volume exchanges, the costal cartilages are sufficiently resilient (elastic or springy) to pull the rib cage downward.

(2) With greater-volume exchanges, musculature can be recruited to aid in lowering the rib cage.

(3) Gravity may also play a role.

b. As the transverse and A-P diameters decrease, the volume of the thoracic cavity also decreases. This increases the pressure of the air inside (Boyle's law). Thus, there is a relatively lower atmospheric pressure outside, and air is forced out of the lungs. (The elasticity (springiness) of tissues within the thoracic cavity also helps to push the air out.)

Section IV. DIAPHRAGMATIC ("ABDOMINAL") BREATHING

7-14. PHYSICAL CHARACTERISTICS OF THE ABDOMINOPELVIC CAVITY

a. The abdominopelvic cavity is a closed system filled with a fluid (water) continuum.

b. The abdominopelvic cavity is inclosed by essentially muscular barriers.

(1) The inferior end is closed off by the pelvic diaphragm.

(2) The cylindrical walls of the abdomen are composed of three muscular sheets. Their orientation is similar to plywood. These muscles are kept taut by their intrinsic tone, but they are capable of additional contraction.

(3) Forming the top of the abdominopelvic cavity is the thoracic diaphragm. We discuss the thoracic diaphragm in the next paragraph.

7-15. THORACIC DIAPHRAGM

The thoracic diaphragm is attached to the inferior margin of the rib cage and to the bodies of the lumbar vertebrae behind. As a muscular membrane, it domes upward into the thoracic cavity. Upon contraction, the fibers of the thoracic diaphragm shorten and pull downward. This downward motion produces a piston-like pressure on the contents of the abdominopelvic cavity.

7-16. DIAPHRAGMATIC INHALATION

a. As the thoracic diaphragm contracts and lowers, the vertical diameter of the thoracic cavity is increased. This increases the volume of the thoracic cavity. Thus, according to Boyle's law, the pressure of the air in the lungs decreases. The relatively higher atmospheric pressure outside pushes the air into the lungs, and the alveoli are inflated.

b. At the same time, the thoracic diaphragm produces a pistol-like pressure upon the noncompressible fluid continuum in the abdominopelvic cavity. By Pascal's law, the resulting pressure is distributed equally to the elastic walls of the cavity. As these walls are stretched by the added pressure, they "store" potential energy.

7-17. DIAPHRAGMATIC EXHALATION

a. When the thoracic diaphragm relaxes, it no longer pushes down upon the contents of the abdominopelvic cavity. The potential energy stored in the stretched muscular walls becomes kinetic energy, and the walls rebound. This energy is sufficient for exhalation during quiet breathing.

b. However, during forced breathing, the muscles of the abdominal wall will contract in accordance with the amount of air to be pushed out.

c. As the muscles in the abdominal wall rebound (and contract in forced breathing), pressure is applied to the fluid continuum in the abdominopelvic cavity. By Pascal's law, this pressure is transferred to the underside of the thoracic diaphragm. The relaxed thoracic diaphragm is thus pushed up into the thoracic cavity. This decreases the vertical diameter and the volume of the thoracic cavity. The decreased volume results in increased pressure within the lungs (Boyle's law). Since the air pressure in the lungs is relatively greater than the outside atmospheric pressure, air is forced out through the respiratory passageways. (This is aided by the elastic rebound of tissues in the thoracic cavity.)

Section V. INTRODUCTION TO THE HUMAN RESPIRATORY SYSTEM

7-18. GENERAL

The human respiratory system consists of a series of organs that form a passageway for the air flowing to and from the alveoli of the lungs. The lungs themselves are discrete organs of the body containing the alveoli and are located in individual serous cavities.

7-19. DIVISIONS

The air passageway can be conveniently divided into three groups of structures. The larynx is the central portion. The other organs are grouped as supra laryngeal or infra-laryngeal.

Section VI. THE SUPRALARYNGEAL STRUCTURES

7-20. GENERAL FUNCTIONS

The general functions of the supra laryngeal structures (Figure 7-3) are to condition the in flowing air and to test it. Conditioning includes cleansing, warming, and moistening.

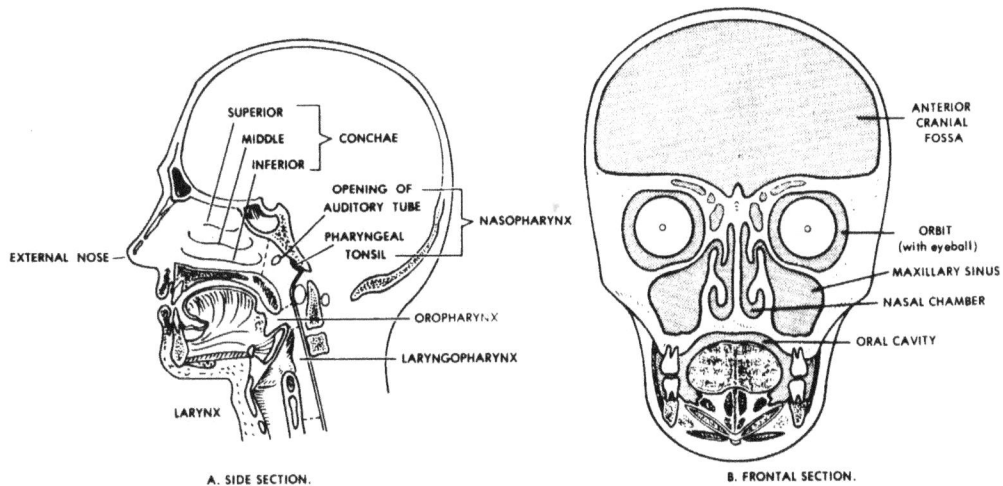

Figure 7-3. Supra laryngeal structures.

7-21. NOSE

The (external) nose is the beginning of the respiratory system in humans. It is located in the center of the front of the face. It is pyramid shaped, with the base facing inferiorly. The base consists of two openings called the nares or nostrils. These open into a pair of vestibules, one on each side. The nares are guarded by stiff nasal hairs. These nasal hairs serve to remove the larger particles (such as lint and cinders) from the inflowing air.

7-22. NASAL CHAMBERS

The vestibules of the nose are continuous posteriorly with the right and left nasal chambers.

a. **Nasal Septum.** Like the vestibules, the nasal chambers are separated by a nasal septum, a vertical wall from front to back. Constructed of bone and cartilage, the nasal septum extends from the floor to the roof and from front to back.

b. **Mucoperiosteal Lining.** Each nasal chamber is lined with a mucoperiosteal lining. This mucoperiosteal lining is a special combination of tissues, which are rich in blood vessels. This excellent supply of blood furnishes moisture and heat. On the surface of the mucoperiosteum are minute hair-like processes called cilia. The cilia continuously drive fluids on the surface to the rear. A part of the fluids secreted on the surface is a mucous material. As a part of the continuous process of cleansing the inflowing air, finer particles are trapped by the mucus.

c. **Conchae.** Thus, the conditioning of the inflowing air depends upon direct contact with the mucoperiosteum. The greater the surface area, the more efficient will be the conditioning. The <u>conchae</u> are three shelf-like projections that extend from the lateral wall of each nasal chamber. Thus, a superior, a middle, and an inferior concha are found on each side. During ordinary breathing, the air enters the vestibules of the nose and passes through the lower portions of the nasal chambers in direct contact with the inferior and middle conchae.

      d. **Olfactory Epithelium.** As the air passes through the nasal chambers, some of the air reaches the superior recesses of the nasal chambers. In these superior recesses is found the <u>olfactory epithelium</u>. The olfactory epithelium contains special hair cells that can detect individual molecules found in the air. Thus, the sense of smell (olfaction), tests the quality of inflowing air.

      e. **Paranasal Sinuses.** Connected with each nasal chamber are cavities found in the middle layer of various skull bones. These cavities are the paranasal sinuses. Like the nasal chambers, they are lined with a continuation of the mucoperiosteum. Each paranasal sinus is named according to the bone in which it is located. The function of the paranasal sinuses is unknown.

7-23. NASOPHARYNX

      The two nasal chambers are continuous posteriorly with a single cavity known as the nasopharynx.

      a. **Pharyngeal Tonsils ("Adenoids").** The pharyngeal tonsils are a pair of lymphoid aggregates in the upper posterior recess of the nasopharynx.

      b. **Auditory (Pharyngeotympanic or Eustachian) Tubes.** On each lateral wall of the nasopharynx is a small mound with a slit-like opening. This is the opening of the <u>auditory tube</u>, which passes laterally to the middle ear cavity. Because of this tube, the air pressures are kept equal on the inner and outer sides of the tympanic membrane (eardrum).

      c. **Soft Palate.** The floor of the nasopharynx is the soft palate. The soft palate is a musculomembranous structure. (Unlike the soft palate, the hard palate is bony. The hard palate forms the floor of the nasal chambers and the roof of the oral cavity.)

7-24. PHARYNX AND FUNCTION OF SOFT PALATE

      The <u>nasopharynx</u> (of the respiratory system) and the <u>oropharynx</u> (of the digestive system) are continuous posteriorly with the <u>pharynx proper</u>. During swallowing, the soft palate is raised like a trap door to close off the upper air passageways. This prevents movement of food into the upper air passageways.

Section VII. LARYNX

7-25. INTRODUCTION

The larynx (voice box; "Adams apple") is located in the lower anterior neck region. In many respects, the larynx is different in men and women (sexual dimorphism).

7-26. LARYNX AS A PART OF THE HYOID COMPLEX

The larynx is suspended from the hyoid bone by a membrane. The root of the tongue is attached to the top anterior portion of the hyoid bone. These three structures--the larynx, the hyoid bone, and the tongue--are together known as the hyoid complex. They always move together as a unit.

7-27. GENERAL FUNCTIONS OF THE LARYNX

The larynx performs several functions in humans.

a. Its primary function is to control the volume of the air passing through the air passageways, to and from the alveoli of the lungs (para 7-28).

b. The larynx also produces selected vibration frequencies in the moving column of air (para 7-29).

c. During swallowing, the hyoid complex is raised into the oral cavity. As this happens, the epiglottis of the larynx acts like a trap door, turning down to cover the entrance of the larynx. This prevents swallowed items from entering the lower air passageway, altogether forming the glottis.

7-28. CONTROL OF VOLUME OF AIR

A pair of folds is found at the bottom of the vestibule of the larynx. These are called the vocal folds or true vocal cords. Extending from front to back, there is one vocal fold on each side. With a special set of muscles, the vocal folds can be drawn apart or pulled together, altogether forming the glottis.

a. Thus, the vocal folds are used to control the size of the opening between them, which is called the rima glottidis. When the rima glottidis is wide, air can flow easily between the upper and lower air passageways. When the vocal cords are drawn so tightly that the rima glottidis is completely closed, no air can flow through.

b. In Valsalva's maneuver (para 7-9b(4), (5)), the lungs are filled with air and the rima glottidis is closed tightly. The muscles of the trunk wall contract strongly to increase the internal pressure of the trunk.

(1) This internal pressure stiffens the trunk into a more rigid structure. Thus, one uses Valsalva's maneuver to provide support for a strenuous effort with the upper members.

(2) When Valsalva's maneuver is followed by a sudden opening of the rima glottidis, the result is a cough. This is used to clear the air passageways.

(3) An individual whose trunk wall muscles are paralyzed cannot do these things.

7-29. PRODUCTION OF HUMAN SPEECH

Human speech is a combination of a number of processes. Essentially, a column of air flows out through the oral cavity, where it is chopped into bits of speech known as phonemes.

a. Speech sounds produced when the oral cavity is not blocked are called vowels. Sounds resulting from the closing or chopping action of the oral cavity are known as consonants.

b. The column of air vibrates at different frequencies (pitch). These vibration frequencies are gained by the air as it passes through the larynx. The pitch is varied by a change in the tension of the vocal cords. The higher the tension, the higher will be the pitch (vibration frequency).

Section VIII. THE "RESPIRATORY TREE" AND PULMONARY ALVEOLI

7-30. INTRODUCTION

The infralaryngeal structures (Figure 7-4) include the "respiratory tree" and the lungs. The respiratory tree is so named because it has the appearance of an inverted tree, with its trunk and branches. It is essentially a tubular structure connecting the larynx to the alveoli of the lungs. This tubular structure is lined with a ciliated epithelium. (Remember, cilia are hair-like projections from cells.) The tubes are kept open (patent) by a series of ring-like structures of cartilage.

7-31. TRACHEA

The "trunk" of the tree is the trachea. The trachea extends from the inferior margin of the larynx, down through the neck, and into the center of the thorax.

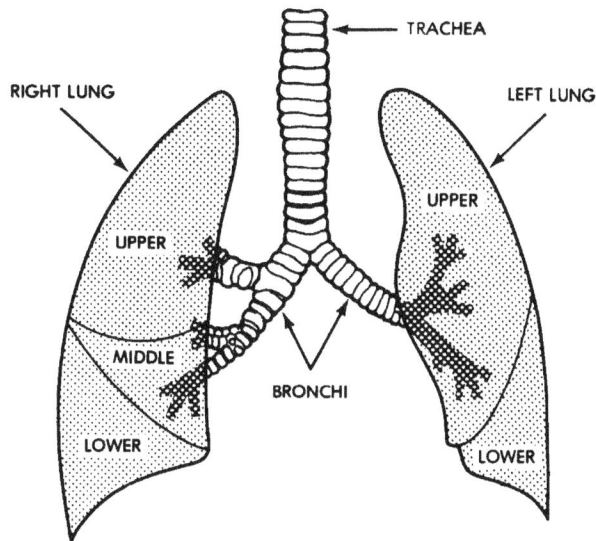

Figure 7-4. Infralaryngeal structures.

7-32. BRONCHI

In the center of the thorax, the trachea divides into right and left primary bronchi. The right is somewhat more vertical than the left. Therefore, when a person accidentally aspirates ("breathes in") a foreign object, it is more likely to be found in the right primary bronchus than the left.

a. Each primary bronchus extends laterally into the substance of the appropriate lung. Within each lung, the tubular structure divides, subdivides, and divides again, up to about 30 times. Thus, the tubes become more and more numerous and smaller and smaller in size. At the terminals of the branching tubes are groups of spherical alveoli. This gives the appearance of a bunch of grapes.

b. A variety of situations may occlude (close or shut off) these tubular air passageways.

(1) A foreign object may be aspirated ("breathed in").

(2) The wall of the tube may constrict in a bronchial spasm.

(3) The lining of the tube may become swollen with fluid and close the passageway.

7-33. "DEAD AIR"

None of the air found in the upper and lower passageways plays a part in actual respiration. Thus, this air is often referred to as "dead air." During quiet breathing, it amounts to about two-fifths of the total air volume exchanged.

7-34. PULMONARY ALVEOLI

External respiration is the exchange of gases between the air and the blood. External respiration takes place in the alveoli (alveolus, singular). The alveoli are small, spherical sacs that are continuous with the terminal elements of the branches of the respiratory tree. As we indicated earlier, external respiration is a surface phenomenon in which the gases pass through the wall of the alveolus.

a. Since there is a critical relationship between volume and surface area, the inflated alveolus is spherical. The alveolus is also of a particular size that is ideal for the efficiency of external respiration.

b. In each lung, there are billions of alveoli.

c. Numerous blood capillaries are adjacent to the walls of the alveoli.

d. To facilitate the exchange of gases between the air in the alveolus and the blood in the capillaries, the wall of the alveolus contains a special chemical known as surfactant.

e. The inner surfaces of the alveoli must be kept wet to make the transfer of gases possible. Because these surfaces are wet, one of the major fluid losses of the body is with the exhaled air.

Section IX. LUNGS AND PLEURAL CAVITIES

7-35. INTRODUCTION

In the thoracic cavity is a pair of lungs. Each lung is an individual organ containing the branching elements of one side of the respiratory tree, the connected alveoli, and the corresponding pulmonary NAVL. As with the other organs, the tissues are held together with fibrous connective tissue (FCT).

a. The lungs are located within individual serous cavities, called the pleural cavities. The lungs with their pleural cavities constitute the major contents of the thoracic cavity. The pleural cavities help to provide lubrication.

b. Located in the middle of the thorax, between the two pleural cavities, is the mediastinum ("I stand between"). The mediastinum is a tissue- and organ-filled space. Within it, the heart (of the blood circulatory system) is located at the same level as the lungs.

7-36. LUNG STRUCTURE

The two lungs occupy their respective sides of the thoracic cavity.

a. The left lung tends to be smaller. This makes room for the extension of the heart into the left side of the thorax.

b. In general, the right lung is divided into three major lobes. The left lung is in two major lobes.

c. Due to the branching pattern of the respiratory tree (and associated NAVL), each lung consists of broncho pulmonary segments--10 in the right lung and 8 in the left lung.

7-37. PLEURAL CAVITIES

Surrounding each lung individually is a serous cavity, called the pleural cavity. The minute quantity of serous fluid in the cavity serves as a lubricant. This serves to minimize friction for the expansion and contraction of the lungs during breathing.

a. Each lung is intimately covered with a serous membrane, the visceral pleura.

b. The outer wall of the pleural cavity is lined with another serous membrane known as the parietal pleura. Areas of the parietal pleura are variously named according to their location.

(1) The mediastinal pleura forms the lateral wall of the mediastinum.

(2) The diaphragmatic pleura covers the superior surface of the diaphragm.

(3) The costal pleura lines the inner surface of the rib cage.

(4) The cupolar pleura is a dome-like extension into the root of the neck. It contains the apex of the lung.

c. When each lung is in its smaller volume, its corresponding diaphragmatic pleura lies close to the lower costal pleura. The slit-like cavity between them is called the costophrenic sinus. Fluids of each pleural cavity tend to collect in this sinus, since it is the lowest area for each. When the diaphragm contracts and flattens out, each costophrenic sinus opens up and the inferior portion of the expanding lung occupies this space.

Section X. THE PULMONARY NAVL

7-38. NERVOUS CONTROL OF BREATHING

As we have seen, breathing is a combination of many factors. These factors are integrated and controlled by the nervous system.

a. Respiratory reflexes are controlled by the <u>respiratory center</u> found in the medullary portion of the hindbrainstem. (See lesson 12). The <u>level of carbon dioxide</u> (CO_2) in the circulating blood is one of the major influences upon the respiratory reflex.

b. The individual <u>intercostal nerves</u> innervate the intercostal muscles.

c. The <u>muscles attached to and moving the rib cage</u> are innervated by their appropriate nerves. (Ultimately, almost every muscle in the body may be mobilized to assist in breathing.)

d. The diaphragm is innervated by its own individual pair of <u>phrenic</u> <u>nerves</u>.

7-39. FUNCTIONAL BLOOD SUPPLY

There are essentially two blood supplies for the lungs--nutrient blood and functional blood. <u>Nutrient blood</u> is carried by the bronchial arteries from the thoracic aorta. Nutrient blood provides nourishment and oxygen to the tissues of the lung. <u>Functional blood</u> is actually involved in the respiratory exchange of gases between the alveoli and the capillaries. Functional blood is brought to and from the lungs by the <u>pulmonary cycle of the cardiovascular system</u>.

a. The pulmonary cycle originates in the <u>right ventricle</u> of the heart. Contraction of the right ventricle forces the blood into the <u>pulmonary arch</u>, which divides into the right and left <u>pulmonary arteries</u> to their respective lungs. Paralleling the branching of the respiratory tree, the arteries divide and subdivide within the lungs. These arteries lead to <u>capillaries</u> in the vicinity of the alveoli. The walls of these capillaries are thin enough to accommodate the passage of gases to and from the alveolus.

b. The blood, now saturated with oxygen, is collected by the <u>pulmonary venous system</u>. The blood is deposited ultimately into the <u>left</u> <u>atrium</u> of the heart.

Section XI. EXCHANGE AND TRANSPORTATION OF GASES: ARTIFICIAL BREATHING/RESUSCITATION

7-40. EXCHANGE AND TRANSPORTATION OF GASES

a. **Gases Involved.** Oxygen and carbon dioxide are the primary gases involved in respiration. Under special circumstances, nitrogen may also be of concern.

b. **Pressure Gradients.** A gas moves from an area where its pressure is greater to an area where its pressure is less. Thus, the movement of gases depends upon such pressure gradients.

c. **External Respiration.** At the alveoli, gases are exchanged between the air inside and the blood in the adjacent capillaries.

d. **Internal Respiration.** Within the body, gases are exchanged between the blood of the capillaries and the individual cells of the body.

e. **Transportation of Gases.** The gases are transported (Figure 7-5) between the alveoli and the individual cells by the cardiovascular system.

(1) Some of the gases are dissolved directly in the plasma of the blood.

(2) However, in humans, the greater percentage of the gases is carried within the substance of the RBCs (red blood cells, erythrocytes). The RBC, found in great numbers in the blood, is specially constructed for transporting the gases. Hemoglobin, a substance found within RBCs, has a great affinity for oxygen. Yet, the hemoglobin can readily give up the oxygen wherever it is needed.

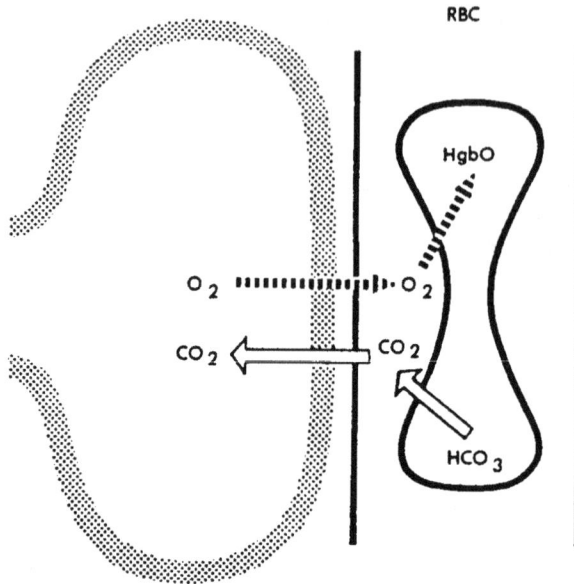

A. AT THE ALVEOLUS (EXTERNAL RESPIRATION).

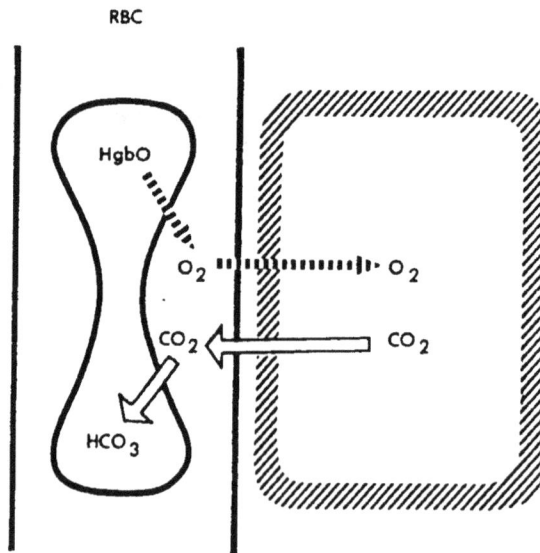

B. AT THE BODY CELL (INTERNAL RESPIRATION).

Figure 7-5. Scheme of the exchange of the gases.

7-41. ARTIFICIAL BREATHING/RESUSCITATION

When an individual stops breathing, he will soon die if the tissues of the body, particularly the brain, do not get a fresh supply of oxygen.

a. Various mechanical devices are sometimes used to maintain breathing. One is the pulmotor.

b. In "mouth-to-mouth" resuscitation, the operator forces air from his own respiratory system into the respiratory system of the patient. Fortunately, the initial air forced into the patient is the "dead air" of the operator and still has its full amount of oxygen.

c. There are also various techniques for manipulating the patient's rib cage to simulate normal function.

d. At times, gravity may be used to assist a patient. In particular postures, a patient may find breathing easier. Also, under certain circumstances, a patient may be positioned to drain accumulated fluids from specific parts of the lungs.

Continue with Exercises

EXERCISES, LESSON 7

REQUIREMENT. The following exercises are to be answered by completing the incomplete statements.

After you have completed all the exercises, turn to "Solutions to Exercises" at the end of the lesson, and check your answers.

1. The processes of respiration and breathing serve to provide _____n to the body cells. This oxygen is used in the process of m_____ o_____, which releases the energy trapped in g_____ e molecules.

Also, the gas _____ n _____ e is removed along with other unwanted gases.

2. In general, respiration is the exchange of _____s. The two kinds of respiration in the human body are e_____l and i_____l respiration. In external respiration, gases are exchanged between the _____d and the surrounding _____. In internal respiration, gases are exchanged between the _____d and the individual _____s of the body.

3. Breathing is the process by which _____r is moved into and out of the _____s. The two types of breathing in humans are _____l breathing and d_____c breathing. In costal breathing, the _____ cage is used. In diaphragmatic breathing, there is reciprocal interaction between the _____m and the abdominal _____l.

When the air flows inward, we call it inh_____ or ins_____. When the air flows outward, we call it exh_____ or exp_____.

4. In respiration and breathing, the movement of air and various gases is due to d_____s in their relative p_____s from one space to another. If the pressure or concentration of a substance is greater in one space than another, then there is a p_____ e g_____t for that substance. As a result, the substance will move from the area of _____er pressure to the area of _____er pressure.

Boyle's Law: If we increase the volume of a closed container, the pressure inside will (increase) (decrease). Likewise, if we decrease the volume, the pressure inside will (increase) (decrease).

Pascal's Law: A pressure applied to the fluid filling a closed container will produce an _____l pressure at each and every point on the inner surface.

More gases can be exchanged or treated as the surface area (increases) (decreases).

5.   Since the wall of the thorax is reinforced by muscles, bones, and cartilages, we can consider the thorax to be a "_____d-walled c_____r" filled with gas.

    The abdominopelvic cavity is filled with a f____d c_____m, the water of the soft tissues.

6.   Breathing is the process of _____ing air into and out of the _____s.

    Breathing involves the pressure gradient between the surrounding at_____ and the _____c cavity. Since atmospheric pressure is relatively constant, breathing depends upon changing the pressure within the t_____ c_____.

7.   The lungs have a certain total volume called the _____l lung _____y. There is a certain portion of air always present in the lungs, called the r_____l_____e. If one inhales as much air as possible and then exhales as much as possible, the volume exhaled is called the _____l_____y.

8.   The breathing cycle includes an i_____n, e_____n, and then a short _____ period. The rate of respiration is the number of breathing _____s per _____. The amount of air exchanged in a given period depends upon the _____e and _____h of breathing, which are adjusted according to physiological _____d.

9.   In ordinary, low-level activity, the breathing cycles are of the _____t type. Occasionally, there will be a breathing cycle with a slightly greater volume exchange, called the _____y cycle.

    The volumes of air exchanged are much greater in _____d breathing. The volume depends upon the _____n demand.

    If one makes an exhalation effort but still holds the air inside the lungs, it is called _____'s maneuver. If one suddenly releases the air, the result is a _____.

10.   Costal breathing is accomplished by moving the r____ ____e as a whole.

11.   In costal inhalation, the lungs are expanded and inflated with air as a result of the _____d movement of the rib cage.

    The "bucket handle" effect increases the _____e diameter of the rib cage. The second type of movement increases the _____r-_____r diameter of the rib cage.

These increased diameters enlarge the volume of the _____c_____y.
Thus, the pressure of the air inside (decreases) (increases). The pressure difference
forces air into the _____y passages and into the a_____i of the lungs.

12.   Costal exhalation is essentially the reverse of ____l_____n. The rib cage
moves _____ward as a whole. There is a decrease in the _____se and __-__
diameters. This ___creases the pressure inside so that it is (greater) (less) than the
pressure outside.

13.   The abdominopelvic cavity is enclosed by essentially _____r barriers.

       The thoracic diaphragm is attached to the inferior margin of the ___ _____
and to the bodies of the lumbar _____e behind. It domes upward into the
_____ cavity. As the diaphragm contracts, it moves _____ward and produces a
piston-like pressure on the contents of the a_____c cavity.

14.   As the thoracic diaphragm contracts and lowers, the vertical _____r of the
thoracic cavity increases. This increases the volume of the _____ cavity. Thus, the
pressure of the air in the lungs (increases)(decreases). Thus, air moves (into) (out of)
the lungs.

       The walls of the abdominopelvic cavity are _____d by the added pressure.
As this happens, the walls store _____ energy.

15.   When the thoracic diaphragm relaxes, the potential energy stored in the
stretched muscular walls becomes _____ energy, and the walls rebound. During
forced breathing, the walls _____t for the amount of air to be pushed out.

       When the abdominal walls rebound or contract, pressure is transferred to the
underside of the _____c_____m. The relaxed thoracic diaphragm is thus pushed
up into the t_____c_____. This decreases the v_____l d_____r and v_____e
of the thoracic cavity. This results in ___creased pressure within the lungs, and air is
forced (out) (in) through the respiratory passageways.

16.   The general functions of the supralaryngeal structures are to condition the
inflowing air and to _____t it. Conditioning includes cl_____ing, w_____ing, and
m_____ing.

17.   The nares are guarded by stiff nasal _____s, which serve to remove (larger)
(smaller) particles from the inflowing air.

18.   The excellent supply of blood to the mucoperiosteal lining of the nasal chambers furnishes _____ e and _____ t.

The cilia continuously drive fluids on the surface to the <u>(front) (rear)</u>.

Finer particles carried by the inflowing air are trapped by the _____. The conditioning of the inflowing air depends upon direct contact with the m_____ m. The conchae serve to increase the s_____ a_____ of the mucoperiosteum in the nasal chambers.

The olfactory epithelium contains special hair cells which can detect individual m_____ s found in the air. Thus, the sense of smell tests the _____ y of inflowing air.

The paranasal sinuses are cavities found in the middle layer of various skull _____ s.

19.   The primary function of the larynx is to control the volume of _____ passing through the air passageways to and from the alveoli. The larynx also produces selected vibration _____ s in the moving column of air. The epiglottis of the larynx acts like a _____ to prevent food items from entering the lower air passageways.

20.   The vocal folds are used to control the size of the _____ g between them, called the r_____ s.

Valsalva's maneuver is used to provide support for a strenuous effort with the _____ r_____ s. When Valsalva's maneuver ends with a sudden opening of the rima glottidis, the result is a _____ h.

21.   A column of air may be chopped into bits of s_____. The frequencies of the vibrations are the _____ h, varied by a change in the _____ n of the vocal cords.

22.   A variety of situations may occlude a bronchus: A foreign _____ may be aspirated. The wall of the tube may constrict in a bronchial _____ m. The lining of the tube may become _____ n with fluid and close the passageway.

23.   The air in the passageways does not take part in actual _____ n. Therefore, it is often called "_____ air."

24.   External respiration is the exchange of gases between the air and the _____.
It takes place in the _____i, which are small, spherical _____s. Adjacent to the walls
of the alveoli are numerous blood _____s. The wall of the alveolus contains a special
chemical known as _____t. To make the transfer of gases possible, the inner
surface of the alveoli must be kept ____t.

25.   The pleural cavities help to provide _____n for the expansion and contraction
of the _____s.

26.   Respiratory reflexes are controlled by the _____y center in the medullary
portion of the h_____m. One of the major influences upon this center is the
level of c_____ d_____ in the circulating blood.

27.   Providing nourishment and oxygen to the tissues of the lung is the _____
blood. Actually involved in the exchange of gases is the _____ blood.

28.   Functional blood is brought to and from the lungs by the _____y cycle of the
cardiovascular system. This cycle includes the right _____, the _____ arch,
the right and left _____ arteries, the _____s in the vicinity of the alveoli,
the pulmonary _____s system, and the (left) (right) atrium.

29.   Gases are transported between the alveoli and the individual cells by the
_____ system. Some of the gases are dissolved directly in the _____ of
the blood. However, in humans, the greater percentage of the gases is carried within
the substance of the _____s. Within these cells, there is a substance which readily
accepts and gives up oxygen; this substance is called _____.

30.   In "mouth-to-mouth" resuscitation, the initial air forced into the patient is the
"_____ air," which still has its full amount of _____.

Check Your Answers on Next Page

SOLUTIONS TO EXERCISES, LESSON 7

1.   The processes of respiration and breathing serve to provide <u>oxygen</u> to the body cells. This oxygen is used in the process of <u>metabolic oxidation</u>, which releases the energy trapped in <u>glucose</u> molecules.

     Also, the gas <u>carbon dioxide</u> is removed along with other unwanted gases. (para 7-1)

2.   In general, respiration is the exchange of <u>gases</u>. The two kinds of respiration in the human body are <u>external</u> and <u>internal</u> respiration. In external respiration, gases are exchanged between the <u>blood</u> and the surrounding <u>air</u>. In internal respiration, gases are exchanged between the <u>blood</u> and the individual <u>cells</u> of the body. (para 7-2a)

3.   Breathing is the process by which <u>air</u> is moved into and out of the <u>lungs</u>. The two types of breathing in humans are <u>costal</u> breathing and <u>diaphragmatic</u> breathing. In costal breathing, the <u>rib</u> cage is used. In diaphragmatic breathing, there is reciprocal interaction between the <u>diaphragm</u> and the abdominal <u>wall</u>.

     When the air flows inward, we call it <u>inhalation</u> or <u>inspiration</u>. When the air flows outward, we call it <u>exhalation</u> or <u>expiration</u>. (para 7-2b)

4.   In respiration and breathing, the movement of air and various gases is due to <u>differences</u> in their relative <u>pressures</u> from one space to another. If the pressure or concentration of a substance is greater in one space than another, then there is a <u>pressure gradient</u> for that substance. As a result, the substance will move from the area of <u>higher</u> pressure to the area of <u>lower</u> pressure.

     Boyle's Law: If we increase the volume of a closed container, the pressure inside will <u>decrease</u>. Likewise, if we decrease the volume, the pressure inside will <u>increase</u>.

     Pascal's Law: A pressure applied to the fluid filling a closed container will produce an <u>equal</u> pressure at each and every point on the inner surface.

     More gases can be exchanged or treated as the surface area <u>increases</u>. (para 7-3)

5.   Since the wall of the thorax is reinforced by muscles, bones, and cartilages, we can consider the thorax to be "<u>solid</u>-walled <u>container</u>" filled with gas.

     The abdominopelvic cavity is filled with a <u>fluid continuum</u>, the water of the soft tissues. (para 7-4)

6.   Breathing is the process of <u>moving</u> air into and out of the <u>lungs</u>.

Breathing involves the pressure gradient between the surrounding <u>atmosphere</u> and the <u>thoracic</u> cavity. Since atmospheric pressure is relatively constant, breathing depends upon changing the pressure within the <u>thoracic cavity</u>.
(paras 7-5, 7-6)

7.   The lungs have a certain total volume called the <u>total</u> lung <u>capacity</u>. There is a certain portion of air always present in the lungs, called the <u>residual volume</u>. If one inhales as much air as possible and then exhales as much as possible, the volume exhaled is called the <u>vital capacity</u>. (para 7-8)

8.   The breathing cycle includes an <u>inhalation</u> (or <u>inspiration</u>), and <u>exhalation</u> (or <u>expiration</u>), and then a short <u>rest</u> period. The rate of respiration is the number of breathing <u>cycles</u> per <u>minute</u>. The amount of air exchanged in a given period depends upon the <u>rate</u> and <u>depth</u> of breathing, which are adjusted according to physiological <u>demand</u>. (para 7-9)

9.   In ordinary, low-level activity, the breathing cycles are of the <u>quiet</u> type. Occasionally, there will be a breathing cycle with a slightly greater volume exchange, called the <u>complementary</u> cycle.

The volumes of air exchanged are much greater in <u>forced</u> breathing. The volume depends upon the <u>oxygen</u> demand.

If one makes an exhalation effort but still holds the air inside the lungs, it is called <u>Valsalva's</u> maneuver. If one suddenly releases the air, the result is a <u>cough</u>.
(para 7-9b)

10.   Costal breathing is accomplished by moving the <u>rib cage</u> as a whole. (para 7-10)

11.   In costal inhalation, the lungs are expanded and inflated with air because of the <u>upward</u> movement of the rib cage.

The "bucket handle" effect increases the <u>transverse</u> diameter of the rib cage. The second type of movement increases the <u>anterior-posterior</u> diameter of the rib cage.

These increased diameters enlarge the volume of the <u>thoracic cavity</u>. Thus, the pressure of the air inside <u>decreases</u>. The pressure difference forces air into the <u>respiratory</u> passages and into the <u>alveoli</u> of the lungs. (para 7-12)

12.   Costal exhalation is essentially the reverse of <u>costal inhalation</u>. The rib cage moves <u>downward</u> as a whole. There is a decrease in the <u>transverse</u> and <u>A-P</u> diameters. This <u>increases</u> the pressure inside so that it is <u>greater</u> than the pressure outside. (para 7-13)

13.   The abdominopelvic cavity is inclosed by essentially muscular barriers.

        The thoracic diaphragm is attached to the inferior margin of the rib cage and to the bodies of the lumbar vertebrae behind. It domes upward into the thoracic cavity. As the diaphragm contracts, it moves downward and produces a piston-like pressure on the contents of the abdominopelvic cavity. (paras 7-14, 7-15)

14.   As the thoracic diaphragm contracts and lowers, the vertical diameter of the thoracic cavity increases. This increases the volume of the thoracic cavity. Thus, the pressure of the air in the lungs decreases. Thus, air moves into the lungs.

        The walls of the abdominopelvic cavity are stretched by the added pressure. As this happens, the walls store potential energy. (para 7-16)

15.   When the thoracic diaphragm relaxes, the potential energy stored in the stretched muscular walls becomes kinetic energy, and the walls rebound. During forced breathing, the walls contract for the amount of air to be pushed out.

        When the abdominal walls rebound or contract, pressure is transferred to the underside of the thoracic diaphragm. The relaxed thoracic diaphragm is thus pushed up into the thoracic cavity. This decreases the vertical diameter and volume of the thoracic cavity. This results in increased pressure within the lungs, and air is forced out through the respiratory passageways. (para 7-17)

16.   The general functions of the supralaryngeal structures are to condition the inflowing air and to test it. Conditioning includes cleansing, warming, and moistening. (para 7-20)

17.   The nares are guarded by stiff nasal hairs, which serve to remove larger particles from the inflowing air. (para 7-21)

18.   The excellent supply of blood to the mucoperiosteal lining of the nasal chambers furnishes moisture and heat.

        The cilia continuously drive fluids on the surface to the rear.

        Finer particles carried by the inflowing air are trapped by the mucus. The conditioning of the inflowing air depends upon direct contact with the mucoperiosteum. The conchae serve to increase the surface area of the mucoperiosteum in the nasal chambers.

        The olfactory epithelium contains special hair cells that can detect individual molecules found in the air. Thus, the sense of smell tests the quality of inflowing air.

        The paranasal sinuses are cavities found in the middle layer of various skull bones. (para 7-22)

19.   The primary function of the larynx is to control the volume of <u>air</u> passing through the air passageways to and from the alveoli. The larynx also produces selected vibration <u>frequencies</u> in the moving column of air. The epiglottis of the larynx acts like a <u>trap door</u> to prevent food items from entering the lower air passageways. (para 7-27)

20.   The vocal folds are used to control the size of the <u>opening</u> between them, called the <u>rima glottidis.</u>

Valsalva's maneuver is used to provide support for a strenuous effort with the <u>upper</u> members. When Valsalva's maneuver ends with a sudden opening of the rima glottidis, the result is a <u>cough</u>. (para 7-28)

21.   A column of air may be chopped into bits of <u>speech</u>. The frequencies of the vibrations are the <u>pitch</u>, varied by a change in the <u>tension</u> of the vocal cords. (para 7-29)

22.   A variety of situations may occlude a bronchus: A foreign <u>object</u> may be aspirated. The wall of the tube may constrict in a bronchial <u>spasm</u>. The lining of the tube may become <u>swollen</u> with fluid and close the passageway. (para 7-32b)

23.   The air in the passageways does not take part in actual <u>respiration</u>. Therefore, it is often called "<u>dead</u> air." (para 7-33)

24.   External respiration is the exchange of gases between the air and the <u>blood</u>. It takes place in the <u>alveoli</u>, which are small, spherical <u>sacs</u>. Adjacent to the walls of the alveoli are numerous blood <u>capillaries</u>. The wall of the alveolus contains a special chemical known as <u>surfactant</u>. To make the transfer of gases possible, the inner surfaces of the alveoli must be kept <u>wet</u>. (para 7-34)

25.   The pleural cavities help to provide <u>lubrication</u> for the expansion and contraction of the <u>lungs</u>. (paras 7-35a, 7-37)

26.   Respiratory reflexes are controlled by the <u>respiratory</u> center in the medullary portion of the <u>hindbrainstem</u>. One of the major influences upon this center is the level of <u>carbon dioxide</u> in the circulating blood. (para 7-38)

27.   Providing nourishment and oxygen to the tissues of the lung is the <u>nutrient</u> blood. Actually involved in the exchange of gases is the <u>functional</u> blood. (para 7-39)

28.   Functional blood is brought to and from the lungs by the <u>pulmonary</u> cycle of the cardiovascular system. This cycle includes the right <u>ventricle</u>, the <u>pulmonary</u> arch, the right and left <u>pulmonary</u> arteries, the <u>capillaries</u> in the vicinity of the alveoli, the pulmonary <u>venous</u> system, and the <u>left</u> atrium. (para 7-39)

29.   Gases are transported between the alveoli and the individual cells by the cardiovascular system. Some of the gases are dissolved directly in the plasma of the blood. However, in humans; the greater percentage of the gases is carried within the substance of the RBCs. Within these cells, there is a substance that readily accepts and gives up oxygen; this substance is called hemoglobin. (para 7-40e)

30.   In "mouth-to-mouth" resuscitation, the initial air forced into the patient is the "dead air," which still has its full amount of oxygen. (para 7-41b)

End of Lesson 7

LESSON ASSIGNMENT

LESSON 8   The Human Urinary System.

LESSON ASSIGNMENT   Paragraphs 8-1 through 8-7.

LESSON OBJECTIVES   After completing this lesson, you should be able to identify the major function of the urinary system.

SUGGESTION   After completing the assignment, complete the exercises at the end of this lesson. These exercises will help you to achieve the lesson objectives.

LESSON 8

THE HUMAN URINARY SYSTEM

Section I. THE KIDNEY

8-1. INTRODUCTION TO THE URINARY SYSTEM

a. The urinary system is a collection of organs to rid the body of nitrogenous wastes. These nitrogenous wastes are created by the metabolism of proteins.

b. The urinary system includes the organs known as the kidney, the ureters, the urinary bladder, and the urethra (Figure 8-1). Together, these organs remove the nitrogenous wastes from the circulating blood, concentrate them into a fluid known as urine, and eliminate the urine from the body.

8-2. GENERAL ANATOMY OF THE KIDNEY

In the human, there are two kidneys, one right and one left.

a. **Location.** Both kidneys are attached high up on the posterior abdominal wall. The left kidney is slightly higher than the right.

b. **Shape.** In the adult, each kidney measures about 1x2x4 inches. The kidneys have a kidney-bean shape. That is, they are notched on the medial side, they have a convex lateral curvature, and their front and rear surfaces are somewhat flat.

c. **Capsule.** Each kidney is surrounded by a dense FCT membrane called a capsule.

d. **Internal Structure.** When a kidney is cut from side to side, the internal structure is similar to that in Figure 8-1. There is a fleshy portion surrounding a central opening. The fleshy portion is divided into an outer cortex layer and an inner medulla.

(1) The medulla consists of a series of pyramids whose apices (peaks) point into the hollow center of the kidney. The apex (peak) of each renal pyramid is known as the papilla.

R ——— KIDNEY ——— L

— URETER —

URINARY
BLADDER

URETHRA

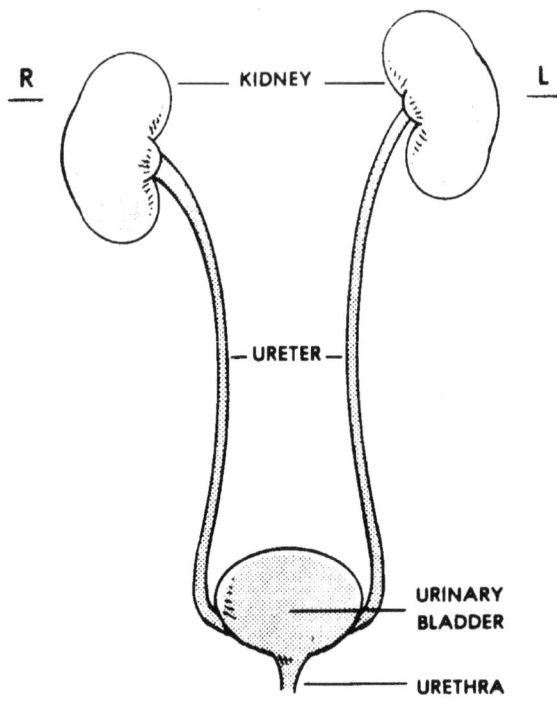

A. GENERAL SCHEME.

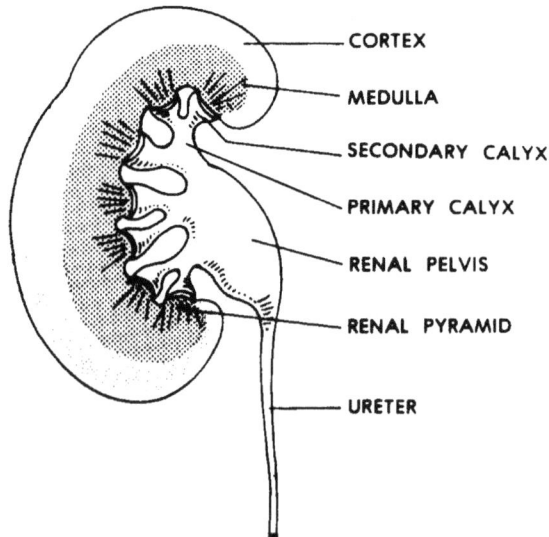

CORTEX

MEDULLA

SECONDARY CALYX

PRIMARY CALYX

RENAL PELVIS

RENAL PYRAMID

URETER

B. FRONTAL SECTION OF A KIDNEY.

Figure 8-1. The human urinary system.

(2) The central cavity of the kidney is known as the renal sinus. Its opening on the medial aspect of the kidney is known as the hilus (or hilum). The sinus contains a number of structures:

(a) The spaces among these structures are filled with loose areolar FCT (fibrous connective tissue) and fat.

(b) The renal NAVL enter the kidney directly from the abdominal aorta, through the hilus, and into the renal sinus. They then continue in a regular pattern throughout the medulla and cortex of the kidneys.

(c) A funnel-shaped, cup-like tube, called a calix (or calyx), surrounds the papilla of each pyramid. All of the calices are continuous with and empty into a hollow structure called the renal pelvis.

e. **Adherence to the Posterior Abdominal Wall.** Each kidney is attached to the posterior abdominal wall on its respective side. Enclosing the kidneys and holding them in place are special perirenal fascial membranes and perirenal fats. During a "crash diet," an individual may lose some of this perirenal fat. This allows the kidney to move with the motions of the body. If the kidney should slump too far down, a kink may form in the ureter. This would prevent the normal flow of urine from the kidney to the bladder.

8-3. THE NEPHRON

The actual unit of kidney function is the structure referred to as the nephron (Figure 8-2). It is estimated that each kidney has about a million nephrons. Each nephron consists of a renal corpuscle and a tubular system.

a. **Renal Corpuscle.** A nephron begins with a renal corpuscle. The renal corpuscle is made up of a double-walled capsule and an arterial capillary network known as the glomerulus. An afferent arteriole supplies blood to the glomerulus, and an efferent arteriole drains blood from the glomerulus.

AFFERENT = carry to

EFFERENT = carry away from

The blood from the afferent arteriole fills the glomerulus. Because of a pressure gradient, a large percentage of fluid in this blood passes through the wall of the glomerular capillary. The fluid then passes through the inner wall of the capsule. This brings the fluid into the hollow space between the inner and outer walls of the capsule.

b. **Tubular System.** The fluid, or filtrate, then passes through the tubular system of the nephron. Here, the majority of the water, glucose, and other valuable substances are reabsorbed from the fluid and returned to the cardiovascular system.

Thus, at the end of the tubular system, the result is a very concentrated fluid containing the nitrogenous wastes. This concentrated fluid is called urine.

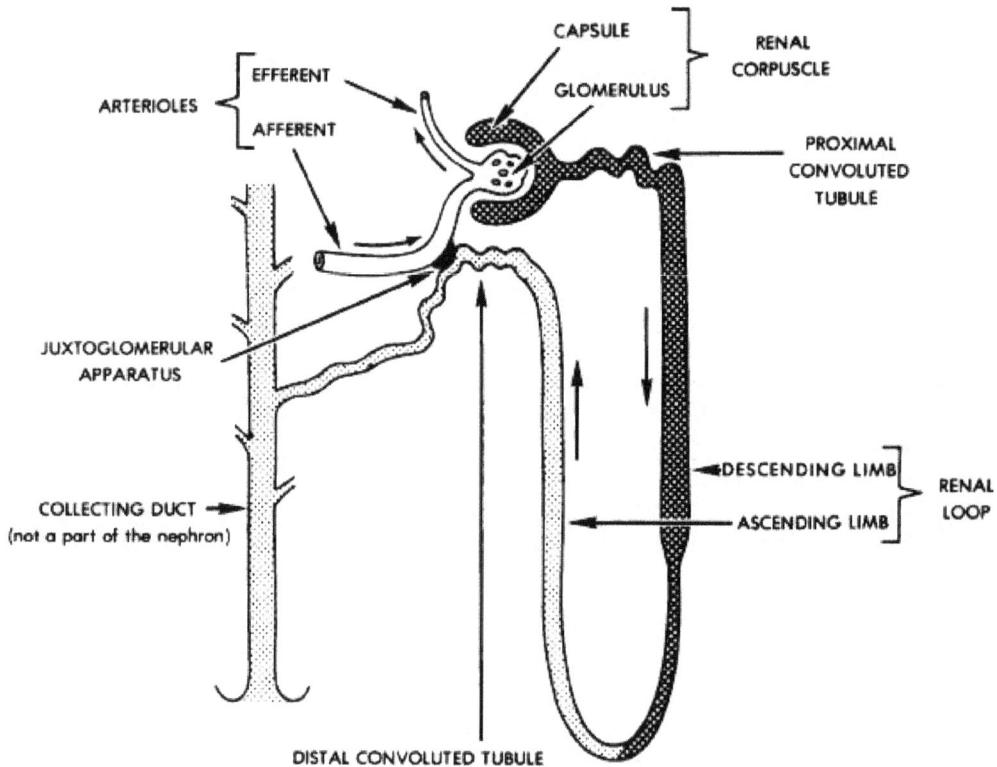

Figure 8-2. A "typical" nephron.

8-4. COLLECTION OF URINE

The urine from each nephron flows into a collecting tubule (straight renal tubule). The collecting tubules merge until they form one of the papillary ducts that open at the papilla of the renal pyramid. At the papilla, the urine empties into the calices. The urine then flows into the renal pelvis in the sinus of the kidney.

Section II. OTHER PARTS OF THE HUMAN URINARY SYSTEM

8-5. THE URETERS

The ureter is a tubular structure that is continuous with the renal pelvis. The ureter of each kidney passes down the posterior abdominal wall on its respective side.

The ureter then enters the pelvic region. The urine moves along the ureters drop by drop, pushed by the wave like muscular contractions (peristalsis) of the tubular wall. In the pelvis, the two ureters enter the posterior inferior corners of the urinary bladder.

8-6. THE URINARY BLADDER

The urinary bladder is an organ that is highly specialized to store urine until it is eliminated from the body.

a. **Trigone.** The base of the urinary bladder is known as the trigone because of its triangular shape. The trigone is fairly solid and nonstretchable.

b. **Stretchable Wall.** The rest of the wall of the urinary bladder is very stretchable and forms a spherical sac when filled.

c. **Transitional Epithelial Lining.** The mucosal lining of the urinary bladder is made up of a unique epithelium, called the transitional epithelium.

(1) Voiding reflex. The transitional epithelium has the capacity to stretch to a certain degree. At the limit of its stretchability, it causes a message to be sent to the spinal cord about the fullness of the urinary bladder. This initiates the voiding reflex, which would cause the urine to pass out of the body.

(2) Increments of stretching and reorganization. Often, however, it is not convenient to void (empty the bladder). Thus, after a short period, the transitional epithelium can reorganize itself and undergo another increment of stretching. Soon, however, the fullness message is somewhat more urgent. There can be several increments of stretching until the limit of the urinary bladder is finally reached. At that limit, the urine must be voided.

8-7. THE URETHRA

The urethra is the single tubular structure that connects the urinary bladder to the outside.

a. **Sexual Dimorphism.** Relatively short and straight, the female urethra opens directly to the outside. However, the male urethra is incorporated into the penis. Since the male urethra has two more-or-less right-angle turns, one permanent and one flexible, the male is more difficult to catheterize than the female.

b. **Urethral Sphincters.** The urethral sphincters are two muscular structures which prevent urine from leaving the urinary bladder. Each urethral sphincter is a circular mass of muscle tissue. Relaxation of the sphincters allows urine to be forced through them.

Continue with Exercises

EXERCISES, LESSON 8

REQUIREMENT. The following exercises are to be answered by completing the incomplete statements. After you have completed all the exercises, turn to "Solutions to Exercises" at the end of the lesson, and check your answers.

1.   The urinary system is a collection of organs to rid the body of n_____ _____s, created by the metabolism of _____s. These organs remove the n_____ _____s from the circulating _____d, concentrate them into a fluid known as _____e, and eliminate the _____e from the body.

2.   A nephron begins with a renal c_____. The renal corpuscle is made up of a double-walled c_____ and an arterial capillary network known as the g_____. Supplying blood to the glomerulus is an _____t arteriole. Draining blood from the glomerulus is an _____t arteriole. Fluid from the blood in the glomerular capillary passes into space between the inner and outer walls of the c_____.

3.   The fluid, called f_____, passes through the tubular system of the n_____. As this fluid passes through the tubular system, substances such as w_____ and g_____ are reabsorbed and returned to the c_____ system. The resulting c_____d fluid is called _____e.

4.   At the papilla, the urine empties into the c_____s. The urine then flows into the renal p_____ in the s_____ of the kidney. The urine then moves along the _____s drop by drop until it reaches the u_____ b_____.

5.   The urinary bladder is highly specialized to _____e urine until it is e_____d from the body. Thus, except for the trigone, the wall of the urinary bladder is very _____ble.

    When the transitional epithelium reaches the limit of its stretchability, a message is sent to initiate the _____ing reflex. There can be several i_____s of stretching until the limit of the urinary _____r is reached.

6.   The urethra is the single tubular structure which connects the urinary bladder to the _____e. The female urethra is relatively s____t and s_____t. The male urethra has two more-or-less r____-a____ turns.

    Two muscular structures preventing urine from leaving the urinary bladder are the u_____ _____s. Urine is forced through them when the sphincters ____x.

Check Your Answers on Next Page

SOLUTIONS TO EXERCISES, LESSON 8

1.   The urinary system is a collection of organs to rid the body of <u>nitrogenous</u> <u>wastes</u>, created by the metabolism of <u>proteins</u>. These organs remove the <u>nitrogenous</u> <u>wastes</u> from the circulating <u>blood</u>, concentrate them into a fluid known as <u>urine</u>, and eliminate the <u>urine</u> from the body. (para 8-1)

2.   A nephron begins with a renal <u>corpuscle</u>. The renal corpuscle is made up of a double-walled <u>capsule</u> and an arterial capillary network known as the <u>glomerulus</u>. Supplying blood to the glomerulus is an <u>afferent</u> arteriole. Draining blood from the glomerulus is an <u>efferent</u> arteriole. Fluid from the blood in the glomerular capillary passes into the space between the inner and outer walls of the <u>capsule</u>. (para 8-3)

3.   The fluid, called <u>filtrate</u>, passes through the tubular system of the <u>nephron</u>. As this fluid passes through the tubular system, substances such as <u>water</u> and <u>glucose</u> are reabsorbed and returned to the <u>cardiovascular</u> system. The resulting <u>concentrated</u> fluid is called <u>urine</u>. (para 8-3b)

4.   At the papilla, the urine empties into the <u>calices</u>. The urine then flows into the renal <u>pelvis</u> in the <u>sinus</u> of the kidney. The urine then moves along the <u>ureters</u> drop by drop until it reaches the <u>urinary</u> <u>bladder</u>. (paras 8-4 and 8-5)

5.   The urinary bladder is highly specialized to <u>store</u> urine until it is <u>eliminated</u> from the body. Thus, except for the trigone, the wall of the urinary bladder is very <u>stretchable</u>.

     When the transitional epithelium reaches the limit of its stretchability, a message is sent to initiate the <u>voiding</u> reflex. There can be several <u>increments</u> of stretching until the limit of the urinary <u>bladder</u> is reached. (para 8-6)

6.   The urethra is the single tubular structure that connects the urinary bladder to the <u>outside</u>. The female urethra is relatively <u>short</u> and <u>straight</u>. The male urethra has two more-or-less <u>right-angle</u> turns.

     Two muscular structures preventing urine from leaving the urinary bladder are the <u>urethral sphincters</u>. Urine is forced through them when the sphincters <u>relax</u>. (para 8-7)

End of Lesson 8

LESSON ASSIGNMENT

LESSON 9   The Human Reproductive (Genital) System.

LESSON ASSIGNMENT   Paragraphs 9-1 through 9-23.

LESSON OBJECTIVES   After completing this lesson, you should be able to:

9-1. Given a list of statements describing functions of the human reproductive system, identify the false statement.

9-2. Match names of subgroups of reproductive organs with their definitions.

SUGGESTION   After completing the assignment, complete the exercises at the end of this lesson. These exercises will help you to achieve the lesson objectives.

LESSON 9

THE HUMAN REPRODUCTIVE (GENITAL) SYSTEM

Section I. INTRODUCTION

9-1. DEFINITION

The human reproduction system is a collection of organs for the production of offspring. Thus, succeeding generations are provided for the continuation of the species.

9-2. TWO DISTINCT SEXES

In humans there are two distinctly separate sexes, male and female. The presence of different anatomical forms of the two sexes is called sexual dimorphism.

DI = two

MORPH = body form

SEXUAL = by virtue of sex

The contribution of hereditary materials by two parents increases the chances for improved genetic recombinations.

9-3. SEX HORMONES

Sex hormones are body chemicals associated with sex and sexual development. They belong to a chemical group called steroids. Sex hormones are formed primarily in two types of organs: the gonads and the adrenal cortex. (The adrenal cortex is the outer layer of the adrenal gland, which rests upon each kidney). The sex hormones of the female are called estrogens and progesterone. The sex hormones of the male are called androgens.

9-4. MAJOR ORGAN SUBGROUPS

In both males and females, the organs of the reproductive system can be grouped according to function. These subgroups are the primary sex organs (gonads), the secondary sex organs, and the secondary sexual characteristics.

9-5. EXTERNAL GENITALIA

In both sexes, there are certain structures at the surface known as the external genitalia.

9-6. COMMON EMBRYONIC ORGANS

In male and female embryos, there is a common origin of the organs of the reproductive system. (The organs of the urinary system share this common origin). The importance of this common origin is that, under certain conditions, females may develop with males characteristics, males may develop with female characteristics, and even true intersexes may occur. (True intersexes possess both male and female gonadal tissue.)

9-7. SEX DETERMINATION

At the moment the egg is fertilized by the sperm, the new genetic combination determines whether the individual will be male or female. Later in development, however, sex hormones play an important role in the production of sexual organs and characteristics.

Section II. GAMETES (SEX CELLS)

9-8. INTRODUCTION

Within the genetic makeup of each individual, there is a pair of chromosomes known as the sex chromosomes. There are two kinds of such chromosomes--X and Y.

9-9. MEIOSIS

Within the gonads, there is a special type of cell division known as meiosis. The usual set of chromosomes is reduced in this reduction division. Thus, the gametes (ova or spermatozoa) have only a single set of chromosomes.

9-10. FERTILIZATION

In the final analysis, the production of a new individual is based upon the union of the male gamete (spermatozoon) with the female gamete (ovum). This process is called fertilization. At this time, a double set of chromosomes is reconstituted.

a. If the zygote (fertilized egg) has two X chromosomes, the individual will be female (XX).

b. If the zygote has one X and one Y chromosome, the individual will be male (XY).

Section III. THE MALE REPRODUCTIVE SYSTEM (FIGURE 9-1)

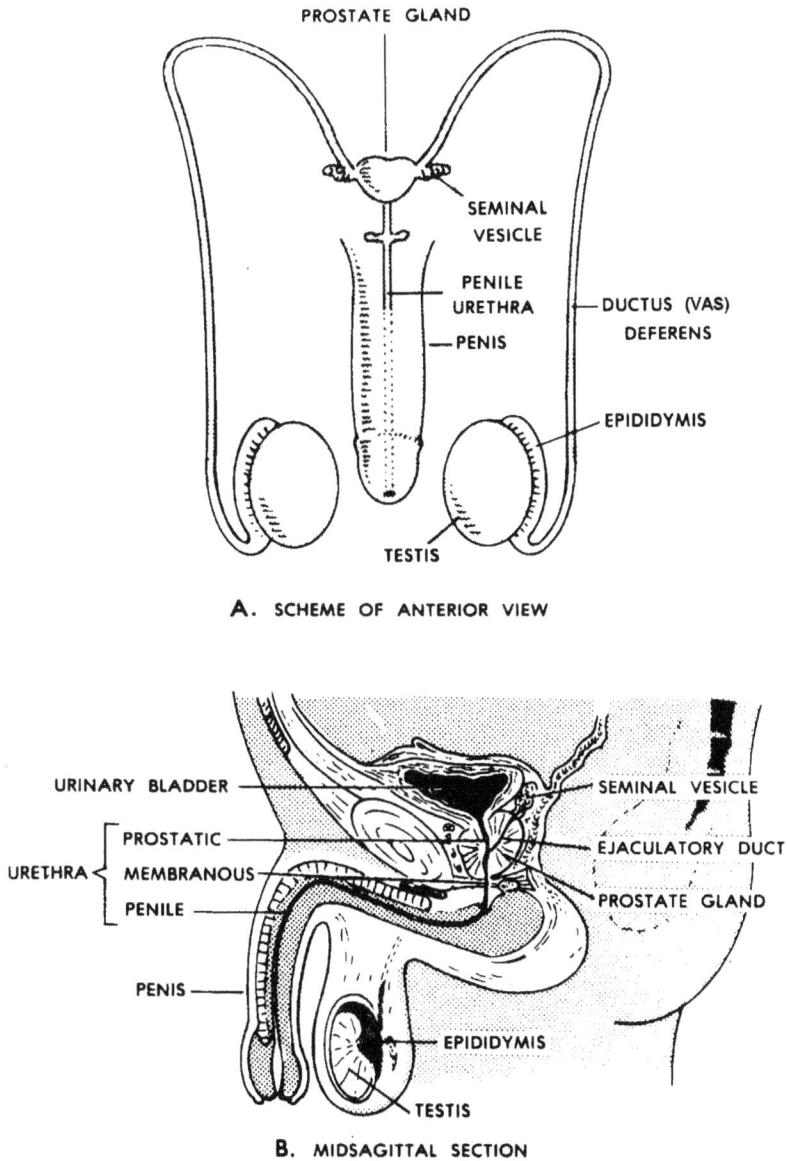

A. SCHEME OF ANTERIOR VIEW

B. MIDSAGITTAL SECTION

Figure 9-1. The human male reproductive (genital) system.

9-11. PRIMARY SEX ORGAN--TESTIS

The testis is the primary sex organ (gonad) of the male

a. **Location.** Each male has a pair of testes located within the scrotum. The scrotum is a sac suspended from the inferior end of the trunk, between the thighs. Each testis is within a separate serous cavity within the scrotum.

(1) Migration. Originally, testes develop within the posterior abdominal region of the body. However, during development, they "migrate" out of the body cavity, through the inguinal canal of the abdominal wall, and into the scrotum.

(2) Temperature control. For the production of mature sperm (spermatozoa), the testes must be at a temperature that is a few degrees lower than that of the body cavity. For this reason, the testes are located outside of the body cavity.

(a) Under cold conditions, each testis is pulled up toward the body by the cremaster muscle. At the same time, the dartos muscle of the scrotal wall contracts and thus reduces the exposed surface area and thickens the wall.

(b) Under warm conditions, these structures are "relaxed." This allows the scrotum with the testes to hang free.

(c) If a boy baby is born with undescended testes (either in the abdominal cavity or inguinal canal) and if nothing is done to bring the testes into the scrotum, he will be sterile.

b. **Production of Spermatozoa.** Millions of spermatozoa (male gametes) are produced by the seminiferous tubules of the testis.

SEMEN = seed

FER = to carry

The male sex hormones (androgens) are also produced by cells of the testes.

9-12. SECONDARY SEX ORGANS

In general, the secondary sex organs of the male are responsible for the transport and care of the spermatozoa.

a. **Epididymis.** The spermatozoa pass from the seminiferous tubules into the tubular structure known as the epididymis. The epididymis is a very long tube, but it is coiled and attached to the surface of the testis in the scrotum. As the spermatozoa pass along the length of the epididymis, they are nurtured by the secretions of the epididymal wall. During this passage through the epididymis, the spermatozoa become mature functioning gametes. They remain in the epididymis until "called for."

b. **Ductus (Vas) Deferens.** During sexual excitement, the spermatozoa leave the epididymis and are carried by another duct known as the ductus deferens. The ductus deferens passes through the inguinal canal, enters the body cavity, and turns into the pelvic cavity.

c. **Seminal Vesicle.** At the posterior surface of the prostate gland, the ductus deferens is joined by another duct called the seminal vesicle. The seminal vesicle is also a long tubular structure, but it is coiled up into a small mass at the back of the prostate gland. The seminal vesicle produces a nutrient fluid that helps to maintain the spermatozoa.

d. **Ejaculatory Duct.** On each side, as the ductus deferens and seminal vesicle join, they form a single tube on the same side, called the ejaculatory duct. Each ejaculatory duct, left and right, carries the seminal vesicle secretion and spermatozoa through the substance of the prostate gland. Each ejaculatory duct empties into the prostatic urethra.

e. **Prostate Gland.** The prostate gland is located in the pelvic cavity immediately under the urinary bladder. The urethra of the urinary system passes through the substance of the prostate gland, where it is known as the prostatic urethra. The prostate gland also adds a secretion. Altogether, the combination of secretions and spermatozoa is known as the semen.

f. **Urethra.** In the male, the urethra is common to both the urinary system and the reproductive system. At different times, it carries either the urine or the semen.

(1) As already mentioned, the initial part of the urethra passes through the prostate gland and is called the prostatic urethra.

(2) Immediately below the prostate gland, the urethra passes through the perineal membrane. Here, it is surrounded by the external urethral sphincter. This short section of the urethra is called the membranous urethra.

(3) That portion of the urethra passing through the penis (discussed below) is known as the penile urethra.

g. **Penis.** The penis is a structure attached to the pubic arch of the bony pelvis and to the underside of the perineal membrane. It is an external structure of the male genital system, which is capable of enlargement and stiffening (erection).

(1) The most favorable position for the deposit of semen (spermatozoa) is the upper recess of the vagina. This is opposite the opening of the cervix of the uterus. For this purpose, the penis is inserted into the female vagina ("sheath").

(2) Covering the glans ("head") of the penis is a fold of skin called the prepuce. In many cultures, the prepuce is removed shortly after birth in the procedure called circumcision. At the base of the glans, there are glands that secrete a lipid-like material called smegma. Thus, there is a need for continual cleanliness.

9-13. SECONDARY SEXUAL CHARACTERISTICS

The secondary sexual characteristics of the male are those features designed to make a male attractive to the female. They help ensure that the two sexes will get together to produce the new generation. Among the more obvious of these features are muscularity, deep voice, and hair distribution.

Section IV. THE FEMALE REPRODUCTIVE SYSTEM (FIGURE 9-2)

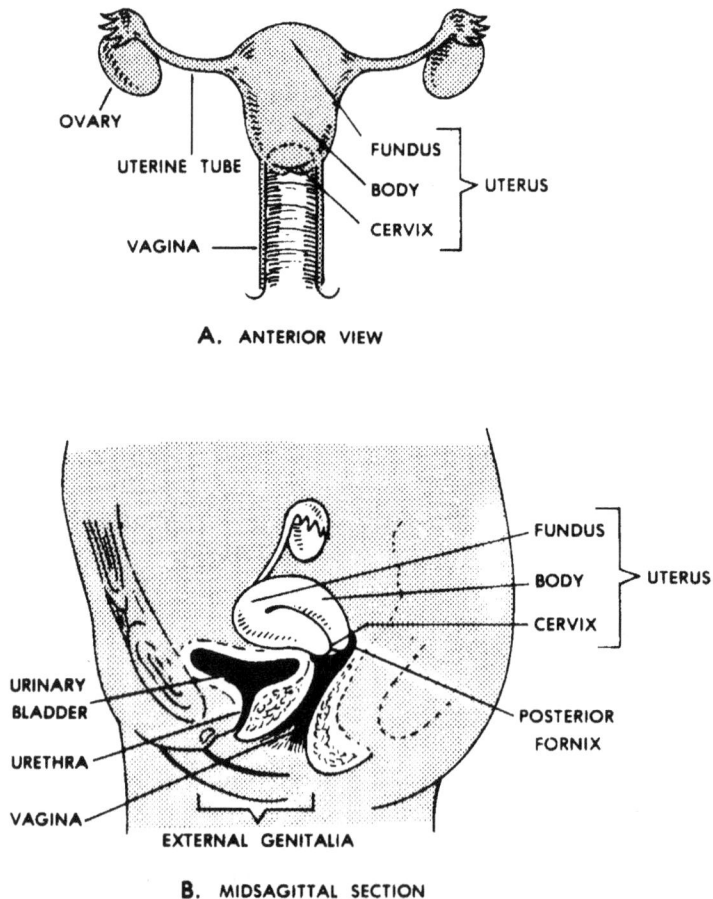

Figure 9-2. The human female reproductive (genital) system.

9-14. PRIMARY SEX ORGAN--OVARY

The ovary is the primary sex organ (gonad) of the female.

a. **Location.** Each female has a pair of ovaries, located in the pelvic cavity. Each ovary is attached to the posterior aspect of the broad ligament on its respective side of the uterus.

b. **Production of the Ovum.** One female gamete (ovum) is released per menstrual cycle (about 28 days).

(1) Within an ovary, one of the germinal cells begins to develop and grows larger as it stores food material. This development takes place within a follicle, a fluid-filled cavity within the ovary.

(2) At midperiod, the mature ovum is expelled from the follicle onto the surface of the ovary. The free ovum is picked up by the uterine tube. (para 9-15a).

c. **Production of Female Sex Hormones.** Initially, the cells of the ovary that form the follicle secrete the hormones called estrogens. After the ovum has been expelled from the follicle, the resulting cavity is filled with a yellowish material known as the corpus luteum. The corpus luteum secretes primarily progesterone, a hormone that helps prepare the uterus for pregnancy. Thus, estrogens are secreted during the first half of the menstrual cycle, and progesterone is added during the second half of the period. This pattern of hormone secretion is a major factor in the menstrual cycle.

9-15. SECONDARY SEX ORGANS

The secondary sex organs of the female serve to transport and care for the ovum and to develop the new individual (embryo and fetus).

a. **Uterine Tube (Oviduct, Fallopian Tube).** The uterine tube picks up the free ovum when it is expelled from the follicle of the ovary. The ovum stays in the uterine tube to await fertilization. If it is fertilized, it goes through the initial stages of embryonic development, and the embryo then passes on to the uterus. On the other hand, if it is not fertilized, its stored food is exhausted in 3 to 5 days; it dies and its remains are absorbed by the uterine tube.

b. **Uterus.** The uterus is a single pear-shaped organ located within the pelvic cavity of the female. The early embryo passes into the uterus from the uterine tube. The embryo continues its development within the uterus.

(1) Endometrium. The inner lining of the uterus is known as the endometrium. The endometrium is an epithelium containing uterine glands and blood vessels. Under the influence of the estrogens and progesterone, the embryo present at

the end of the menstrual cycle, the endometrium breaks down. (This produces a "flow" of blood and cellular elements (menses) in a process known as menstruation.)

(2) Amniotic sac and placenta. When the embryo passes into the uterine cavity from the uterine tube, it "burrows" into the endometrium. Later, a fluid-filled sac (the amniotic sac) surrounds the embryo. The embryo floats free, surrounded by amniotic fluid. The embryo has an umbilical cord that originates in the center of its anterior abdomen. The umbilical cord is attached to the wall of the uterus by a special structure known as the placenta.

(3) Cervix. The cervix, the inferior end of the uterus, is inserted into the top of the vagina. Through the center of the cervix is the cervical canal. Its wall consists primarily of circular muscle tissue, which holds the opening closed until time for parturition (giving birth). During the initial stage of parturition, the cervical musculature dilates (stretches) to form an opening for the passage of the newborn (to be).

c. **Vagina.** The vagina is a tubular structure that extends from the cervix of the uterus to the exterior of the perineum. After the vagina receives the male penis, the semen is discharged into the upper recess opposite the opening of the cervix. At parturition, the vagina forms the birth canal through which the newborn passes to the outside.

d. **External Genitalia.** The opening of the vagina and of the urethra are covered by the external genitalia. Included among the external genitalia are two pairs of folds--the major and minor labia. Also included is the clitoris, a small structure comparable to the male penis but without the urethra.

9-16. SECONDARY SEXUAL CHARACTERISTICS

The secondary sexual characteristics of the female are those features designed to make a female attractive to the male. These features include a higher-pitched voice, hair distribution, and body softness and shape.

9-17. THE FEMALE BONY PELVIS

The female bony pelvis is an important consideration in childbirth.

a. Several studies have been concerned with the spatial relationships of the female bony pelvis. One of the most extensive is the Caldwell-Moloy Classification of Female Pelvis. This study categorizes female pelvis by shape. It illustrates those types that are better and those that are less well suited for childbirth.

b. Just before childbirth, the phenomenon of "relaxation" occurs. In this phenomenon, the ligaments of the bony pelvis and perineum become quite stretchable. This increases the diameters of the birth canal.

9-18. THE MAMMARY GLAND

The mammary glands are cutaneous glandular structures of the female.

a. **Location.** The mammary glands are located in the upper pectoral regions. On occasion, a mammary gland may be found elsewhere along the "milk line." The milk line extends from the axilla above to the inguinal region below.

b. **Structure.** Each mammary gland is made up of glandular tissue and associated ducts. These structures are embedded in FCT and fat.

c. **Lactation.** During pregnancy, the mammary glands respond to the estrogens and progesterone with additional growth. Toward the end of pregnancy, it begins to form a fluid substance, colostrum. Within 2 or 3 days after the baby is born, the breasts begin to secrete large quantities of milk instead of colostrum.

d. **Importance of Nursing.** One cannot overemphasize the importance of nursing (breast-feeding) the newborn.

(1) Human milk is the natural food of the newborn infant.

(2) Strong psychological effects accompany nursing. This is true for both the child and the mother.

(3) Initially after childbirth, the mammary gland secretes colostrum. Colostrum is not primarily a food item. In fact, the baby loses birth weight. Colostrum consists most importantly of antibodies that protect the newborn during the first 6 months of life.

(4) A baby may develop an upper respiratory infection. During suckling, it will inject some of the microorganisms into the milk ducts of the mammary gland. By the next feeding, the mammary gland has produced the antibodies appropriate for that infection.

e. **Self-Examination.** The female breast (mammary gland) is often a location for tumor growth. Thus, it is important for a woman to be able to examine her own breasts. During this self-examination, she must remember that a portion of the breast extends up into the axilla. (This portion is called the "axillary tail.")

Section V. INTRAUTERINE DEVELOPMENT

9-19. GENERAL

The site of fertilization (when it occurs) is usually in the uterine tube. Initial development of the embryo also takes place in the uterine tube. However, most development is intrauterine (within the uterus).

a. **Embryo.** During the first 8 weeks of development, the developing individual is called an embryo. The processes by which the embryo develops are studied in embryology.

b. **Fetus.** During the remainder of the intrauterine period, the developing individual is known as the fetus. During this latter period, the details of structure and function develop.

9-20. SUPPORT OF THE EMBRYO AND FETUS

In paragraph 9-15b(2), we discussed the amniotic sac, umbilical cord, and placenta. During intrauterine development, the embryo/ fetus is within the amniotic sac. Floating free in the amniotic fluid, it is connected to the placenta by the umbilical cord. The placenta is the specific area of exchange between the maternal blood and the fetal blood. By this exchange, the fetus gets rid of waste materials and acquires food, oxygen, and other needed substances from the mother.

Section VI. PARTURITION

9-21. DEFINITION

Parturition is the process of childbirth.

9-22. INITIAL PHASE

The initial phase includes dilation (stretching) of the uterine cervix. At the appropriate moment, the amniotic membranes rupture and release the amniotic fluid.

9-23. PASSAGE OF THE FETUS

The release of amniotic fluid is followed by the passage of the fetus through the birth canal.

a. During this passage, the newborn makes two partial rotations to accommodate the diameters of the relaxed bony pelvis.

b. In the birthing process, there are several reflexes occurring at appropriate times. Natural childbirth (without anesthetics or similar devices) allows these reflexes to occur normally. Since the uterine wall musculature (myometrium) is not capable of expelling the fetus by itself, the mother must learn how to utilize the abdominal wall musculature in coordination with the uterine wall musculature to effect a normal childbirth.

c. The head of the newborn presents itself in the perineum. If the central tendon of the perineum has not relaxed sufficiently, an episiotomy may be performed. This procedure involves cutting the posterior margin of the vagina to prevent tearing. Proper repair of the central tendon is essential to the proper recovering of the pelvis and perineum.

d. After the birth of the newborn, the placenta and amniotic membranes ("afterbirth") are delivered. These are accompanied by a significant flow of blood.

Continue with Exercises

EXERCISES, LESSON 9

REQUIREMENT. The following exercises are to be answered by completing the incomplete statements.

       After you have completed all the exercises, turn to "Solutions to Exercises" at the end of the lesson, and check your answers.

1.   Sex hormones belong to a chemical group called _____s. Sex hormones are formed primarily by the _____ds and the _____l cortex. The sex hormones of the female are called _____s and _____e. The sex hormones of the male are called _____s.

2.   Whether an individual will be male or female is determined at the moment the egg is _____d by the sperm. This is determined by the new _____c combination. Substances that later influence the production of sexual organs and characteristics are the sex _____s.

3.   The two kinds of sex chromosomes are ___ and ___.

       Within the gonads, there is a special type of cell division known as m_____s. The gametes, formed with this type of cell division, have a <u>(single) (double)</u> set of chromosomes.

       The production of a new individual is based upon the union of two _____s, that is, a s_____n and an _____m. This process is called f_____n. This produces a zygote with a <u>(single) (double)</u> set of chromosomes. If the zygote has two X chromosomes (XX), the individual will be a _____. If the zygote has one X and one Y chromosome (XY), the individual will be a _____.

4.   During development, the testes "migrate" out of the body cavity, through the _____l canal of the abdominal wall, and into the _____. The testes are generally cooler than the body cavity to ensure production of _____e sperm. If undescended testes remain uncorrected, the male will be _____e.

       Produced within each testis are millions of _____a and a_____s.

5.   The secondary sex organs of the male are responsible for the transport and care of the _____a.

       As the spermatozoa pass along the length of the epididymis, they are _____d by the secretions of the epididymal wall.

The seminal vesicle produces a n_____t fluid, which helps to maintain the
_____a.

In the male, the combination of secretions and spermatozoa is known as
the _____n.

6.   The penis is capable of _____n. The most favorable position in the vagina
for the deposit of semen is the upper recess of the _____a, opposite the opening of
the _____x of the _____s.

7.   The secondary sexual characteristics of the male are those features designed to
make a male _____ve to a female.

8.   One ovum is released per _____l cycle.

The development of a germinal cell takes place within a_____e, a fluid-filled
cavity within the _____y.

At midperiod, the mature ovum is expelled from the _____e onto the surface of
the ovary and is then picked up by the _____e tube.

9.   Initially, the cells of the ovary that form the follicle secrete the hormones called
_____s. After the ovum has been expelled from the follicle, the resulting cavity is
filled with a yellowish material known as the _____s _____m, which secretes
primarily _____e. This hormone prepares the _____s for pregnancy.
Thus, during the first half of the menstrual period _____s are secreted; during the
second half of the menstrual period _____e is added.

10.   The secondary sex organs of the female serve to transport and care for
the _____ and to develop the e_____ and _____s.

The uterine tube picks up the free _____ when it is expelled from the
_____e of the ovary. The ovum stays in the uterine tube to await _____n. If
it is fertilized, it goes through the initial stages of development as an _____o, which
then passes on to the _____s. If it is not fertilized within 3 to 5 days, its stored
_____ is exhausted and it _____.

11.   The embryo continues its development within the _____, whose inner lining is known as the _____ m. This inner lining contains _____e glands and blood vessels. To receive the early embryo, the endometrium is d_____d. If there is no embryo present at the end of the menstrual cycle, the _____m breaks down. Thus, a "flow" of blood and cellular elements occurs in a process known as _____n.

        When the embryo passes into the uterus from the uterine tube, it "burrows" into the _____. Later, the fluid-filled _____c sac surrounds the embryo. The embryo floats free, surrounded by _____c fluid. The embryo has an _____l cord that originates in the center of its anterior _____n. This cord is attached to the wall of the uterus by a special structure known as the _____a.

        The circular muscle tissue in the wall of the cervix holds the opening closed until time for _____n, when the musculature d_____s to form an _____g for the passage of the _____n to be.

12.   After the vagina receives the male penis, the semen is discharged into the upper recess opposite the opening of the _____x. At parturition, the vagina forms the _____h _____l through which the newborn passes to the outside.

        The openings of the vagina and urethra are covered by the external _____a.

13.   The secondary sexual characteristics of the female are those features designed to make a female _____ve to the male.

14.   When the female bony pelvis "relaxes" for childbirth, the ligaments of the bony _____s and _____m become quite stretchable. This increases the d_____s of the birth canal.

15.   The mammary glands respond to the estrogens and progesterone with additional _____h. Towards the end of the pregnancy, the breasts begin to form a fluid substance, _____m. Within 2 to 3 days after the birth, the breasts begin to secrete large quantities of _____.

        Human milk is the natural _____ of the newborn infant.

        Accompanying nursing, for both the child and the mother, are strong p_____l effects.

        Initially after childbirth, the mammary gland secretes _____m, consisting most importantly of _____s, which protect the infant during the first 6 _____s of life.

Later, the mother's milk contains _____s for specific infections of the child.

It is important for a woman to be able to _____e her own breasts.

16.   The placenta is the specific area of exchange between the maternal _____d and the _____l_____. By this exchange, the fetus gets rid of _____ materials and acquires _____d, _____n, and other needed substances from the mother.

17.   Parturition is the process of c_____h.

The initial phase includes s_____g of the uterine cervix. At the appropriate moment, the _____c membranes rupture and release the _____ fluid.

During its passage through the birth canal, the newborn makes two partial r_____s to accommodate the diameters of the relaxed bony pelvis.

In natural childbirth, there are several _____xes occurring normally at appropriate times.

The head of the newborn presents itself in the _____m.

After the birth of the newborn, the _____a and _____c m_____s are delivered.

Check Your Answers on Next Page

SOLUTIONS TO EXERCISES, LESSON 9

1.　　Sex hormones belong to a chemical group called <u>steroids</u>. Sex hormones are formed primarily by the <u>gonads</u> and the <u>adrenal</u> cortex. The sex hormones of the female are called <u>estrogens</u> and <u>progesterone</u>. The sex hormones of the male are called <u>androgens</u>. (para 9-3)

2.　　Whether an individual will be male or female is determined at the moment the egg is <u>fertilized</u> by the sperm. This is determined by the new <u>genetic</u> combination. Substances that later influence the production of sexual organs and characteristics are the sex <u>hormones</u>. (para 9-7)

3.　　The two kinds of sex chromosomes are <u>X</u> and <u>Y</u>.

　　Within the gonads, there is a special type of cell division known as <u>meiosis</u>. The gametes, formed with this type of cell division, have a <u>(single)</u> set of chromosomes.

　　The production of a new individual is based upon the union of two <u>gametes</u>, that is, a <u>spermatozoon</u> and an <u>ovum</u>. This process is called <u>fertilization</u>. This produces a zygote with a <u>double</u> set of chromosomes. If the zygote has two X chromosomes (XX), the individual will be a <u>female</u>. If the zygote has one X and one Y chromosome (XY), the individual will be a <u>male</u>. (paras 9-8 thru 9-10)

4.　　During development, the testes "migrate" out of the body cavity, through the <u>inguinal</u> canal of the abdominal wall, and into the <u>scrotum</u>. The testes are generally cooler than the body cavity to ensure production of <u>mature</u> sperm. If undescended testes remain uncorrected, the male will be <u>sterile</u>.

　　Produced within each testis are millions of <u>spermatozoa</u> and <u>androgens</u>. (para 9-11)

5.　　The secondary sex organs of the male are responsible for the transport and care of the <u>spermatozoa</u>.

　　As the spermatozoa pass along the length of the epididymis, they are <u>nurtured</u> by the secretions of the epididymal wall.

　　The seminal vesicle produces a <u>nutrient</u> fluid that helps to maintain the <u>spermatozoa</u>.

　　In the male, the combination of secretions and spermatozoa is known as the <u>semen</u>. (para 9-12)

6.　　The penis is capable of <u>erection</u>. The most favorable position in the vagina for the deposit of semen is the upper recess of the <u>vagina,</u> opposite the opening of the <u>cervix</u> of the <u>uterus</u>. (para 9-12g(1))

7.   The secondary sexual characteristics of the male are those features designed to make a male <u>attractive</u> to a female. (para 9-13)

8.   One ovum is released per <u>menstrual</u> cycle.

        The development of a germinal cell takes place within a <u>follicle</u>, a fluid-filled cavity within the <u>ovary</u>.

        At midperiod, the mature ovum is expelled from the <u>follicle</u> onto the surface of the ovary and is then picked up by the <u>uterine</u> tube. (para 9-14b)

9.   Initially, the cells of the ovary that form the follicle secrete the hormones called <u>estrogens</u>. After the ovum has been expelled from the follicle, the resulting cavity is filled with a yellowish material known as the <u>corpus luteum</u>, which secretes primarily <u>progesterone</u>. This hormone prepares the <u>uterus</u> for pregnancy. Thus, during the first half of the menstrual period <u>estrogens</u> are secreted, during the second half of the menstrual period <u>progesterone</u> is added. (para 9-14c)

10.   The secondary sex organs of the female serve to transport and care for the <u>ovum</u> and to develop the <u>embryo</u> and <u>fetus</u>.

        The uterine tube picks up the free <u>ovum</u> when it is expelled from the <u>follicle</u> of the ovary. The ovum stays in the uterine tube to await <u>fertilization</u>. If it is fertilized, it goes through the initial stages of development as an <u>embryo</u>, which then passes on to the <u>uterus</u>. If it is not fertilized within 3 to 5 days, its stored <u>food</u> is exhausted and it <u>dies</u>. (para 9-15)

11.   The embryo continues its development within the <u>uterus</u>, whose inner lining is known as the <u>endometrium</u>. This inner lining contains <u>uterine</u> glands and blood vessels. To receive the early embryo, the endometrium is <u>developed</u>. If there is no embryo present at the end of the menstrual cycle, the <u>endometrium</u> breaks down. Thus, a "flow" of blood and cellular elements occurs in a process known as <u>menstruation</u>.

        When the embryo passes into the uterus from the uterine tube, it "burrows" into the <u>endometrium</u>. Later, the fluid-filled <u>amniotic</u> sac surrounds the embryo. The embryo floats free, surrounded by <u>amniotic</u> fluid. The embryo has an <u>umbilical</u> cord that originates in the center of its anterior <u>abdomen</u>. This cord is attached to the wall of the uterus by a special structure known as the <u>placenta</u>.

        The circular muscle tissue in the cervix holds the opening closed until time for <u>parturition</u>, when the musculature <u>dilates</u> to form an <u>opening</u> for the passage of the <u>newborn</u> to be. (para 9-15b)

12.   After the vagina receives the male penis, the semen is discharged into the upper recess opposite the opening of the cervix. At parturition, the vagina forms the birth canal through which the newborn passes to the outside.

The openings of the vagina and urethra are covered by the external genitalia. (paras 9-15c, d)

13.   The secondary sexual characteristics of the female are those features designed to make a female attractive to the male. (para 9-16)

14.   When the female bony pelvis "relaxes" for childbirth, the ligaments of the bony pelvis and perineum become quite stretchable. This increases the diameters of the birth canal. (para 9-17)

15.   The mammary glands respond to the estrogens and progesterone with additional growth. Towards the end of the pregnancy, the breasts begin to form a fluid substance, colostrum. Within 2 to 3 days after the birth, the breasts begin to secrete large quantities of milk.

Human milk is the natural food of the newborn infant.

Accompanying nursing, for both the child and the mother, are strong psychological effects.

Initially after childbirth, the mammary gland secretes colostrum, consisting most importantly of antibodies, which protect the infant during the first 6 months of life.

Later, the mother's milk contains antibodies for specific infections of the child.

It is important for a woman to be able to examine her own breasts. (para 9-18)

16.   The placenta is the specific area of exchange between the maternal blood and the fetal blood. By this exchange, the fetus gets rid of waste materials and acquires food, oxygen, and other needed substances from the mother. (para 9-20)

17.   Parturition is the process of childbirth.

The initial phase includes stretching of the uterine cervix. At the appropriate moment, the amniotic membranes rupture and release the amniotic fluid.

During its passage through the birth canal, the newborn makes two partial rotations to accommodate the diameters of the relaxed bony pelvis.

In natural childbirth, there are several reflexes occurring normally at appropriate times.

The head of the newborn presents itself in the perineum.

After the birth of the newborn, the placenta and amniotic membranes are delivered. (paras 9-21 thru 9-23)

End of Lesson 9

LESSON ASSIGNMENT

LESSON 10

Cardiovascular and Other Circulatory Systems of the Human Body.

LESSON ASSIGNMENT

Paragraphs 10-1 through 10-45.

LESSON OBJECTIVE

After completing this lesson, you should be able to identify functions of the cardiovascular and lymphatic systems; including functions of their parts.

SUGGESTION

After completing the assignment, complete the exercises at the end of this lesson. These exercises will help you to achieve the lesson objectives.

LESSON 10

CARDIOVASCULAR AND OTHER CIRCULATORY SYSTEMS OF THE HUMAN BODY

Section I. INTRODUCTION

10-1. NEED FOR A CIRCULATORY SYSTEM

In simple organisms such as unicellular and one-or two-layer organisms, materials can be transferred among cells by simple processes of diffusion. However, in large organisms, a system is needed for the distribution and collection of materials. This is because diffusion does not occur fast enough to carry the large volumes of materials necessary through the greater distances required.

10-2. DISTRIBUTION OF SUBSTANCES

a. **Products of the Digestive System.** Some of the substances distributed to the body cells are products of the digestive system. These materials meet individual cell requirements for energy, growth, repair, synthesis of new materials, and storage for later use.

b. **Oxygen.** In the lungs, oxygen is obtained by the blood through the process of external respiration. Oxygen is then transported to the individual body cells, where it is used in metabolic oxidation. This provides energy for production of ATP (adenosine triphosphate), which is necessary for carrying on the life processes of the body.

10-3. COLLECTION OF SUBSTANCES

Some substances are collected from the body cells for elimination. These include carbon dioxide, nitrogenous wastes, and other potentially harmful substances that are carried to organs like the lungs, liver, or kidneys for elimination from the body.

10-4. HORMONES AND OTHER CONTROL SUBSTANCES

Hormones are the products of endocrine glands (see lesson 11). Hormones and other control substances are distributed throughout the body by circulatory systems. The tissues or organs affected by these substances are usually called target organs. In turn, substances released by the target organs often affect the original endocrine gland. This results in a feedback system.

10-5. CONTINUOUS RENEWAL AND REMOVAL OF FLUIDS

Secretory processes continuously renew the various fluid systems of the human body. At the same time, the volume of fluid in each system is kept at a constant level through the removal of excess fluids. Should the removal processes be interrupted, the volume of fluid will increase. The resulting increase in pressure can have serious consequences. Depending on the system involved, the consequences might include deafness, hydrocephalus, or pulmonary edema.

10-6. COMPONENTS OF ANY CIRCULATORY SYSTEM

Any circulatory system has three general components:

a. **Vehicle.** The vehicle is a fluid (flowing) medium. The materials being carried are dissolved or suspended in this fluid. This is the blood, lymph, or cerebrospinal fluid.

b. **Conduits.** Conduits are like pipes. They contain the fluids in which materials are transported to and from the various parts of the body. These are the blood vessels or lymph vessels.

c. **Motive Forces.** Motive forces act upon the vehicle to make it flow through the conduits. These are provided by the heart.

10-7. EXAMPLES OF CIRCULATORY SYSTEMS

Some circulatory systems of the human body are the cardio-vascular system, the lymphatic system, and the CSF (cerebrospinal fluid) system. The lesser systems include the aqueous humor of the bulbus oculi (eyeball) and the endolymph and perilymph, which are fluids of the inner ear.

10-8. INTRODUCTION TO THE CARDIOVASCULAR SYSTEM

The cardiovascular system (Figure 10-1) is the primary circulatory system of the human body. It includes a heart, blood, and blood vessels.

a. One function of the cardiovascular system is transport. Some substances carried by the cardiovascular system are dissolved or suspended in the fluid portion of the blood. Others are bound up in special cellular elements (RBCs).

b. The cardiovascular system also provides protection against foreign substances. This function involves active attack by white blood cells as well as more subtle processes of the immune system.

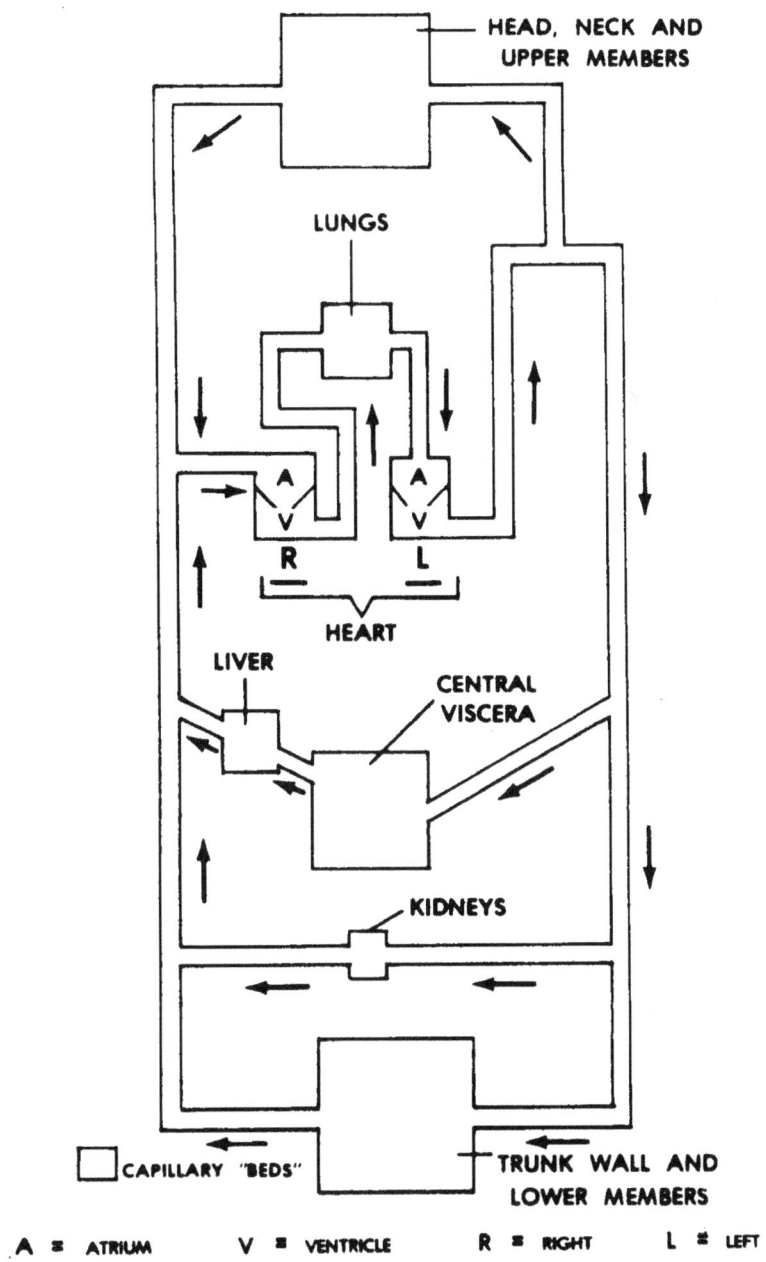

Figure 10-1. Diagram of the human cardiovascular (cirulatory) system.

Section II. THE BLOOD--THE VEHICLE OF THE CARDIOVASCULAR SYSTEM

10-9. DEFINITION

Blood is the vehicle of the cardiovascular system. Thus, the component actually transports substances.

10-10. PLASMA

Plasma makes up about 55 percent of the total blood volume.

a. **Water.** The major constituent of plasma is water. The physical characteristics of water make it a very good vehicle.

(1) Since water is <u>fluid</u>, it can flow through the conduits.

(2) Since most substances can be dissolved in water, it is often known as the "<u>universal solvent</u>."

(3) At ordinary pressures, water is essentially <u>non-compressible</u>.

(4) In addition, water has important <u>temperature characteristics</u>.

(a) Water has an ample <u>heat-carrying capacity</u>. It can carry heat readily throughout the body.

(b) Some of this heat is transferred to the water of the sweat glands. Since water can dissipate great quantities of heat through evaporation, excess heat can be efficiently disposed of at the surface of the skin.

b. **Dissolved and Suspended Substances.** To some extent, all transported substances are dissolved or suspended in the water of the plasma. These substances include various gases, end products of digestion, various control substances, and waste products. Also, there are three major <u>plasma proteins</u>--albumin, globulins, and fibrinogen. Together with dissolved salts (electrolytes), these plasma proteins help to maintain the tonicity of the plasma. In addition, fibrinogen is important to blood clotting.

10-11. FORMED ELEMENTS

The remainder of the blood volume consists of the formed elements--the red blood cells, the white blood cells, and the platelets. In adults, these formed elements normally make up 40 percent to 45 percent of the total blood volume. (This measure is called the <u>hematocrit</u>.)

a. **Red Blood Cells (RBCs; Erythrocytes).** The primary function of RBCs is to contain the protein called hemoglobin, which in turn carries oxygen. Thus, RBCs carry the majority of the oxygen to the individual cells of the body.

(1) Structure. The normal, mature red blood cell is a biconcave disc. The biconcave shape results from the loss of the nucleus just before the final maturation of the RBC. Since this shape increases the surface area of the disc, there is an increase in the capacity for the flow of substances into and out of the RBC.

(2) Hemoglobin. Within the cytoplasm of the RBC is a special protein called hemoglobin. Because of its iron atoms, hemoglobin has a great affinity for oxygen. It will readily pick up oxygen until it is saturated. At the same time, however, hemoglobin will readily give up oxygen in areas of low concentration.

(3) Life cycle of the RBC. Because of the loss of its nucleus, the RBC has a limited life period (about 120 days). At the end of this period, the spleen removes the "worn out" RBC, and the liver salvages the "pieces," particularly the iron.

b. **White Blood Cells (WBCs; Leukocytes).** The white blood cells are also formed elements of the blood. There are several types.

(1) Neutrophils and other phagocytic WBCs. The phagocytic WBCs can move independently out of the capillaries and penetrate into the tissues of the body. There, they actively attack foreign substances and engulf them in a process called phagocytosis. When these WBCs are overcome by foreign substances and die, their bodies accumulate to form a substance called pus.

(2) Lymphocytes. The lymphocytes are involved with the immune system of the body, including the production of antibodies.

c. **Platelets.** The platelets are the third type of formed element in the blood. Platelets are fragments of former cells. They are very important in the clotting process.

10-12. SERUM

After blood has been treated to remove the formed elements and the protein fibrinogen, there is a clear light-straw-colored fluid remaining. This fluid is called serum.

10-13. TRANSPORT OF GASES

One very important transport function of the blood is to carry gases back and forth between the lungs and the individual cells of the body. The alveoli and the individual body cells are the sites of exchange of gases to and from the blood. At these sites, the gases move according to the directions of pressure of concentration gradients. That is, each gas moves from an area where it is in higher concentration to an area of lesser concentration.

a. **Oxygen.** Oxygen is in the air filling the alveolus of the lung. The oxygen passes through the walls of the alveolus and capillary to become dissolved in the plasma of the blood. Most of the dissolved oxygen is rapidly picked up by the hemoglobin of the RBCs. Thus, the RBC is the main transporting element for oxygen in the blood.

b. **Carbon Dioxide.** Carbon dioxide is produced during metabolic oxidation within the individual cell. It passes through the cell membrane and the wall of the capillary to become dissolved in the plasma of the blood. Through action of an enzyme in the RBCs, most of the carbon dioxide (CO_2) is transformed into bicarbonate ions (HCO_3).

10-14. TRANSPORT OF OTHER SUBSTANCES

Other substances, such as the end products of digestion, are also carried by the blood. They are either dissolved or suspended in the plasma.

10-15. IMPORTANCE OF BLOOD IN ENERGY MOBILIZATION

The life processes cannot continue in the body cells without sources of energy. From glucose, energy is released to produce ATP, the driving force of the life processes of the body.

a. When a specific portion of the cerebral cortex is active, more blood is delivered to that portion. This is an example of how more blood can be delivered to the body parts where it is most needed.

b. When the hormone epinephrine (Adrenalin) is secreted by the adrenal gland, it is delivered to all parts of the body by the cardiovascular system. Among other effects, epinephrine increases the rate of metabolism of all cells of the body. This helps to mobilize energy during a "fight-or-flight" stress reaction.

c. In periods when much energy is required, the body can use its stores of fat as a source of energy. As we have seen in the chapter on the digestive system, the lymphatic circulatory system picks up the end products of lipid (fat) digestion and carries them to the cardiovascular system.

(1) This fat is generally deposited throughout the body, particularly the subcutaneous layer, as yellow fat. In a rapid turnover, the high energy content of the fat is released for use throughout the body.

(2) In infants, there is often brown fat at the junctions of the major blood vessels. In periods of high-energy requirements, this brown fat releases energy into the blood stream immediately.

10-16. RESPONSES TO HEMORRHAGE

A blood vessel may be damaged by transection (cutting across) or rupture. At such points, a volume of whole blood can flow out of the blood vessels. This escape of blood from the blood vessels is called hemorrhage.

HEMO = blood

RRHAGE = excessive flow ("bursting forth")

a. **Vascular contraction.** The first response to a cut or ruptured vessels is contraction (spasm) of the blood vessel itself. This may considerably reduce the volume of blood loss.

b. **Platelet Plug.** If the hole is small, a plug formed by clumping of the platelets may be adequate to stop the bleeding.

c. **Blood Clotting.** There is a complicated process for sealing off holes or ends of blood vessels after a cut or rupture. By this process, called coagulation or clotting, the blood forms a solid mass to seal the opening where the blood is escaping. The mass is called a blood clot. After many intermediate steps, the protein fibrinogen of the blood is converted into sticky strands of fibrin. These sticky strands adhere to the wall of the opening and form a meshwork in the opening, which traps RBCs and plasma. Thus, the opening is sealed.

d. **Hematoma.** A hematoma is a collection of blood, usually clotted, in an organ, space, or tissue. When found immediately beneath the skin, it will produce a purplish spot or mark. With time, as the clot is broken down and resorbed, the hematoma changes color and becomes smaller.

e. **Mobilization of Blood Reservoirs.** Certain areas of the body contain enough blood that they can be used as reservoirs to maintain the circulating blood volume. This is important when a volume of blood has been lost through hemorrhage. Among these are the spleen and the liver, whose sinuses together can release several hundred milliliters of blood. Also important are several groups of veins, including the large abdominal veins, which can also provide several hundred milliliters of blood.

10-17. BLOOD TRANSFUSIONS AND BLOOD MATCHING

a. **Transfusions.** In cases where an individual has lost whole blood by hemorrhaging, it is often necessary to give transfusions of whole blood. Whole blood transfusions continue the functions of the RBCs. On the other hand, if an individual has suffered burns causing a loss of fluid but not the loss of formed elements, plasma or a plasma substitute will often be used.

b. **Blood Matching.** There are a number of substances (antigens) on the surfaces of RBCs that vary among individuals. The blood of other individuals may contain or develop antibodies to these antigens. Before blood transfusions, the blood of the recipient and the donor must be matched to avoid potentially fatal reactions. Important systems of such antigens include the ABO system and the Rh system.

Section III. THE BLOOD VESSELS--THE CONDUITS OF THE CARDIOVASCULAR SYSTEM

10-18. INTRODUCTION

The blood vessels are tubular structures throughout the entire body. Since this tubular system is continuous (without interruption or opening), we sometimes refer to it as a closed system.

10-19. TYPES OF BLOOD VESSELS AND THEIR CONSTRUCTION

In general, there are three types of blood vessels--arteries, veins, and capillaries. We use the following abbreviations:

A. = artery   V. = vein

Aa. = arteries   Vv. = veins

NAVL = nerve(s), artery(ies), vein(s), lymphatic(s)

a. **Three General Layers.** In general, a blood vessels has a wall composed of three layers.

(1) Intima. The innermost layer is the intima. The intima is a simple epithelium made up of a single layer of flat epithelial cells.

(2) Media. The main portion of the wall is the media. It is made up of a combination of FCT and smooth muscle tissue.

(3) Adventitia. The outer surface of the blood vessel is the adventitia. It is an FCT layer.

b. **Comparison of the Structures of Arteries and Veins.** Given an artery and a vein with similar inner diameters, the artery will have a thicker wall than the vein. This greater thickness is due to the presence of more smooth muscle tissue and the presence of elastic FCT as a significant element.

c. **Capillary Structure.** Capillary walls have only one layer--the intima. Capillary networks (beds) are the exchange areas for the cardiovascular system. This includes the internal exchange areas between the blood and the individual cells of the body. Since the capillary wall consists of flat single cells, substances can move readily between the body cells and the blood.

10-20. SPECIAL SITUATIONS

This paragraph describes several special situations associated with the blood vascular system.

a. **Nutrient Versus Functional Blood Supplies.** The lungs, liver, and heart actually have two blood supplies. The <u>functional</u> blood supply provides blood to be worked upon by the organ. The <u>nutrient</u> blood supply provides blood for the usual exchange of materials between body cells and the blood.

b. **Collateral Circulation.** A <u>collateral circulation</u> is a special organization of blood vessels around a major joint of other area of the body. Its purpose is to provide a continuing supply of blood even if one of the vessels is damaged. Several blood vessels are included so that there will be an alternate route when needed.

c. **End Arteries.** There are other areas of the body where a single artery is the sole supply of blood. Such an artery is called an <u>end artery</u>. When an end artery is damaged and can no longer supply blood to an area, the tissues of the areas will die. End arteries are most common in the brain and the heart.

d. **Portal Veins.** A <u>portal vein</u> is a venous blood vessel that begins with capillaries in one area and ends in capillaries of another area. The most important portal vein in the human body is the hepatic portal vein. The <u>hepatic portal vein</u> extends from the capillaries of the digestive system to the capillaries/sinusoids of the liver.

10-21. LOCATIONS OF BLOOD VESSELS TYPES

In the human body, blood vessels are located differently according to their types.

a. **Arteries.** If an artery is injured, the threat to life is greater than with other types of blood vessels. For protection, arteries tend to be located deep within the structures of the body. Only the very smallest of arteries, especially the cutaneous arteries, come close to the surface of the body.

b. **Veins.** There are both deep veins and cutaneous veins. The <u>deep veins</u> accompany the arteries side by side. The <u>cutaneous veins</u> are found in the subcutaneous layer of the body. The cutaneous veins drain into the deep veins at specific locations (especially the inguinal region and the axillary region).

c. **Capillaries.** The capillaries are located throughout all tissues of the body. No individual cell is more than two cells away from a capillary. The networks of capillaries in the tissues are often called capillary beds.

10-22. PATTERNS OF BLOOD CIRCULATION

Blood vessels make up a closed system, since there is no place in the system where whole blood can leave.

a. **Direction of Flow of Arteries and Veins.** Arteries carry blood from the chambers of the heart to the tissue of the body. Veins carry blood from the tissues to the chambers of the heart. (Coronary arteries carry blood from the chambers of the heart inside to the walls of the heart outside.)

b. **Two-Cycle System.** It is also a two-cycle system (Figure 10-2). It involves both the pulmonary cycle and the systemic cycle. Blood circulates through two circuits. In the pulmonary cycle, blood circulates from the heart to the lungs and back to the heart. In the systemic cycle, blood circulates from the heart to the rest of the body and back to the heart.

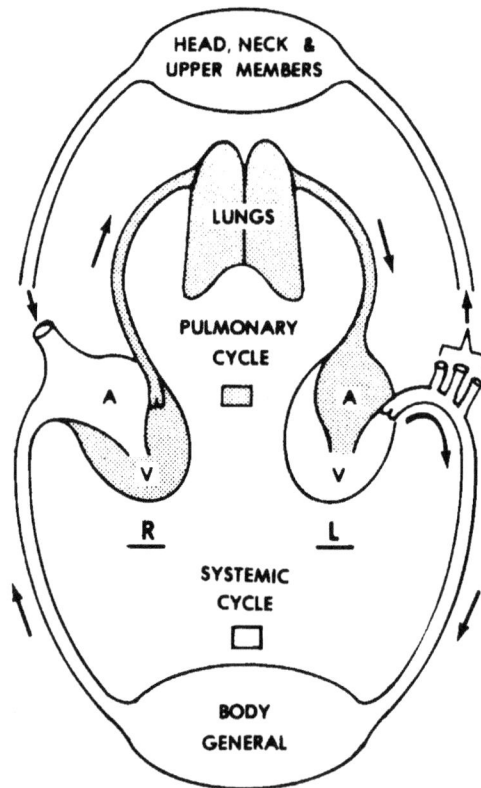

Figure 10-2. Cardiovascular circulatory pattern.

c. **Fetal Circulation.** Since the fetus is located within the uterus, its lungs do not take in air. Therefore, the pulmonary cycle does not function in the fetus. Essentially, fetal blood flows to and from the placenta. There are certain bypasses in the heart to avoid the pulmonary cycle. At the time of birth, the fetal circulation is changed to the normal pattern.

Section IV. THE HEART--THE PRIMARY MOTIVE FORCE OF THE CARDIOVASCULAR SYSTEM

10-23. INTRODUCTION

In humans, the heart is the primary motive force for driving the blood along the arterial vessels. The heart consists of four separate chambers. Two chambers function as a "right heart," and two function as a "left heart." The muscular walls (myocardium) of the chambers apply force to the blood within and force the blood to move out of the chambers. (See Figure 10-3.)

10-24. CHAMBERS OF THE HUMAN HEART

a. **Atria.** Two chambers are called the atria (singular: atrium). Down the middle, an interatrial septum separates the two atria.

(1) The muscular walls of the atria tend to be relatively thin.

(2) Attached to each atrium is an earlike appendage called an auricle. The auricles of the atria tend to have somewhat thicker walls.

b. **Ventricles.** The other two chambers are the right and left ventricles. Between the ventricles is the interventricular septum.

(1) The left ventricle tends to be cylindrical in shape. It has a relatively thick wall.

(2) The right ventricle has a somewhat semilunar (half-moon) cross section, since it is wrapped around one side of the left ventricle.

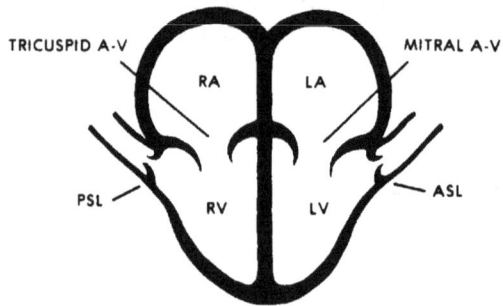

A. SCHEME OF HEART STRUCTURE.

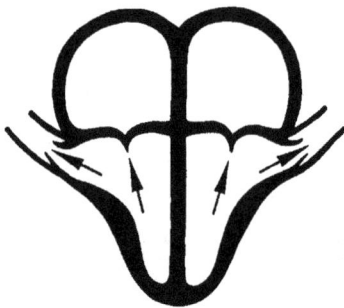

(1.) VENTRICULAR SYSTOLE

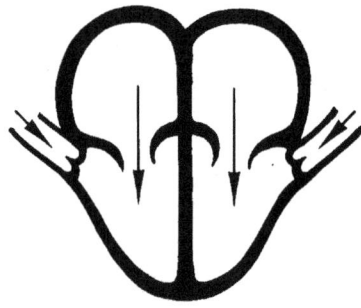

(2.) VENTRICULAR DIASTOLE

B. DIAGRAMATIC HEART ACTION.

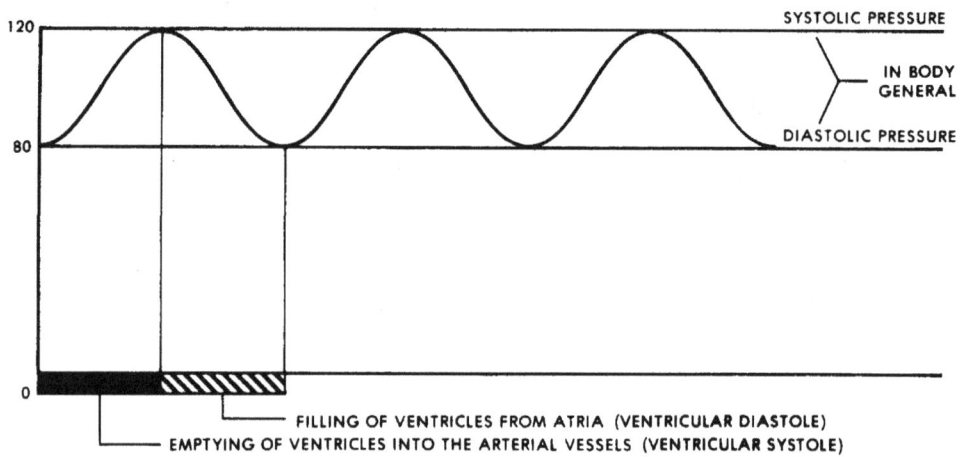

C. FUNCTION

Figure 10-3. The human heart function.

10-25. FIBROUS SKELETON OF THE HEART

There is an FCT structure within the substance of the heart. This structure is known as the fibrous skeleton of the heart. This fibrous skeleton serves two general purposes: (1) as sites of attachment for muscle tissues and (2) as supporting structures for the cardia valves. All of the fibrous structures are continuous and form the fibrous skeleton of the heart.

a. **Fibrous Portion of the Interventricular Septum.** The uppermost portion (also called the membranous portion) of the interventricular septum is a part of the fibrous skeleton of the heart.

b. **Atrioventricular (AV) Rings.** Each atrioventricular valve of the heart is surrounded by a dense fibrous ring. This ring maintains the valve opening.

c. **Cylinders at Bases of Great Arteries.** Each of the semilunar valves of the heart is located within a short fibrous cylinder. This cylinder maintains the structure and function of the valve.

10-26. WALL STRUCTURE

The walls of the chambers of the heart are in three layers.

a. The chambers themselves are lined with a simple epithelium known as the endocardium.

b. Likewise, a simple epithelium surrounds the outside of the heart. It is known as the epicardium. The epicardium is the same as the visceral pericardium, which we shall discuss later.

c. By far the most important is the myocardium, the middle layer. It is made up of cardiac muscle tissue.

(1) Cardiac muscle tissue consists of fibers formed by the fusion of many individual cells (syncytium). These cardiac fibers are striated and branched.

(2) The myocardium is thicker in the walls of the ventricles than the atria. This is because greater pressures are needed for the ventricles to perform their function. The wall of the left ventricle is especially thick, since it has to drive the blood throughout the body.

(3) The inner surfaces of the ventricular walls have ridges of muscle known as the trabeculae carneae, with spaces between them.

(4) When the musculature within a chamber wall contracts, the lumen (cavity) decreases in diameter. This is particularly true of the left ventricle. There is

also a twisting or wringing action of the left ventricle that causes the apex of the heart to hit against the inner surface of the chest wall--the apex beat.

(5) The stroke volume is the amount of blood forced out of each ventricle in one contraction. The cardiac output is the volume of blood pumped out of the ventricles (RT into the lungs, LT into the systemic circulation) in one minute (expressed in liters per minute). These volumes will change according to the needs of the body.

10-27. CARDIAC VALVES

Valves are structures that ensure that fluids will pass through them in only one direction. That is, a valve will open to allow fluids to pass in one direction but will close to prevent fluids from passing in the other direction. There are two sets of cardiac valves--the atrioventricular (AV) valves and the semilunar valves. Although the two sets of valves are quite different in design, they both function passively in response to the flow of the blood.

a. **AV Valves.** The AV valves are found between the atria and the ventricles. The AV valves consist of flaps, known as cusps. The outer margin of each flap is attached to the inner surface of a fibrous ring. The inner edge of each flap is free.

(1) On the right side is the tricuspid valve. On the left side is the mitral valve. ("Might is never right.")

(a) Thus, the tricuspid valve is between the right atrium and the right ventricle. It is named for its three cusps.

(b) The mitral valve is located between the left atrium and the left ventricle. Since it has two cusps, it is sometimes called the "bicuspid" valve.

(2) The contraction of the atrial walls forces the blood from the atria through the AV valves and into the ventricles (atrial systole).

(3) When the atria relax (atrial diastole) and the ventricles contract, the pressure would tend to drive the blood back into the atria. However, each opening is sealed when the cusps of each AV valve meet in the valve center. This prevents blood from flowing further back into the atria.

(4) A special anatomic arrangement helps prevent backward flow into the atria. Chordae tendineae are fibrous cords attached to the ventricular side of the cusps. Since these cords of dense FCT have a fixed length, they cannot be stretched or shortened. The other ends of these cords are attached to the papillary muscles. The papillary muscles are special extensions of the muscular walls of the ventricles. As the ventricles contract and become smaller, these muscles take up the slack in the cords.

b. **Semilunar (Aortic and Pulmonary) Valves.** As mentioned before, the bases of the two great arteries (the pulmonary arch and the aortic arch) begin at their respective ventricles as short cylinders of the fibrous skeleton. Within each of these cylinders are three cuplike cusps, which make up each semilunar valve. When the ventricles contract (ventricular systole) and the AV valves have closed, the blood moves out into the great arteries through the semilunar valves. When the ventricles relax (ventricular diastole), the back pressure of the blood in the great arteries forces the cusps of the semilunar valves to the center and seals off each opening.

10-28. NAVL OF THE HEART

a. **Controls of Heart Function.**

(1) Extrinsic controls. A number of cardiac nerves arise from both the sympathetic and parasympathetic portions of the nervous system (chapter 12). The sympathetic portion accelerates the action of the heart, while the parasympathetic portion slows it down. These portions are both controlled by cardiovascular centers in the medulla of the hind-brainstem. In addition, as everyone is well aware, various emotional states can affect the actions of the heart.

(2) Intrinsic controls. Within the substance of the heart, certain fibers of the myocardium have been transformed from contracting muscle tissue to impulse-transmitting fibers. These are called Purkinje's fibers. Together, these fibers provide intrinsic control for the action of the heart.

(a) The sinoatrial (SA) node is a collection of these fibers in the interatrial septum. The SA node is often called the pacemaker of the heart because it initiates each cycle of the contractions of the heart chambers.

(b) The atrioventricular (AV) node is another group of these fibers just above the interventricular septum.

(c) Descending from the AV node is the bundle of His, which branches into the right and left septal bundles. These branches pass down on either side of the interventricular septum.

(d) Impulse begin in the SA node, pass to the AV node, and then descend through the septal bundles to stimulate the myocardium of the ventricular walls to contract.

(3) Humoral control. Apparently, some substances transported by the blood can accelerate or slow the action of the heart. This situation is called the humoral control of heart action.

b. **Coronary Arteries.** Previously, we have described the flow of blood through the chambers of the heart. This blood, upon which the heart acts, is called functional blood. Now, we wish to discuss the supply of nutrient blood to the heart. This blood nourishes the tissues of the heart. The nutrient blood supplies oxygen and food materials to the tissues of the heart and removes waste materials. This nutrient blood is supplied to the walls of the heart by the right and left coronary arteries.

    (1) The openings leading into the coronary arteries are located in the base of the ascending aorta, just above (behind the cusps of) the semilunar valve (aortic valve). When this valve is open, its cusps cover the openings of the coronary arteries. When the valve is closed, the backpressure of the blood in the aorta fills the coronary arteries with blood. The coronary arteries then distribute the blood to all of the tissues of the relaxed heart.

    (2) Many of the branches of the coronary arteries are of the end artery type. This means that such a branch is the sole supply of nutrient blood to a specific area of the heart. If the branch should be closed for any reason, the tissue in that area will die for lack of oxygen and nourishment.

    c. **Cardiac Veins and Coronary Sinus.** The blood from the tissues of the heart is collected by the cardiac veins. These veins empty into the coronary sinus, a vessel, which in turn empties into the right atrium.

    d. **Thebesian Veins.** The thebesian veins are many minute sinuses found in the myocardium of the ventricles. They extend from the lumen into the myocardium of each ventricle.

10-29. HEART SOUNDS

    When the valves of the heart close, they produce audible sounds. First, the closing of the AV valves produces a noticeable "LUB." When the semilunar valves subsequently close, another sound "DUB" is produced to complete the cycle. These are referred to as the heart sounds--"LUB DUB, LUB DUB," etc.

10-30. ELECTROCARDIOGRAM (EKG)

    Since the myocardial tissue is living material, its activity produces electrical impulses. With an electrocardiogram, the pattern of these electrical impulses can be recorded.

10-31. THE PERICARDIUM

    a. **General.** The heart is an active organ of the human body. Its pumping action, which begins in the very early embryo, continues without stopping until death. During each cycle of its activity, the heart changes in shape and size and tends also to rotate. (The number of cycles per minute is called heart rate.) To reduce the amount of friction resulting from this activity, the heart is includes within a serous sac, called the pericardium, or pericardial sac.

b. **Serous Space and Two Serous Pericardia.** As in all serous cavities, there is a serous space between two serous membranes.

(1) The visceral pericardium intimately covers the surface of the heart. Earlier, we referred to this as the epicardium.

(2) The parietal pericardium is the outer serous membrane.

(3) Between the two serous pericardia is a very thin space containing a thin film of pericardial fluid. This lubricating fluid makes the action of the heart much less strenuous.

c. **Fibrous Pericardium.** The parietal pericardium is covered with a very dense fibrous envelope. This envelope forms the outer portion of the pericardial sac.

Section V. MOTIVE FORCES INVOLVED IN DRIVING THE BLOOD THROUGH THE SYSTEM

10-32. INTRODUCTION

The blood (vehicle for transporting material) is driven through the blood vessels (conduits) by a variety of motive forces.

10-33. ARTERIAL BLOOD FLOW

Blood is driven through the arteries by a combination of forces. First, there is the force produced by the contraction of the ventricular walls. Second, there is the elastic recoil of the arterial walls.

a. **Systole.** When the left ventricle contracts (systole), it forces the blood into the aortic arch. Above the base cylinder, the wall of the aortic arch is mainly elastic FCT. As the blood fills the aortic arch, the walls are stretched.

b. **Diastole.** When the ventricle relaxes (diastole), the wall of the arch recoils and presses against the blood. With the closing of the aortic semilunar valve, the blood is forced to move out along the arteries in a pressure pulse. Since the elasticity of the arterial walls produces a continuous pressure, the blood moves continuously throughout the system.

c. **Arterial Pressures.** The highest pressure is called the systolic pressure, and the lowest pressure is the diastolic pressure.

d. **Vasoconstriction.** Vasoconstriction is the actual contraction of the arterial walls. Vasoconstriction can further increase the pressure on the blood in the arteries.

e. **Gravity.** Gravity helps to move blood to the trunk and lower members. However, it is a hindrance in moving blood to the head and neck.

10-34. VENOUS BLOOD FLOW

There is usually a low level of pressure in the veins. There are valves in the veins that ensure that blood flows continuously toward the heart. Therefore, as pressure is applied to a vein, there will be a pump effect.

a. **Pressure from Arteries.** The muscular compartments of the upper and lower limbs tend to be full in healthy persons. Therefore, as blood enters the arteries within these compartments, a volume of blood must leave through the veins.

b. **Pressure from Muscular Contractions.** During muscular activity, additional forces press against the veins and produce a "milking action." Again, blood moves through the veins back toward the heart.

c. **Gravity.** In the head and neck, gravity helps to move the blood down through the veins. In the trunk and lower limbs, the valves help to prevent a backward flow of blood in the veins.

Section VI. CAPILLARIES

10-35. INTRODUCTION

The capillary beds make up the greatest cross-sectional area of the cardiovascular system. In the capillary beds, the actual exchange of materials takes place between the blood and the cells of the body.

10-36. FILTRATION PHENOMENON

The wall of the capillary consists of a single layer of flat cells. The minute spaces surrounding the capillaries and the individual cells of the body make up the tissue space (interstitial/ extracellular space). Fluid passes from the capillary into the tissue space and carries with it various substances. Some of this fluid returns to the capillary on the venous side.

10-37. CAPILLARY SPHINCTERS

The capillary beds are provided with precapillary sphincters that can reduce or completely stop the flow of blood into the capillaries. At the other end of the capillary bed are postcapillary sphincters; when these close, there is a backpressure and more fluid flows into the tissue space.

Section VII. TEMPERATURE CONTROL BY MEANS OF THE BLOOD

10-38. ELIMINATION OF EXCESS HEAT

Heat is produced as a by-product by various activities of the human body, particularly muscular contractions. When excess heat is accumulated, it must be eliminated from the body to maintain a healthy condition.

a. The water of the blood has a great heat-carrying capacity.

b. There are superficial capillary beds in the subcutaneous layer, close to the surface of the body. When the blood flows through these beds, some of its heat can radiate directly to the surrounding environment.

c. The sweat glands take water from the blood and secrete it onto the surface of the skin. Here, even more calories of heat are lost during the evaporation of the water.

10-39. CONSERVATION OF BODY HEAT

On the other hand, if the body has an insufficient amount of heat, heat loss must be reduced. For this purpose, the superficial capillary beds can be closed down. Then, the fat in the subcutaneous layer serves as insulation.

10-40. CORE TEMPERATURE CONTROL

Unlike the peripheral portions of the body, whose temperatures may vary considerably, the center of the body must be maintained at a certain temperature within very narrow limits.

a. **Control.** There are special temperature detectors in the hypothalamus of the forebrainstem. These continuously monitor the temperature of the blood flowing through the brain.

b. **Counter-Current Mechanism.** The peripheral blood in the limbs is several degrees cooler than the blood in the center of the body. Therefore, it must be warmed as it returns toward the heart. As previously described, the arteries and veins of the limbs are located side by side as they extend from the trunk and through the length of the limbs. As it returns to the trunk, cool venous blood is gradually warmed by the arterial blood flowing in the opposite direction.

10-41. COOLING OF ORGANS WITH A HIGH METABOLIC RATE

Certain organs of the body, such as the brain and the liver, have a relatively high metabolic rate. Because of this, they produce excessive heat. Part of the blood supply to these organs is specifically designed to remove the excess calories of heat.

10-42. WARMING OF INFLOWING AIR

As blood flows through the arteries of the mucoperiosteum of the nasal chambers, the inflowing air is warmed.

10-43. ERYTHEMA

At the site of an infection or injury, the most common reaction observed is redness (erythema). This indicates that extra blood and heat are available for healing.

Section VIII. OTHER CIRCULATORY SYSTEMS

10-44. THE LYMPHATIC SYSTEM

In general, the lymphatic system is a drainage system that picks up tissue fluids and returns them to the cardiovascular system. The tissue fluids are picked up in the interstitial spaces. They are eventually returned to the veins.

a. **Lymphatic Capillaries and Vessels.**

(1) Within the tissue spaces, the lymphatic system begins with lymph capillaries. A lymph capillary begins with a blind end (cul-de-sac).

(2) The capillaries eventually come together to form lymphatic vessels, which gradually join and become larger and larger. Physiologically, lymphatic vessels are very similar to veins. Like veins, they have low pressure and possess valves.

(3) The thoracic duct is a major collecting vessel of the lymphatic system that empties into the deep veins of the neck. It begins in the upper posterior abdomen with a collection of sacs called the cisterna chyli. The cisterna chyli is a receiving area for lymph from three other major lymphatic vessels. From the cisterna chyli, the thoracic duct passes upward through the thorax and into the root of the neck. There, it empties into the deep veins of the neck.

b. **Lymph Nodes.** Along the lymphatic vessels at various intervals are small structures known as lymph nodes. The lymph nodes function as sieves for the lymph passing through them. In healthy individuals, the lymph nodes usually draw no attention. However, in chronic diseases, the lymph nodes become enlarged and hardened (indurated). In the axilla, the inguinal region, and the neck, certain lymph nodes are large enough to be palpated even in health. <u>Tonsils</u> are aggregates of lymphatic tissue.

c. **Lymphocytes.** Associated with the lymphatic system are special cells known as lymphocytes. The lymphocytes become part of the formed elements of the blood. They are primarily involved in the immune reactions of the body.

10-45. CIRCULATORY SYSTEMS OF LESSER VOLUME

In addition to the cardiovascular and lymphatic circulatory systems, there are other circulatory systems of lesser volume.

a. The <u>cerebrospinal fluid (CSF) system</u> is involved with the central nervous system. CSF is formed with fluid from the arteries and eventually returned to venous vessels.

b. The <u>bulbus oculi</u> (eyeball) and the <u>inner ear</u> are fluid-filled hollow organs. Such organs have their own internal circulatory systems. In the case of the bulbus oculi, the fluid is the aqueous humor. In the case of the inner ear, the fluid is the endolymph/perilymph. In such cases, the fluids are produced from fluids of arterial vessels and then are picked up by venous vessels. Should the drainage pattern be interrupted, fluids will accumulate and cause increased pressure within the hollow organ. The increased pressure will interfere with the organ functions; examples are glaucoma of the eye and deafness of the ear.

Continue with Exercises

EXERCISES, LESSON 10

REQUIREMENT. The following exercises are to be answered by completing the incomplete statements.

After you have completed all the exercises, turn to "Solutions to Exercises" at the end of the lesson, and check your answers.

1.   The three general components of any circulatory system are the v_____, c_____s, and the motive _____s.

2.   The primary circulatory system of the human body is the c_____lar system. It includes a _____t, _____d, and blood _____s.

One function of the cardiovascular system is t_____t. Some substances carried by the cardiovascular system are d_____ed or s_____ed in the fluid portion of the blood. Others are bound up in special cellular elements, the ____s.

The cardiovascular system also provides p_____n against foreign substances. This function involves active attack by _____e blood cells as well as other processes of the immune system.

3.   Blood is the _____e of the cardiovascular system. Thus, it is the component which actually t_____s substances.

4.   Making up about 55 percent of the total blood volume is _____a. Its major constituent is ____r.

5.   The physical characteristics of water make it a very good _____e. Since water is fluid, it can ____w through the conduits. Since it can dissolve many substances, it is often called the "universal _____." Water is essentially non-compressible. Also, water has important t_____e characteristics. Water has an ample ____t-carrying capacity. Water can dissipate great quantities of heat through e_____n.

6.   Many substances are dissolved or suspended in the water of the plasma. These substances include various g____s, end products of _____n, various control substances, and waste products. Also, there are three major plasma proteins--_____min, _____lins, and _____gen. The tonicity of the plasma proteins and dissolved salts are called e_____s. In addition, fibrinogen is important to ____ing.

7. In adults, the formed elements make up about 40 percent to 45 percent of the total blood _____ e.

8. The primary function of RBCs is to contain the protein called _____ bin, which in turn carries _____ n.

The shape of the RBC increases its capacity for the _____ w of substances into and out of the cell.

Within the cytoplasm of the RBC is a special protein called _____ n. Because of its iron atoms, it has a great affinity for _____ n.

At the end of its life period, the "worn out" RBC is removed by the _____ n and the "pieces," particularly the iron, are salvaged by the _____.

9. The second category of formed elements of the blood is the _____ e blood cells.

Phagocytic WBCs actively attack foreign substances and engulf them in a process called _____ s. When the WBCs are overcome and die, their bodies accumulate to form a substance called _____.

The lymphocytes are involved with the i_____ e system of the body, including the production of _____ ies.

10. The third type of formed element in the blood is the _____ s. These are fragments of former _____ s. They are very important in the _____ing process.

11. After the formed elements and fibrinogen are removed from the blood, the remaining fluid is called _____.

12. One very important transport function of the blood is to carry gases back and forth between the _____ s and the individual _____ s of the body. The sites of exchange are the _____ i and the individual body _____ s. At these sites, a gas moves from the area where its concentration is _____ er to the area where its concentration is _____ er.

Near the alveoli, most of the dissolved oxygen is rapidly picked up by the h_____ n of the ___ s. Therefore, the RBC is the main transporting element for _____.

Produced during metabolic oxidation is _____ n _____ e. It passes through the cell membrane and the capillary wall to become dissolved in the _____ a of the blood. Through the action of an enzyme, most of this gas is transformed into _____ate ions.

13.   The escape of blood from damaged blood vessels is called _____rrh_____.

        The first response to a cut or ruptured vessel is contraction (spasm) of the blood _____ itself.

        If the hole is small, a plug formed by clumping of the _____s may stop the bleeding.

        A complicated process for sealing off holes or ends of blood vessels is called _____n or _____ing. In this process, the blood forms a solid mass call a blood _____. After a number of steps, the protein fibrinogen is converted into sticky strands of _____n. The resulting meshwork traps ____s and _____a and thus seals the opening.

        Within the body a collection of blood, usually clotted and resulting from hemorrhage, is called a _____a.

        The spleen, the liver, and large abdominal veins serve as blood r_____s, which can be mobilized to maintain the circulating blood _____e.

14.   If an individual has lost whole blood by hemorrhaging, it is often necessary to give trans_____s of whole blood. Whole blood transfusions continue the functions of the ___s. When fluid but few formed elements have been lost, _____a or a _____ substitute will often be used.

        On the surfaces of RBCs, there are a number of substances called _____ns. The blood of other individuals may contain _____ies to these substances. The blood of the recipient and the blood of the donor must be _____ed to avoid potentially fatal _____s. Important systems of such antigens include the ___O system and the ___ system.

15.   The lungs, liver, and heart have two blood supplies. Blood to be worked upon by the organ is called _____l blood. Blood for the usual exchange of materials between body cells and the blood is called _____t blood.

16.   An end artery is the ____e supply of blood to an area of the body. End arteries are most common in the _____n and the _____t. If an end artery is damaged and can no longer supply blood to its corresponding area, the tissues of that area will ____.

17.   Cycles of blood circulation include the _____y cycle and the _____c cycle.

In the first of these, blood circulates from the _____t to the _____s and back to the _____. In the second, blood circulates from the _____ to the rest of the body and back to the _____.

18.   The primary motive force for driving the blood along the arteries is the _____, which consists of four separate _____ s.

19.   Why is the wall of the left ventricle especially thick?

The amount of blood forced out of each ventricle in one contraction is called the s_____e v_____e. The amount of blood pumped out of the ventricles in a minute is called the c_____ c o_____t.

20.   Structures ensuring that fluids pass through them in only one direction are called _____ s.

The contraction of the atrial walls forces the blood from the atria through the ___ valves and into the _____ s. When the ventricles contract, the openings between the atria and the ventricles are sealed by the _____ of the ____ valves.

When the ventricles relax, the openings between the great arteries and the ventricles are sealed by the cuplike _____s of the _____ valves.

21.   The action of the heart is accelerated by the _____thetic portion of the nervous system. It is slowed down by the _____thetic portion.

The sinoatrial (SA) node is often called the pacemaker of the heart because it _____.Impulses begin in the ___node, pass to the ____ node, and then descend through the _____l bundles to stimulate the m_____m of the ventricular walls to contract.

22.   Nutrient blood is supplied to the walls of the heart by the right and left _____y arteries.

The openings leading into the coronary arteries are located in the base of the ascending _____, just behind the cusps of the _____ valve. When this valve is open, its cusps cover the openings of the _____y_____s. When the valve is closed, the backpressure within the aorta fills the _____ _____s with blood. The coronary arteries then distribute the blood to all of the tissues of the relaxed _____.

Many of the branches of the coronary arteries are of the ___d artery type. If such a branch is closed for any length of time, the tissue in the area supplied will ____.

23.   The blood from the tissues of the heart is collected by the _____c veins. These veins empty into the _____y sinus, a vessel that in turn empties into the right _____.

24.   The pumping action of the heart continues without stopping until _____. During each cycle, the heart changes in sh____ and s___ and tends to r_____. The number of cycles per minute is called the heart ____. To reduce friction, the heart is enclosed within a _____s sac, called the p_____m.

25.   Intimately covering the surface of the heart is the v_____l pericardium, also called the e_____. The outer serous membrane is the p_____ pericardium. The pericardial fluid provides l_____n and reduces the amount of work done by the _____.

26.   In addition to the force provided by contraction of the ventricular walls, blood is also driven by the e_____ c r_____l of the arterial walls.

The highest arterial pressure is called the ___stolic pressure, and the lowest is called the ___stolic pressure.

Pressure on the blood in the arteries can be further increased by vaso_____ and _____y.

27.   Structures that ensure that blood flows in only one direction in the veins, are the _____s. When a vein is subjected to pressure, the result is a ____p effect. Veins receive pressure from the _____ies, muscular _____ns, and _____y.

28.   Capillary beds are provided with pre_____ sphincters and post-_____ sphincters. The first can stop the flow of blood into the _____s. When the postcapillary sphincters close, more fluid flows into the t_____ ____ce.

29.   As it returns to the trunk, cool venous blood is gradually warmed by the _____l blood flowing in the opposite direction.

30.   In general, the lymphatic system is a _____ge system that picks up tissue ____s and returns them to the cardiovascular system. These are picked up in the in_____l spaces.

A lymph capillary begins with a _____d end.

These capillaries join to form _____c vessels.

A major collecting vessel of the lymphatic system is the _____c duct, which empties into the deep _____s of the neck.

The lymph nodes function as sieves for the _____ passing through them.

The lymphocytes are primarily involved in the _____e reactions of the body.

31.   An additional circulatory system is the _____l fluid system.

Two fluid-filled hollow organs are the _____ll and the _____r___r.

Check Your Answers on Next Page

SOLUTIONS TO EXERCISES, LESSON 10

1.   The three general components of any circulatory system are the <u>vehicle,</u> <u>conduits</u>, and the motive <u>forces</u>. (para 10-6)

2.   The primary circulatory system of the human body is the <u>cardiovascular</u> system. It includes a <u>heart</u>, <u>blood</u>, and <u>blood vessels</u>.

      One function of the cardiovascular system is <u>transport</u>. Some substances carried by the cardiovascular system are <u>dissolved</u> or <u>suspended</u> in the fluid portion of the blood. Others are bound up in special cellular elements, the <u>RBCs</u>.

      The cardiovascular system also provides <u>protection</u> against foreign substances. This function involves active attack by <u>white</u> blood cells as well as other processes of the immune system. (para 10-8)

3.   Blood is the <u>vehicle</u> of the cardiovascular system. Thus, it is the component that actually <u>transports</u> substances. (para 10-9)

4.   Making up about 55 percent of the total blood volume is <u>plasma</u>. Its major constituent is <u>water</u>. (para 10-10)

5.   The physical characteristics of water make it a very good <u>vehicle</u>. Since water is fluid, it can <u>flow</u> through the conduits. Since it can dissolve many substances, it is often called the "universal <u>solvent</u>." Water is essentially non-compressible. In addition, water has important <u>temperature</u> characteristics. Water has an ample <u>heat</u>-carrying capacity. Water can dissipate great quantities of heat through <u>evaporation</u>. (para 10-10a)

6.   Many substances are dissolved or suspended in the water of the plasma. These substances include various <u>gases</u>, end products of <u>digestion</u>, various control substance, and waste products. Also, there are three major plasma proteins--<u>albumin</u>, <u>globulins</u>, and <u>fibrinogen</u>. The tonicity of the plasma proteins and dissolved salts are called <u>electrolytes</u>. In addition, fibrinogen is important to <u>clotting</u>. (para 10-10b)

7.   In adults, the formed elements make up about 40% to 45% of the total blood <u>volume</u>. (para 10-11)

8.   The primary function of RBCs is to contain the protein called <u>hemoglobin</u>, which in turn carries <u>oxygen</u>.

      The shape of the RBC increases its capacity for the <u>flow</u> of substances into and out of the cell.

      Within the cytoplasm of the RBC is a special protein called <u>hemoglobin</u>. Because of its iron atoms, it has a great affinity for <u>oxygen</u>.

At the end of its life period, the "worn out" RBC is removed by the <u>spleen</u> and the "pieces," particularly the iron, are salvaged by the <u>liver</u>. (para 10-11a)

9.   The second category of formed elements of the blood is the <u>white</u> blood cells.

Phagocytic WBCs actively attack foreign substances and engulf them in a process called <u>phagocytosis</u>. When the WBCs are overcome and die, their bodies accumulate to form a substance called <u>pus</u>.

The lymphocytes are involved with the <u>immune</u> system of the body, including the production of <u>antibodies</u>. (para 10-11b)

10.   The third type of formed element in the blood is the <u>platelets</u>. These are fragments of former <u>cells</u>. They are very important in the <u>clotting</u> process. (para 10-11c)

11.   After the formed elements and fibrinogen are removed from the blood, the remaining fluid is called <u>serum</u>. (para 10-12)

12.   One very important transport function of the blood is to carry gases back and forth between the <u>lungs</u> and the individual <u>cells</u> of the body. The sites of exchange are the <u>alveoli</u> and the individual body <u>cells</u>. At these sites, a gas moves from the area where its concentration is <u>higher</u> to the area where its concentration is <u>lesser</u>.

Near the alveoli, most of the dissolved oxygen is rapidly picked up by the <u>hemoglobin</u> of the <u>RBCs</u>. Thus, the RBC is the main transporting element for <u>oxygen</u>.

Produced during metabolic oxidation is <u>carbon dioxide</u>. It passes through the cell membrane and the capillary wall to become dissolved in the <u>plasma</u> of the blood. Through the action of an enzyme, most of this gas is transformed into <u>bicarbonate</u> ions. (para 10-13)

13.   The escape of blood from damaged blood vessels is called <u>hemorrhage</u>.

The first response to a cut or ruptured vessel is contraction (spasm) of the blood <u>vessel</u> itself.

If the hole is small, a plug formed by clumping of the <u>platelets</u> may stop the bleeding.

A complicated process for sealing off holes or ends of blood vessels is called <u>coagulation</u> or <u>clotting</u>. In this process, the blood forms a solid mass call a blood <u>clot</u>. After a number of steps, the protein fibrinogen is converted into sticky strands of <u>fibrin</u>. The resulting meshwork traps <u>RBCs</u> and <u>plasma</u> and thus seals the opening.

Within the body, a collection of blood, usually clotted and resulting from hemorrhage, is called a hematoma.

The spleen, the liver, and large abdominal veins serve as blood reservoirs, which can be mobilized to maintain the circulating blood volume. (para 10-16)

14. If an individual has lost whole blood by hemorrhaging, it is often necessary to give transfusions of whole blood. Whole blood transfusions continue the functions of the RBCs. When fluid but few formed elements have been lost, plasma or a plasma substitute will often be used.

On the surfaces of RBCs, there are a number of substances called antigens. The blood of other individuals may contain antibodies to these substances. The blood of the recipient and the blood of the donor must be matched to avoid potentially fatal reactions. Important systems of such antigens include the ABO system and the Rh system. (para 10-17)

15. The lungs, liver, and heart have two blood supplies. Blood to be worked upon by the organ is called functional blood. Blood for the usual exchange of materials between body cells and the blood is called nutrient blood. (para 10-20a)

16. An end artery is the sole supply of blood to an area of the body. End arteries are most common in the brain and the heart. If an end artery is damaged and can no longer supply blood to its corresponding area, the tissues of that area will die. (para 10-20c)

17. Cycles of blood circulation include the pulmonary cycle and the systemic cycle.

In the first of these, blood circulates from the heart to the lungs and back to the heart. In the second, blood circulates from the heart to the rest of the body and back to the heart. (para 10-22)

18. The primary motive force for driving the blood along the arteries is the heart, which consists of four separate chambers. (para 10-23)

19. Why is the wall of the left ventricle especially thick? It has to drive the blood throughout the body.

The amount of blood forced out of each ventricle in one contraction is called the stroke volume. The amount of blood pumped out of the ventricles in a minute is called the cardiac output. (para 10-26c(2), (5))

20.   Structures ensuring that fluids pass through them in only one direction are called valves.

The contraction of the atrial walls forces the blood from the atria through the AV valves and into the ventricles. When the ventricles contract, the openings between the atria and the ventricles are sealed by the cusps of the AV valves.

When the ventricles relax, the openings between the great arteries and the ventricles are sealed by the cuplike cusps of the semilunar valves. (para 10-27)

21.   The action of the heart is accelerated by the sympathetic portion of the nervous system. It is slowed down by the parasympathetic portion.

The sinoatrial (SA) node is often called the pacemaker of the heart because it initiates each cycle of the contractions of the heart chamber. Impulses begin in the SA node, pass to the AV node, and then descend through the septal bundles to stimulate the myocardium of the ventricular walls to contract. (para 10-28a)

22.   Nutrient blood is supplied to the walls of the heart by the right and left coronary arteries.

The openings leading into the coronary arteries are located in the base of the ascending aorta, just behind the cusps of the semilunar valve. When this valve is open, its cusps cover the openings of the coronary arteries. When the valve is closed, the backpressure within the aorta fills the coronary arteries with blood. The coronary arteries then distribute the blood to all of the tissues of the relaxed heart.

Many of the branches of the coronary arteries are of the end artery type. If such a branch is closed for any length of time, the tissue in the area supplied will die. (para 10-28b)

23.   The blood from the tissues of the heart is collected by the cardiac veins. These veins empty into the coronary sinus, a vessel which in turn empties into the right atrium. (para 10-28c)

24.   The pumping action of the heart continues without stopping until death. During each cycle, the heart changes in shape and size and tends to rotate. The number of cycles per minute is called the heart rate. To reduce friction, the heart is enclosed within a serous sac, called the pericardium. (para 10-31a)

25.   Intimately covering the surface of the heart is the visceral pericardium, also called the epicardium. The outer serous membrane is the parietal pericardium. The pericardial fluid provides lubrication and reduces the amount of work done by the heart. (para 10-31b)

26. In addition to the force provided by contraction of the ventricular walls, blood is also driven by the elastic recoil of the arterial walls.

The highest arterial pressure is called the systolic pressure, and the lowest is called the diastolic pressure.

Pressure on the blood in the arteries can be further increased by vasoconstriction and gravity. (para 10-33)

27. Structures that ensure that blood flows in only one direction in the veins, are the valves. When a vein is subjected to pressure, the result is a pump effect. Veins receive pressure from the arteries, muscular contractions, and gravity. (para 10-34)

28. Capillary beds are provided with precapillary sphincters and post-capillary sphincters. The first can stop the flow of blood into the capillaries. When the postcapillary sphincters close, more fluid flows into the tissue space. (para 10-37)

29. As it returns to the trunk, cool venous blood is gradually warmed by the arterial blood flowing in the opposite direction. (para 10-40b)

30. In general, the lymphatic system is a drainage system that picks up tissue fluids and returns them to the cardiovascular system. These are picked up in the interstitial spaces.

A lymph capillary begins with a blind end.

These capillaries join to form lymphatic vessels.

A major collecting vessel of the lymphatic system is the thoracic duct, which empties into the deep veins of the neck.

The lymph nodes function as sieves for the lymph passing through them.

The lymphocytes are primarily involved in the immune reactions of the body. (para 10-44)

31. An additional circulatory system is the cerebrospinal fluid system.

Two fluid-filled hollow organs are the eyeball and the inner ear. (para 10-45)

End of Lesson 10

LESSON 11	The Human Endocrine System.
LESSON ASSIGNMENT	Paragraphs 11-1 through 11-18.
LESSON OBJECTIVES	After completing this lesson, you should be able to:

11-1. Given a hormone, identify the endocrine organ that produces it.

11-2. Match the names or types of hormones with the body functions affected.

SUGGESTION	After completing the assignment, complete the exercises at the end of this lesson. These exercises will help you to achieve the lesson objectives.

LESSON 11

THE HUMAN ENDOCRINE SYSTEM

Section I. INTRODUCTION

11-1. ENDOCRINE ORGANS

ENDO = within

CRINE = secrete

The endocrine system (Figure 11-1) is a loose collection of organs called <u>endocrine glands</u>.

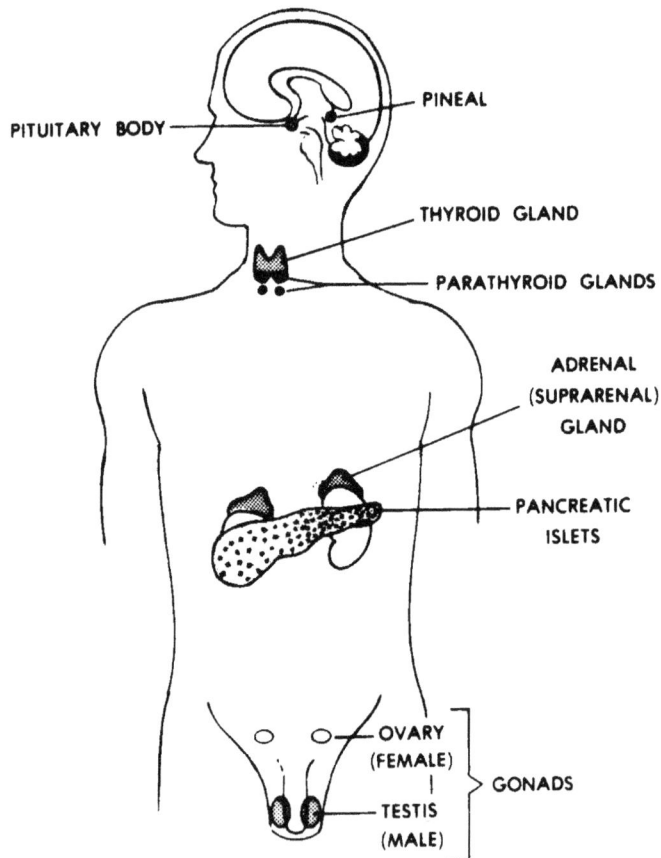

Figure 11-1. The endocrine glands of the human body and their locations.

a. The endocrine glands are organs of internal secretion. Since they lack a duct system, they are often referred to as ductless glands.

b. Since their secretions pass into the blood, they are usually well supplied with blood vessels.

11-2. HORMONE

The secretion of an endocrine organ is called a hormone. The hormone is a chemical required in very small amounts for the proper development and/or functioning of the body. (Note the similarity of this definition to that of a vitamin. However, the hormone is produced within the body, and the vitamin is acquired from without.)

11-3. TARGET ORGAN AND FEEDBACK MECHANISM

When the hormone is secreted by the endocrine organ, it is carried by the blood to the appropriate organ, the target organ. In addition, the level of activity of the target organ often affects the activity of the endocrine organ. Thus, there is a feedback mechanism that causes the endocrine organ to secrete just the right amount of hormone.

Section II. THE PITUITARY BODY

11-4. GENERAL

a. The pituitary body is located immediately under the brain. It is in a special hollow of the floor of the cranial cavity. The pituitary body is actually two glands: the posterior pituitary gland and the anterior pituitary gland.

b. As a whole, the pituitary body produces a large number of hormones. These affect many tissues of the body. Many of these hormones are referred to as tropins (or trophins) because they cause development or activity of the tissues.

11-5. POSTERIOR PITUITARY GLAND

In the embryo, the posterior pituitary gland develops as an outcropping (hypophysis) of the inferior part of the brain. Later in life, the posterior pituitary gland remains connected to the forebrain-stem. There is a series of nuclei in the fore-brainstem which are together referred to as the hypothalamus. The hormones of the posterior pituitary gland are actually produced in the hypothalamus. The hormones pass from the hypothalamus to the posterior pituitary gland by way of neurosecretory fibers. From the posterior pituitary gland, the hormones are secreted into the blood. The main hormones of the posterior pituitary gland are:

a. **Antidiuretic hormone (ADH).** ADH is involved with the resorption or salvaging of water within the kidneys. Antidiuretic hormone is produced under thirst conditions.

b. **Oxytocin.** Oxytocin has several specific effects, particularly upon smooth muscle. It is involved with contractions of smooth muscle in the uterus and with milk secretion.

11-6. ANTERIOR PITUITARY GLAND

In the embryo, the anterior pituitary gland develops from the roof of the pharynx. Eventually, it lies in front of and attached to the posterior pituitary gland. Certain cells of the hypothalamus produce specific secretions called releasing factors. A special venous portal system carries these releasing factors to the anterior pituitary gland. There, they stimulate the cells of the anterior pituitary gland to secrete their specific hormones.

a. **Somatotropin (Somatotrophic Hormone; Growth Hormone).** Somatotropin stimulates the growth of the body in general. When this hormone is deficient, dwarfism results. When it is present in excess amounts, giantism results.

b. **Thyrotropin.** Thyrotropin stimulates the thyroid gland to produce its hormones.

c. **Adrenocorticotropic Hormone (ACTH).** Adrenocorticotropic hormone stimulates the adrenal (suprarenal) cortex to produce its hormones.

d. **Luteinizing Hormone (LH).** Luteinizing hormone stimulates ovulation and luteinization of ovarian follicles in females and promotes testosterone production in males.

e. **Follicle-Stimulating Hormone (FSH).** Follicle-stimulating hormone stimulates ovarian follicle growth in females and stimulates spermatogenesis in males.

f. **Prolactin.** Prolactin stimulates milk production and maternal behavior in females.

Section III. THE PINEAL GLAND

11-7. LOCATION

The pineal gland is located just above the brainstem. It is between the cerebral hemispheres.

11-8. FUNCTIONS

The details of the secretions and functions of the pineal gland are still not fully understood. Apparently, they are associated with sexual drive and reproduction. At least in lower animals, the pineal gland is influenced by the cumulative number of hours of light passing into the eyes each day.

Section IV. THE THYROID AND PARATHYROID GLANDS

11-9. THE THYROID GLAND

a. **Location and Structure.** The thyroid gland is located around the trachea, just below the larynx. It consists of two lobes, left and right. They are connected across the front of the trachea by an isthmus.

b. **Hormones.**

(1) <u>Thyroxin</u>. The most important hormone produced by the thyroid gland is thyroxin. Thyroxin affects the basal metabolic rate (BMR), the level of activity of the body. Since iodine is an important element in the structure of thyroxin, the dietary intake of iodine is very important. When the gland is not functioning properly, it may become enlarged (goiter). Insufficient or excess thyroxin has serious effects on the body.

(2) <u>Calcitonin</u>. A second hormone of the thyroid gland is calcitonin. It is involved with calcium metabolism in the body.

11-10. THE PARATHYROID GLANDS

On the posterior side of each thyroid lobe is a pair (2 + 2 = 4) of tiny bodies called the <u>parathyroid glands</u>. The hormone of the parathyroid glands is <u>parathoromone</u>. It is important in maintaining the calcium levels of the body. When excess thyroid tissue is removed in surgery, the surgeon takes care not to remove the parathyroid glands.

Section V. THE PANCREATIC ISLETS (ISLANDS OF LANGERHANS)

11-11. LOCATION AND STRUCTURE

There are small groups of cells, known as <u>islets</u>, distributed through the substance of the pancreas. These cells function independently of the pancreas and produce their own hormones.

11-12. HORMONES

Insulin and glucagon are two important hormones of the islets. These hormones are concerned with the glucose levels in the body.

Section VI. THE ADRENAL (SUPRARENAL)GLANDS

11-13. LOCATION AND STRUCTURE

As seen in a previous lesson, the kidneys are attached to the upper posterior abdominal wall by a combination of fat and fascia. The adrenal (suprarenal) gland is embedded in the fat immediately above each kidney. Each is triangular or crescent shaped. Each adrenal gland has a central medulla and an outer cortex.

11-14. HORMONES OF THE ADRENAL MEDULLA

The central portion of the adrenal gland produces two hormones: epinephrine (Adrenalin) and norepinephrine (noradrenalin). These hormones mobilize the energy-producing organs of the body and immobilize the others. This is important during the stress reaction ("fight or flight").

11-15. HORMONES OF THE ADRENAL CORTEX

The outer portion (the cortex) of the adrenal gland produces a variety of hormones which can be grouped into three categories:

a. Mineralocorticoids (for example, aldosterone), which are concerned with the electrolyte and water balance of the body.

b. Glucocorticoids (for example, cortisol), which are concerned with many metabolic functions. They are especially known for their anti-inflammatory effects.

c. Sex Hormones (adrenal androgens and estrogens).

Section VII. THE GONADS AS ENDOCRINE GLANDS

11-16. GENERAL

We have already seen that the primary sex organs (gonads) produce sex hormones in addition to sex cells (gametes). These hormones help to determine an individual's actual sex (male or female) and promote the sexual development of the individual.

11-17. MALE SEX HORMONES

In the male, certain cells of the testes produce the male sex hormones, known as <u>androgens</u> (for example, testosterone). Androgens are concerned with male sexuality.

11-18. FEMALE SEX HORMONES

The sex hormones of the female are known as the <u>estrogens</u> and <u>progesterone</u>. In the female, these hormones are secreted in a cyclic sequence, the menstrual cycle. During this cycle, the hormones affect a number of tissues of the female body. These tissues include the endometrium of the uterus, the milk-producing portions of the mammary glands, and so forth. During pregnancy, the placenta continues the production of progesterone.

Continue with Exercises

EXERCISES, LESSON 11

REQUIREMENT. The following exercises are to be answered by completing the incomplete statements.

  After you have completed all the exercises, turn to "Solutions to Exercises" at the end of the lesson, and check your answers with the Academy solutions.

1. The endocrine glands are organs of internal _____n. Since they lack a duct system, they are often called _____less glands. They are usually well supplied with blood vessels to facilitate the release of their secretions into the _____d.

2. A hormone is a chemical required in very small amounts for the proper _____ment or f_____g of the body. Unlike a vitamin, a hormone is produced within the body.

  The blood carries each hormone to its t_____ organ, whose level of activity in turn affects the _____e organ. Thus, to ensure the secretion of just the right amount of hormone, there is a _____k mechanism.

3. Many of the hormones of the pituitary body are called "tropins" because they cause _____ment or _____y of the tissues.

4. Antidiuretic hormone (ADH) and oxytocin are produced by the _____s and released from the _____r pituitary gland.

  Antidiuretic hormone is involved with the r_____ption or sal_____g of water within the kidneys. Antidiuretic hormone is produced under t_____t conditions.

  Oxytocin is involved with _____s of smooth muscle in the uterus and with _____k secretion.

5. Somatotropin, thyrotropin, and adrenocorticotropic hormone (ACTH) are produced by the _____r pituitary gland.

  Somatotropin stimulates the _____th of the body in general.

  Thyrotroin stimulates the _____d gland to produce its hormones.

  ACTH stimulates the a_____ cortex to produce its hormones.

6. The pineal gland is apparently associated with _____l drive and _____n.

7. Thyroxin and calcitonin are secreted by the _____d gland.

    Thyroxin affects the b____ m_____ rate.

    Calcitonin is involved with _____m metabolism.

8. The hormone of the parathyroid gland is parat_____, important in maintaining the _____m levels of the body.

9. Two important hormones of the pancreatic islets are i____in and g____on. These hormones are concerned with the _____se levels in the body.

10. Epinephrine and norepinephrine are produced by the adrenal _____. These hormones mobilize the _____y-producing organs and _____ze the others. This is important during the stress reaction, "_____t or _____t."

11. Mineralocorticoids, glucocorticoids, and some sex hormones are produced by the adrenal _____. Mineralocorticoids are concerned with e_____s of the body. Glucocorticoids are known for their anti-_____y effects.

12. The testes produce male sex hormones, known as _____s.

    The female sex hormones are the _____s and _____e. The tissues affected by female sex hormones include the _____m of the uterus and the milk-producing portions of the _____y glands. During pregnancy, the placenta continues the production of _____e.

Check Your Answers on Next Page

SOLUTIONS TO EXERCISES, LESSON 11

1.   The endocrine glands are organs of internal <u>secretion</u>. Since they lack a duct system, they are often called <u>ductless</u> glands. They are usually well supplied with blood vessels to facilitate the release of their secretions into the <u>blood</u>. (para 11-1)

2.   A hormone is a chemical required in very small amounts for the proper <u>development</u> or <u>functioning</u> of the body. Unlike a vitamin, a hormone is produced within the body.

    The blood carries each hormone to its <u>target</u> organ, whose level of activity in turn affects the <u>endocrine</u> organ. Thus, to ensure the secretion of just the right amount of hormone, there is a <u>feedback</u> mechanism. (paras 11-2, 11-3)

3.   Many of the hormones of the pituitary body are called "tropins" because they cause <u>development</u> or <u>activity</u> of the tissues. (para 11-4b)

4.   Antidiuretic hormone, (ADH) and oxytocin are produced by the <u>hypothalamus</u> and released from the <u>posterior</u> pituitary gland.

    ADH is involved with the <u>resorption</u> or <u>salvaging</u> of water within the kidneys. ADH is produced under <u>thirst</u> conditions.

    Oxytocin is involved with <u>contractions</u> of smooth muscle in the uterus and with <u>milk</u> secretion. (para 11-5)

5.   Somatotropin, thyrotropin, and adrenocorticotropic hormone (ACTH) are produced by the <u>anterior</u> pituitary gland.

    Somatotropin stimulates the <u>growth</u> of the body in general.

    Thyrotropin stimulates the <u>thyroid</u> gland to produce its hormones.

    ACTH stimulates the <u>adrenal</u> cortex to produce its hormones. (para 11-6)

6.   The pineal gland is apparently associated with <u>sexual</u> drive and <u>reproduction</u>. (para 11-8)

7.   Thyroxin and calcitonin are secreted by the <u>thyroid</u> gland.

    Thyroxin affects the <u>basal metabolic</u> rate.

    Calcitonin is involved with <u>calcium</u> metabolism. (para 11-9)

8.   The hormone of the parathyroid gland is <u>parathormone</u>, important in maintaining the <u>calcium</u> levels of the body. (para 11-10)

9. Two important hormones of the pancreatic islets are insulin and glucagon. These hormones are concerned with the glucose levels in the body. (paras 11-11, 11-12)

10. Epinephrine and norepinephrine are produced by the adrenal medulla. These hormones mobilize the energy-producing organs and immobilize the others. This is important during the stress reaction, "fight or flight." (para 11-14)

11. Mineralocorticoids, glucocorticoids, and some sex hormones are produced by the adrenal cortex. Mineralocorticoids are concerned with electrolytes of the body. Glucocorticoids are known for their anti-inflammatory effects. (para 11-15)

12. The testes produce male sex hormones, known as androgens.

The female sex hormones are the estrogens and progesterone. The tissues affected by female sex hormones include the endometrium of the uterus and the milk-producing portions of the mammary glands. During pregnancy, the placenta continues the production of progesterone. (paras 11-17, 11-18)

End of Lesson 11

LESSON 12	The Human Nervous System.
LESSON ASSIGNMENT	Paragraphs 12-1 through 12-38.
LESSON OBJECTIVES	After completing this lesson, you should be able to:

12-1. Identify the major subdivisions of the human nervous system.

12-2. Match terms related to the human nervous system with their definitions.

12-3. Identify body functions and classes of organs and tissues which are the concern of major subdivisions of the human nervous system.

12-4. Given a list of statements about one of the following topics, identify the false statement.

    a.   Electrochemical transmission of neuron impulses.

    b.   General sensory and motor pathways.

    c.   Levels of control in the human nervous system.

SUGGESTION   After completing the assignment, complete the exercises at the end of this lesson. These exercises will help you to achieve the lesson objectives.

LESSON 12

THE HUMAN NERVOUS SYSTEM

Section I. INTRODUCTION

12-1. THE NEURON

The neuron (nerve cell) is the conducting unit of the nervous system. It is specialized to be irritable and transmit signals, or impulses. The neurons are held together and supported by another nervous tissue known as neuroglia, or simply glia.

12-2. MAJOR SUBDIVISIONS OF THE NERVOUS SYSTEM

The human nervous system can be considered in three major subdivisions:

a. The central nervous system (CNS).

b. The peripheral nervous system (PNS).

c. The autonomic nervous system (ANS).

12-3. DEFINITIONS

a. **Neuron.** A neuron (Figure 12-1) is the nerve cell body plus all of its processes and coverings.

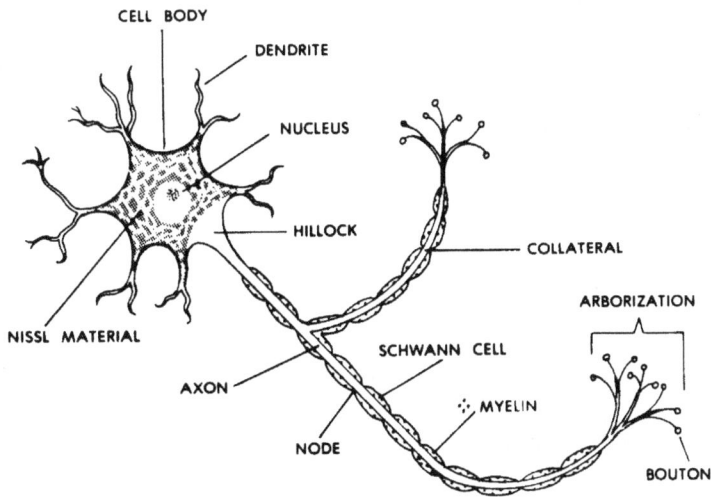

Figure 12-1. A "typical" neuron.

b. **Nerve.** A nerve is a collection of neuron <u>processes</u> together and <u>outside</u> of the CNS.

c. **Fiber Tract.** A fiber tract is a collection of neuron <u>processes</u> together and <u>within</u> the CNS.

d. **Ganglion.** A ganglion is a collection of nerve cell <u>bodies</u> together and <u>outside</u> of the CNS.

e. **Nucleus.** A nucleus is a collection of nerve cell <u>bodies</u> together and <u>within</u> the CNS.

f. **General Versus Special.** If a nervous element is found throughout the body, it is said to be <u>general</u>. A nervous element located in just one part of the body, such as the head, is said to be <u>special</u>. For example, there are <u>general</u> senses, such as pain and temperature, and there are <u>special</u> sense organs, such as the eyes and the ears.

g. **Somatic Versus Visceral.**

(1) The term <u>somatic</u> refers to the peripheral part of the body. Thus, when we speak of <u>somatic innervation</u>, we are talking about the nerve supply to the trunk wall, upper and lower members, head, and neck.

SOMA = body, body wall

(2) The term <u>visceral</u> refers to the visceral organs. These include hollow organs with smooth muscle (such as the intestines and the blood vessels) as well as sweat glands. Thus, <u>visceral innervation</u> refers to the nerve supply for these organs. Note that the visceral organs are located within both the trunk and periphery of the body. Those in the periphery include the blood vessels and the sweat glands.

12-4. OVERVIEW OF THE HUMAN NERVOUS SYSTEM

The human nervous system is an integrated, connected circuitry of nervous tissues.

a. It is supplied with special junctions called <u>synapses</u>. The synapses ensure the flow of information along the circuitry in the proper direction.

b. In general terms, the human nervous system can be compared to a computer. There is <u>input</u>--the sensory information. There is <u>central</u> <u>collation</u> of input along with previously stored information.

COLLATE = collect, compare, and arrange in order

Once a decision has been reached by the central portion, there is an <u>output</u> of commands to the effector organs (muscles and/or glands).

c. There are various control systems to be found within the body. Of these, the nervous system is the most rapid and precise in responding to specific situations.

Section II. THE CENTRAL NERVOUS SYSTEM

12-5. INTRODUCTION

a. **Centrality.** The central nervous system (CNS) (Figure 12-2) is central in both location and function.

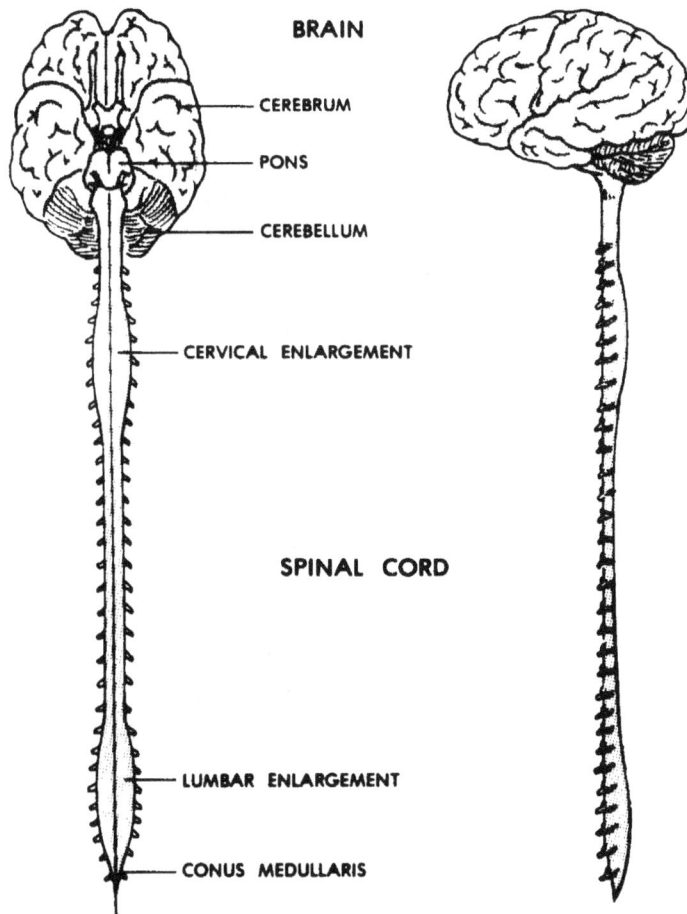

Figure 12-2. The human central nervous system (CNS).

b. **Major Subdivisions.** The fully formed CNS can be considered in two major subdivisions: the brain and the spinal cord.

12-6. THE HUMAN BRAIN

The human brain (Figures 12-3 and 12-4) has three major subdivisions: brainstem, cerebellum, and cerebrum.

a. **The Brainstem.** The brainstem is the core of the brain. We consider it in three parts--the hindbrainstem, the midbrainstem, and the forebrainstem. In general, the brainstem is made up of many nuclei and fiber tracts. It is a primary coordinating center of the human nervous system.

b. **The Cerebellum.** Over the hindbrainstem is the cerebellum. The cerebellum is connected to both the midbrainstem and the hindbrainstem. The cerebellum is the primary coordinating center for muscle actions. Here, patterns of movements are properly integrated. Thus, information is sent to the appropriate muscles in the appropriate sequences. Also, the cerebellum is very much involved in the postural equilibrium of the body.

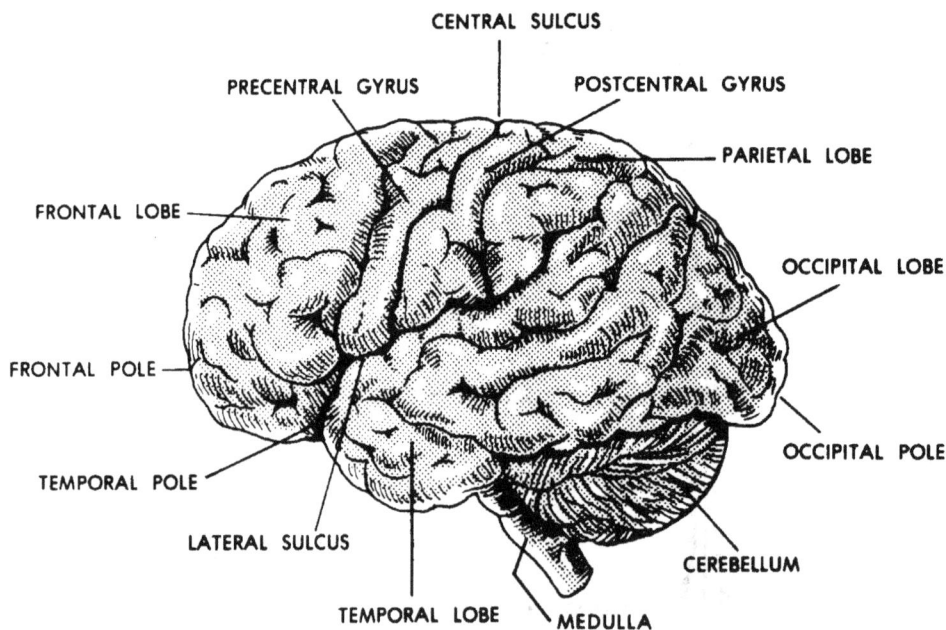

Figure 12-3. Human brain; sideview.

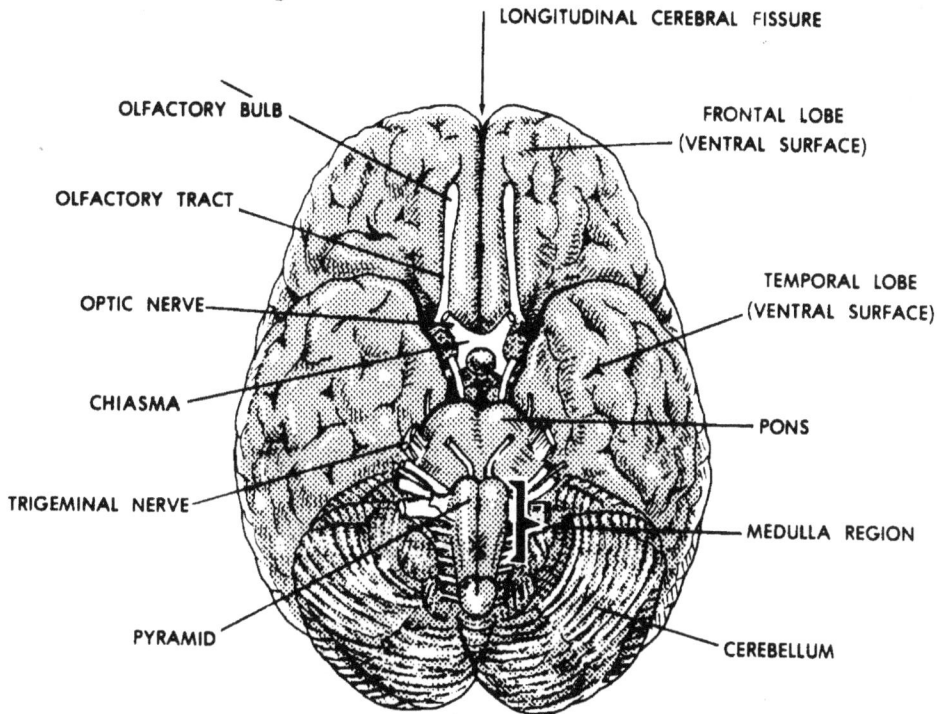

Figure 12-4. Human brain; bottom view.

    c. **The Cerebrum.** Attached to the forebrainstem are the two cerebral hemispheres (Figure 12-5). Together, these two hemispheres make up the cerebrum. Among related species, the cerebrum is the newest development of the brain.

    (1) Cerebral hemispheres. The cerebrum consists of two cerebral hemispheres, right and left. They are joined together by a very large fiber tract known as the corpus callosum (the great commissure).

    (2) Lobes. Each hemisphere can be divided into four lobes. Each lobe is named after the cranial bone it lies beneath--parietal, frontal, occipital, and temporal. (Actually, there are five lobes. The fifth is hidden at the bottom of the lateral fissure. It is known as the insula or insular lobe. It is devoted mainly to visceral activities.)

    (3) Gyri and sulci. The cerebral cortex, the thin layer at the surface of each hemisphere, is folded. This helps to increase the amount of area available to neurons. Each fold is called a gyrus. Each groove between two gyri is called a sulcus.

    (a) The lateral sulcus is a cleft separating the frontal and parietal lobes from the temporal and occipital lobes. Therefore, the lateral sulcus runs along the lateral surface of each hemisphere.

(b)   The <u>central sulcus</u> is a cleft separating the frontal from the parietal lobe. Roughly, each central sulcus runs from the left or right side of the cerebrum to top center and over into the medial side of the cerebrum.

(c)   There are two gyri that run parallel to the central sulcus. Anterior to the central sulcus is the <u>precentral gyrus</u>. Posterior to the central sulcus is the <u>postcentral gyrus</u>.

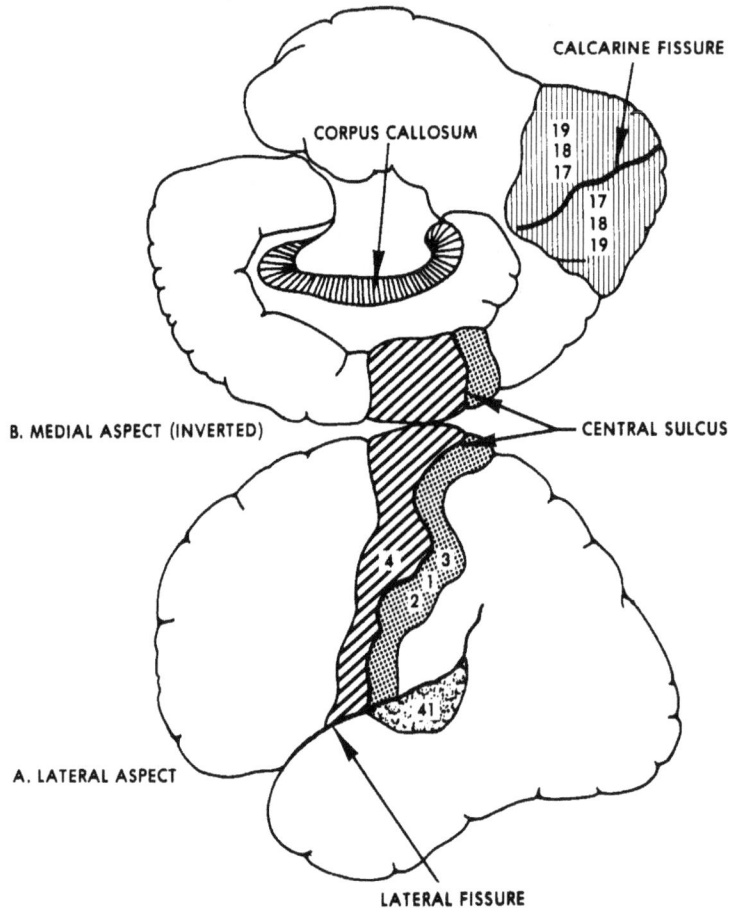

BRODMANN NO.	GYRUS	CONSCIOUS SENSATION
3-1-2	POSTCENTRAL	CONSCIOUS SENSORY
4	PRECENTRAL	VOLITIONAL MOTOR
17-18-19	"CALCARINE"	CONSCIOUS VISION (SIGHT)
41	SUP. TEMPORAL	CONSCIOUS HEARING (AUDITORY)

Figure 12-5. Left cerebral hemisphere.

12-7. THE HUMAN SPINAL CORD

Extending inferiorly from the brain is the spinal cord (Figure 12-6).

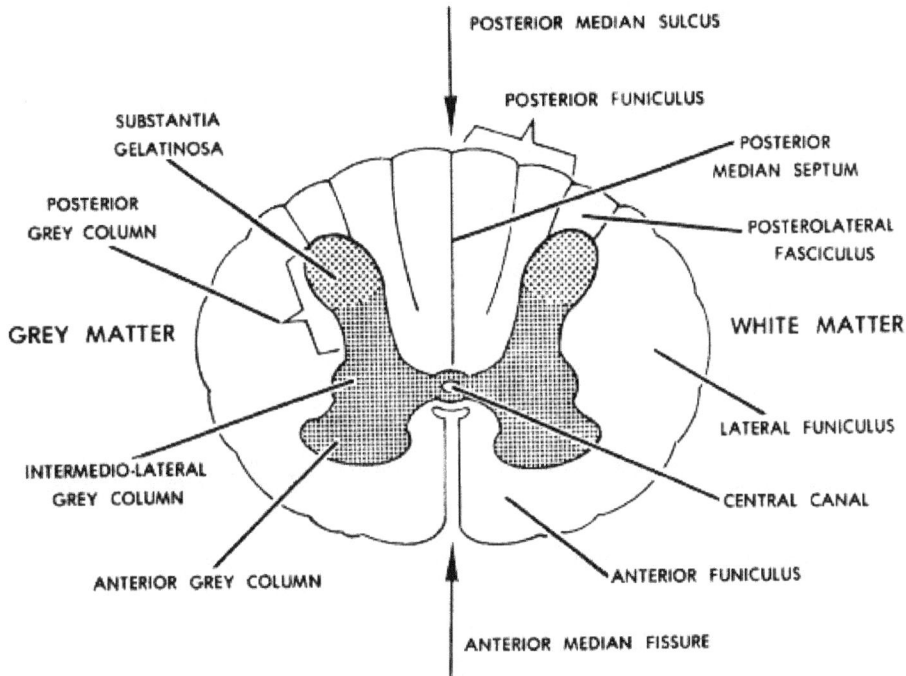

Figure 12-6. A cross section of the spinal cord.

a. The spinal cord is continuous with the brainstem. Together, the spinal cord and the brainstem are called the neuraxis. The foramen magnum is taken as the point that divides the brainstem from the spinal cord. Thus, the brainstem is within the cranial cavity of the skull, and the spinal cord is within the vertebral (spinal) canal of the vertebral column.

b. The spinal cord has a central portion known as the gray matter. The gray matter is surrounded by the white matter.

(1) The gray matter is made up of the cell bodies of many different kinds of neurons.

(2) The white matter is made up of the processes of neurons. The white color is due to their myelin sheaths. These processes serve several purposes: Many make a variety of connections within the spinal cord. Many ascend the neuraxis to carry information to the brain. Many descend the neuraxis to carry commands from the brain.

Section III. THE PERIPHERAL NERVOUS SYSTEM (PNS)

12-8. PERIPHERAL NERVES

Connecting the CNS to all parts of the body are individual organs known as nerves. A <u>nerve</u> is a collection of neuron processes together and outside of the CNS. <u>Peripheral nerves</u> are nerves which pass from the CNS to the periphery of the body. Together, they are referred to as the <u>peripheral nervous system</u>.

a. These nerves are bilateral and segmental.

(1) <u>Bilateral</u>. This means that the peripheral nerves occur in pairs. In each pair, there is one nerve to the right and one to the left.

(2) <u>Segmental</u>. The pairs of peripheral nerves occur in intervals, corresponding to the <u>segments</u> of the human embryo.

b. Peripheral nerves connected to the brainstem are called <u>cranial nerves</u>. They are numbered from I through XII and also have individual names.

c. Peripheral nerves connected to the spinal cord are called <u>spinal nerves</u>. They are identified by a letter representing the region of the vertebral column and a number representing the sequence in the region:

(1) Cervical: C-1 through C-8.

(2) Thoracic: T-1 through T-12.

(3) Lumbar: L-1 through L-5.

(4) Sacral: S-1 through S-5.

(5) Coccygeal.

Thus, there are 31 pairs of spinal nerves.

12-9. A "TYPICAL" SPINAL NERVE (FIGURE 12-7)

In the human body, every spinal nerve has essentially the same construction and components. By learning the anatomy of one spinal nerve, you can understand the anatomy of all spinal nerves. Like a tree, a typical spinal nerve has roots, a trunk, and branches (rami).

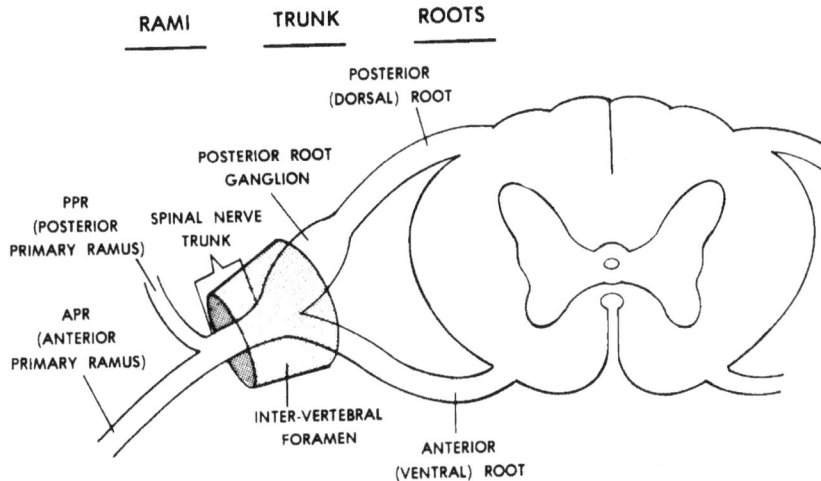

Figure 12-7. A typical spinal nerve, with a cross section of the spinal cord.

a. Coming off of the posterior and anterior sides of the spinal cord are the posterior (dorsal) and anterior (ventral) roots of the spinal nerve. An enlargement on the posterior root is the posterior root ganglion. A ganglion is a collection of neuron cell bodies, together, outside the CNS.

b. Laterally, the posterior and anterior roots of the spinal nerve join to form the spinal nerve trunk. The spinal nerve trunk of each spinal nerve is located in the appropriate intervertebral foramen of the vertebral column. (An intervertebral foramen is a passage formed on either side of the junction between two vertebrae.)

c. Where the spinal nerve trunk emerges laterally from the intervertebral foramen, the trunk divides into two major branches. These branches are called the anterior (ventral) and posterior (dorsal) primary rami (ramus, singular). The posterior primary rami go to the back. The anterior primary rami go to the sides and front of the body, and to the upper and lower members.

Section IV. THE AUTONOMIC NERVOUS SYSTEM

12-10. CONTROL OF VISCERAL ACTIVITIES

The autonomic nervous system (ANS) is that portion of the nervous system concerned with commands for smooth muscle tissue, cardiac muscle tissue, and glands.

a. The term visceral organs may be used to include:

(1) The various <u>hollow organs</u> of the body whose walls have smooth muscle tissue in them. Examples are the blood vessels and the gut.

(2) The glands.

b. The visceral organs are innervated by the ANS. This results in a "visceral motor system." For most of us, the control of the visceral organs is automatic, that is, without conscious control. However, recent research demonstrates that conscious control of some of the visceral organs is possible after proper training.

12-11. TWO MAJOR SUBDIVISIONS

The ANS is organized into two major subdivisions--the sympathetic and the parasympathetic nervous systems.

a. The neurons of the <u>sympathetic nervous system</u> originate in the thoracic and lumbar regions of the spinal cord. Thus, it is also known as the <u>thoraco-lumbar outflow</u>.

b. Some of the neurons of the <u>parasympathetic nervous system</u> originate in nuclei of the brainstem. Others originate in the sacral region of the spinal cord. Thus, the parasympathetic nervous system is also known as the <u>cranio-sacral outflow</u>.

c. In the ANS, there are always two neurons (one after the other) connecting the CNS with the visceral organ. The cell bodies of the second neurons form a collection outside the CNS, called a ganglion. Processes of these <u>postganglionic neurons</u> extend to the visceral organs. Those processes going to peripheral visceral organs are included with the peripheral nerves.

12-12. EQUILIBRIUM

Under ordinary circumstances, the sympathetic and parasympathetic nervous system have opposite effects upon any given visceral organ. That is, one system will stimulate the organ to action, and the other system will inhibit it. The interplay of these two systems helps visceral organs to function within a stable equilibrium. This tendency to produce an equilibrium is called <u>homeostasis</u>.

12-13. RESPONSE TO STRESS

Under conditions of stress, the sympathetic nervous system produces a "fight-or-flight" response. In other words, it mobilizes all of the energy producing structures of the body. Simultaneously, it inhibits those structures that do not contribute to the mobilization of energy. For example, the sympathetic nervous system makes the heart beat faster. Later, as equilibrium is restored, the parasympathetic nervous system slows the heart down.

Section V. ELECTROCHEMICAL TRANSMISSION OF NEURON IMPULSES

2-14. INTRODUCTION

a. The functional elements of the human nervous system are the <u>neurons</u>. The neurons are alined in sequences, one neuron after the other, to form circuits. The transmission of information along the length of a neuron is electrochemical in nature.

b. An important fact is that "connecting" neurons do not actually touch each other. Instead, there is a space between the end of one and the beginning of the next ("continuity without contact"). A specified chemical, called a neurotransmitter, is required to cross the gap between one neuron and the next.

12-15. RESTING POTENTIAL

As a part of their life processes, neurons are able to produce a concentration of negative ions inside and a concentration of positive ions outside of the cell membrane. The difference in the concentration of ions produces an electrical potential across the membrane. This condition is often referred to as <u>polarization</u>. When the neuron is not actually transmitting, this electrical potential across the membrane is known as the <u>resting potential</u>.

12-16. ACTION POTENTIAL (DEPOLARIZATION AND REPOLARIZATION)

Where a stimulus is applied to the neuron, the polarity of the ions is disrupted at the same location. Thus, that location is said to be <u>depolarized</u>. The ions in adjacent areas along the neuron then attempt to restore the original polarity at the location of the stimulus. However, as <u>repolarization</u> occurs in the area of the stimulus, the adjacent areas themselves become <u>depolarized</u>. This results in a wavelike progression of <u>depolarization/repolarization</u> along the length of the neuron. By this means, information is transferred along the neuron.

12-17. EFFECT OF THE THICKNESS OF THE NEURON PROCESSES

The speed with which an impulse travels is proportional to the thickness of the neuron process. The thickest processes (A fibers) have the fastest transmission (about 120 meters/second). The thinnest processes (C fibers) are the slowest (as slow as 1/2 meter/second). The B fibers (thicker than C fibers and thinner than A fibers) are faster than C fibers and slower than A fibers.

12-18. THE SYNAPSE

The gap between successive neurons is wide enough that impulses do not travel from one neuron to the next in the same way as along a single neuron. Information travels from one neuron to the next by means of a chemical neurotransmitter. Together, the gap and the "connecting" membranes of the neurons are called the synapse (Figure 12-8). The gap is called the synaptic cleft.

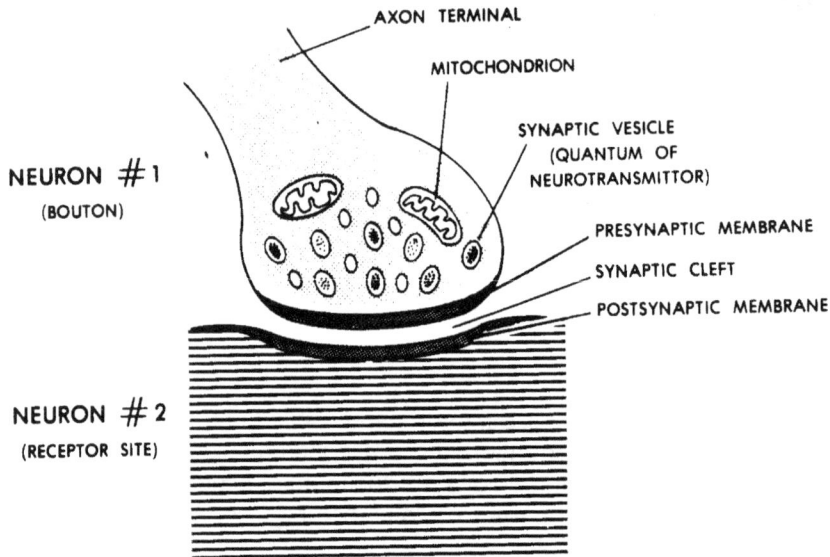

Figure 12-8. A synapse.

a. Many synaptic vesicles (bundles of neurotransmitters) are found in the terminal bulb (bouton) of the first neuron. Each vesicle contains a quantum, a specific amount, of neurotransmitter or a substance used to make the neurotransmitter.

b. When the impulse reaches the bouton, these vesicles are stimulated to release their neurotransmitter. The neurotransmitter then passes out of the bouton, through the presynaptic membrane, into the synaptic cleft. On the other side of the synaptic cleft is the postsynaptic membrane. This is the receptor site of the second neuron.

c. The neurotransmitter is located only in the terminal bulb of the first neuron. For this reason, impulses travel in only one direction through the synapse, from the first to the second neuron. Since this process consumes much energy, there are many well-developed mitochondria in the bouton, or terminal bulb.

12-19. THE NEUROMUSCULAR JUNCTION

While the synapse is the "connection" between two neurons, the neuromuscular junction (Figure 12-9) is the "connection" between a motor neuron and a striated muscle fiber.

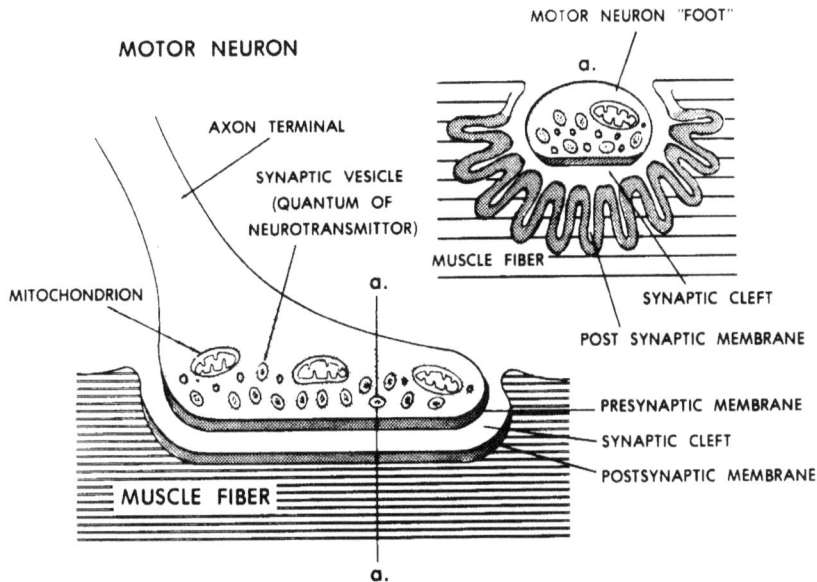

Figure 12-9. A neuromuscular junction.

a. In general terms, the neuromuscular junction and the synapse are physiologically identical. Synaptic vesicles in the enlarged bouton of the motor neuron contain the neurotransmitter acetylcholine (ACH). As an impulse reaches the bouton, ACH is released and passes through thepresynaptic membrane into the synaptic cleft. However, the surface of the postsynaptic membrane is in a series of longitudinal folds. This greatly increases the surface area receptive to the ACH.

b. The motor unit is the group of striated muscle fibers innervated by the terminal arborization (tree-like branching) of one motor neuron. The fewer the muscle fibers found per motor unit, the more the muscle is capable of finer movements. As the number in the motor unit increases, the muscle action is coarser. When a muscle is to be used, the nervous system recruits just enough motor units to supply the strength needed for the work to be done.

Section VI. THE GENERAL REFLEX AND THE REFLEX ARC

12-20. THE GENERAL REFLEX

The simplest reaction of the human nervous system is the reflex. A reflex is defined as an automatic reaction to a stimulus.

12-21. THE GENERAL REFLEX ARC

The pathway followed by the stimulus (impulse) from beginning to end is the reflex arc. The general reflex arc (Figure 12-10) of the human nervous system has a minimum of five components:

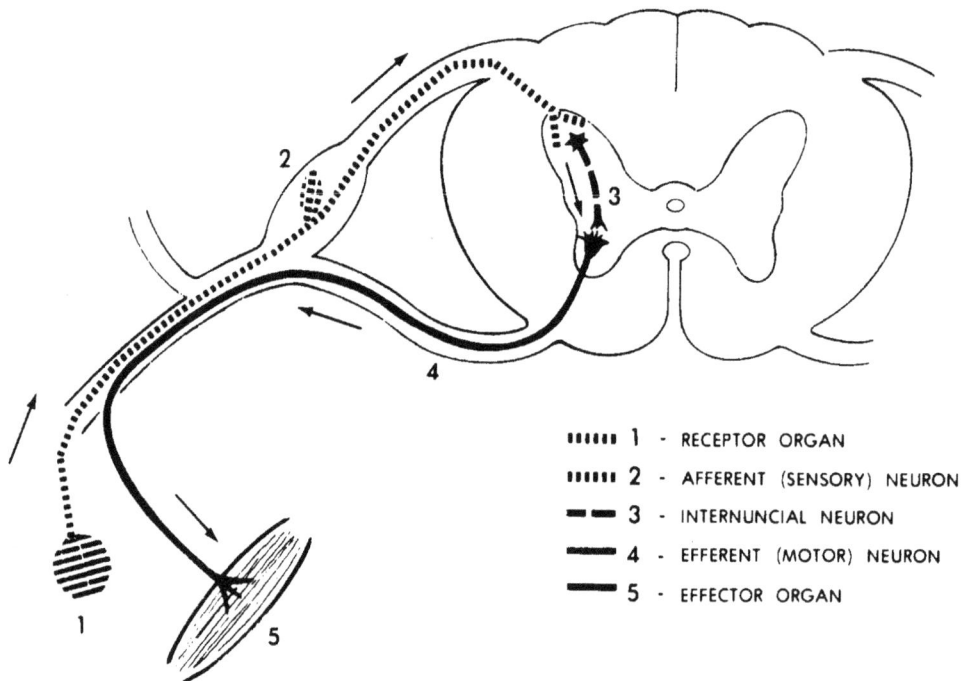

Figure 12-10. The general reflex arc.

a. The stimulus is received by a receptor organ specific to that stimulus.

b. From the receptor organ, the stimulus is carried to the CNS by way of an afferent (sensory) neuron within the appropriate peripheral nerve. The cell body of this afferent neuron is located in the posterior root ganglion of a spinal nerve or the individual ganglion of a cranial nerve.

c. Within the spinal cord or brainstem, the terminal of the afferent neuron synapses with the interneuron, or internuncial neuron.

INTER = between

NUNCIA = messenger

In turn, the internuncial neuron synapses with the cell body of the efferent (motor) neuron.

d. In the spinal cord, the cell bodies of the efferent (motor) neurons make up the anterior column of the gray matter. In the brainstem, the motor neurons make up the individual nuclei of the cranial nerves. The axon of the motor neuron passes out of the CNS by way of the appropriate peripheral nerve. Command information is thus carried away from the CNS.

e. The information is then delivered by the motor neuron to the effector organ. Somatic motor neurons lead to striated muscle fibers, particularly in skeletal muscles. Autonomic (visceral) motor neurons lead to smooth muscle tissue, cardiac muscle tissue, or glands.

Section VII. GENERAL SENSORY PATHWAYS OF THE HUMAN NERVOUS SYSTEM

12-22. INTRODUCTION TO PATHWAYS

A pathway of the human nervous system is the series of neurons or other structures used to transmit an item of information. In general, we consider two major types of pathways--the general sensory pathways and the motor pathways.

a. **Ascent or Descent Through the Neuraxis**. The general sensory pathways ascend through the neuraxis to the brain. The motor pathways descend through the neuraxis from the brain. The neuraxis includes both the spinal cord and the brainstem. The pathways are included in various fiber tracts of the neuraxis.

b. **Crossing to the Opposite Side (Decussation)**. At some specific level in the neuraxis, all of these pathways cross to the opposite side of the midline of the CNS. (Each crossing is called a decussation.) Thus, the right cerebral hemisphere of the brain communicates with the left half of the body. The left cerebral hemisphere communicates with the right half of the body.

12-23. INTRODUCTION TO GENERAL SENSORY PATHWAYS

a. **The General Senses.** The general senses detect those specific stimuli which are received throughout the body (general distribution). When these general senses are perceived at the conscious level (in the cerebral cortex), they are known as sensations. The general senses of humans include pain, touch, temperature, and proprioception ("body sense").

b. **Neurons of a General Sensory Pathway.** A general sensory pathway extends from the point where the stimulus is received to the postcentral gyrus of the cerebral hemisphere (para 12-6c(3)(c)). The postcentral gyrus is the site of conscious sensation of a stimulus. Between the point of stimulus reception and the postcentral gyrus, there is a minimum of three neurons in series.

(1) The first neuron is the afferent (sensory) neuron. It picks up the information from the sensory receptor organ and carries it to the CNS via the appropriate peripheral nerves.

(2) The second neuron is the interneuron, located within the spinal cord or brainstem. It crosses the midline of the CNS to the opposite side. It then ascends the neuraxis to the forebrainstem, where it reaches a mass of gray matter called the thalamus. In the thalamus, the interneuron synapses with the cell body of the third neuron.

(3) The axon of the third neuron projects up through the cerebral hemisphere to the appropriate location in the postcentral gyrus.

c. **Homunculus of Conscious Sensations.** There is a specific location in the postcentral gyrus which corresponds to each location in the body. For example, a location in the postcentral gyrus near the midline of the brain (at the top of the cerebral hemisphere) receives information from the hip region. On the other hand, information from the tongue and the pharynx projects to the lowest part of the postcentral gyrus, just above the lateral sulcus.

d. **Visceral Sensory Inputs.** Visceral sensory inputs follow pathways different from those of other general sensory pathways. The inputs for visceral reflex actions usually travel via the parasympathetic nerves. The visceral inputs for pain usually travel via the sympathetic nerves.

12-24. PAIN--A GENERAL SENSE

Pain is an ancient protective mechanism which generally helps us to avoid injury. However, tolerance for pain varies from one individual to another.

a. **Means of Reducing Pain (Analgesia).**

(1) Endorphins ("morphine from within"). Endorphins are chemicals found naturally within the body which tend to block the sensation of pain.

(2) Drugs. Clinically, a number of drugs are used to block or reduce the sensation of pain.

(3) Competing inputs. Competing pain stimuli tend to minimize each other. The body usually recognizes one pain stimulus at a time. Thus, an individual may "bite his lip" when he anticipates a painful experience.

b. **Pain Receptor.** The pain receptor is not a specific receptor organ, as with most senses. This receptor is referred to as a free nerve ending.

c. **Excessive Stimulation.** If any of the other senses receives excessive stimulus, pain results. Examples are excessive light and excessive noise.

d. **Pain Reflex Arc.** Generally, a pain sensory input causes a reflex action long before the information reaches the cerebral cortex and the pain is consciously perceived. For example, you will remove your hand from a hot object before you realize you have been burned.

e. **Pathway for Conscious Sensation of Pain.** As usual, the pathway leading to conscious sensation of pain consists of three neurons.

(1) The first neuron is the afferent (sensory) neuron from the free nerve ending. Within the CNS, it synapses with the interneuron.

(2) The axon of the interneuron crosses to the opposite side of the CNS. It then ascends the neuraxis in a fiber tract known as the lateral spinothalamic tract. This tract is found in the lateral funiculus (see Figure 12-6). In the thalamus, the interneuron synapses with the third neuron.

(3) The third neuron projects to the appropriate location of the postcentral gyrus of the cerebral hemisphere. Here, this information is interpreted or recognized as a pain sensation from a particular part of the body.

12-25. TEMPERATURE -- GENERAL SENSES

There are two categories of temperature in the body--warmth and cold.

a. However, these are relative entities. For example, a given temperature seems cool when compared to a much higher temperature and seems hot when compared to a much lower temperature.

b. In addition, the body has two different mechanisms for sensing temperature.

(1) Specific sensory receptors detect warmth and especially cold in the periphery of the body.

(2) Special heat-sensitive neurons in the hypothalamus detect increases in the temperature of the blood that flows through the hypothalamus (portion of the forebrainstem). By this means, the body monitors the core temperature, the temperature in the central part of the body.

c. Neurons for the general sense of temperature use pathways similar to those discussed for pain (para 12-24e). They include both nerves and fiber tracts.

12-26. TOUCH -- GENERAL SENSES

Throughout the body are a variety of sensory receptors which detect varying degrees of pressure. For example, the pacinian corpuscles are typical of the receptors which detect deep pressure. In addition, an individual can usually identify the location of a touch on his body; in fact, he can usually distinguish two simultaneous touches to adjacent areas (the "two-touch test"). As usual with the general senses, sensory inputs for touch can also result in immediate reflex actions.

a. **Pathway for Conscious Sensation of Light Touch.**

(1) The pathway for the conscious sensation of light touch begins with the usual afferent (sensory) neuron as the first neuron. The afferent neuron carries the information to the CNS by way of the appropriate nerve.

(2) In the CNS, the afferent neuron synapses with the interneuron, the second neuron of the pathway. After crossing to the opposite side of the CNS, the interneuron ascends the neuraxis in the fiber tract known as the anterior spinothalamic tract. This is in the anterior funiculus of the spinal cord (Figure 12-6).

(3) In the thalamus, the second neuron synapses with the third neuron. The axon of the third neuron then projects to the appropriate location in the postcentral gyrus of the cerebral hemisphere. There, it is interpreted as the conscious sensation, light touch.

b. **Pathway for Conscious Sensation of Deep Touch.** The pathway for deep touch is quite different from that for light touch.

(1) Still, the first neuron is the afferent neuron from the deep touch receptor to the CNS via the appropriate nerve. When the axon of the afferent neuron enters the CNS, it turns upward and ascends the neuraxis in the posterior funiculus (Figure 12-6) of the same side that it entered. In other words, it does not yet cross the midline of the CNS.

(2) In the lower hindbrainstem, the axon of the first neuron synapses with the cell body of the second neuron. The axon of the second neuron then crosses to the opposite side of the brainstem. This axon then continues the ascent through the neuraxis to the thalamus, where it synapses with the third neuron.

(3) Again, the axon of the third neuron projects to the appropriate location in the postcentral gyrus of the cerebral hemisphere. There, impulses are interpreted as conscious sensations of deep touch.

12-27. "BODY SENSE"

a. **General.** Body sense is the combined information from a number of sensory inputs. Second by second, these inputs keep the brain informed of the specific posture of the body and its parts. Some of the senses involved include:

(1) Muscle sense (proprioception).

(2) Joint capsule sense.

(3) Integument senses.

(4) Special senses (eye, ear, etc.).

b. **Proprioception (Muscle Sense).**

(1) For proprioception, there is a very special receptor organ to monitor the degree of stretch of the muscle. These receptor organs, called muscle spindles or stretch receptors, are distributed within the fleshy belly of each skeletal muscle. In effect, the muscle spindles are parallel to striated muscle fibers of the skeletal muscles. Therefore, as the muscle fibers contract or are stretched, the muscle spindle detects relative muscle length.

(a) The afferent neuron from the muscle spindle is known as the annulospiral neuron because its terminal is coiled. Due to this coiling, it is a spring-like apparatus which can be stretched or compressed according to the condition of the muscle. The annulospiral neuron travels to the CNS by way of the appropriate nerve. It continuously carries information about the specific state of the muscle.

(b) An annulospiral neuron from a muscle in one of the limbs, in particular, synapses directly on the motor neuron that carries commands back to the same muscle. This motor neuron is called the alpha motor neuron. Together, the annulospiral neuron and the alpha motor neuron make up the stretch (monosynaptic) reflex. Due to this reflex, there is a proportionate increase in the tension of a muscle as it stretches.

(2) Another stretch receptor associated with the skeletal muscle is the Golgi tendon organ. As its name implies, this organ is located within the tendon of the muscle. The Golgi tendon organ is located in the tendon near its attachment to the muscle fibers. Thus, it detects relative muscle tension. Its threshold is higher than that of the muscle spindles; in other words, there must be proportionately more contraction before it puts out a signal. Thus, when the muscle has been stretched excessively and might be subject to injury, its afferent neuron carries the message to the CNS. This results in relaxation of the muscle.

(3) The pathway for the conscious sensation of these stretches uses the same structures as the deep touch general sense.

Section VIII. MOTOR PATHWAYS IN THE HUMAN NERVOUS SYSTEM

12-28. INTRODUCTION

The CNS receives information through the sensory pathways and collates this information against information stored in memory. This results in a decision. If the decision is to do something, then the CNS sends out commands through the motor pathways to the effector organs (muscles, glands, etc.).

a. The motor pathways descend in the neuraxis and transmit the commands to the motor neurons. The processes of motor neurons leave the CNS by way of the peripheral nerves. The somatic motor neurons activate striated muscle fibers. The visceral motor neurons activate smooth muscle tissue, cardiac muscle tissue, and glands.

b. We usually consider two general motor pathways--the pyramidal motor pathways and the extrapyramidal motor pathways.

12-29. PYRAMIDAL MOTOR PATHWAYS

A pyramidal motor pathway is primarily concerned with volitional (voluntary) control of the body parts, particularly with the fine movements of the hands. Since such a pathway is concerned with volitional actions, it is suitable for neurological screening and testing.

a. **Cerebral Motor Cortex.** The pyramidal motor pathway begins in the precentral gyrus of the cerebral hemisphere. As we have already seen with the sensory pathways, the neurons making up the cerebral cortex of the precentral and postcentral gyri are arranged in a pattern (motor homunculus) corresponding to the various parts of the body to which they are connected.

b. **Motor Neurons.** From the precentral gyrus, the axons of these upper motor neurons (UMN) pass into the neuraxis of the CNS and descend. At the level of the appropriate segmental nerve, the UMN synapses either directly or indirectly with a lower motor neuron of the segmental nerve. Direct synapses (monosynaptic) provide the most rapid reactions. Such direct synapses are used in particular for the fine movements of the hands.

c. **Corticospinal Pathways.** The medulla is the lowest part of the brainstem. On the underside of the medulla, the axons of the UMNs form a pair of structures known as the pyramids. Immediately below the pyramids, at the beginning of the spinal cord, the axons cross to the opposite side of the CNS (spinal cord). The axons then descend as the lateral corticospinal tract, within the lateral funiculus (Figure 12-6). Thus, the left cerebral hemisphere commands the right side of the body, and the right cerebral hemisphere controls the left side of the body.

12-30. EXTRAPYRAMIDAL MOTOR PATHWAYS

The extrapyramidal motor pathways are concerned with automatic (nonvolitional) control of body parts. This particularly includes patterned, sequential movements or actions. Thus, the major command system of the human nervous system uses these pathways. There are several extrapyramidal motor pathways. Having multisynaptic circuits throughout the CNS, they use many intermediate relays before reaching the effector organs. The cerebellum of the brain plays a major role in extrapyramidal pathways; the cerebellum is the major center for coordinating the patterned sequential actions of the body, such as walking.

Section IX. LEVELS OF CONTROL IN THE HUMAN NERVOUS SYSTEM

12-31. INTRODUCTION

a. **General Concept.** The human nervous system can be thought of as a series of steps or levels (Figure 12-11). Each level is more complex than the level just below. No level is completely overpowered by upper levels, but each level is controlled or guided by the next upper level as it functions.

b. **Changes With Development or Injury.**

(1) Babinski's reflex involves dorsiflexion of the big toe when the sole of the foot is stimulated. It can be normally observed in infants up to 18 months of age. As the pyramidal motor pathways develops completely, this reflex disappears. However, if the pyramidal motor system is injured, the Babinski reflex tends to return.

(2) Thus, it is possible to evaluate the extent of development of an individual by identifying the highest level of control. In the case of injury, the highest active level of control helps determine the site of the injury.

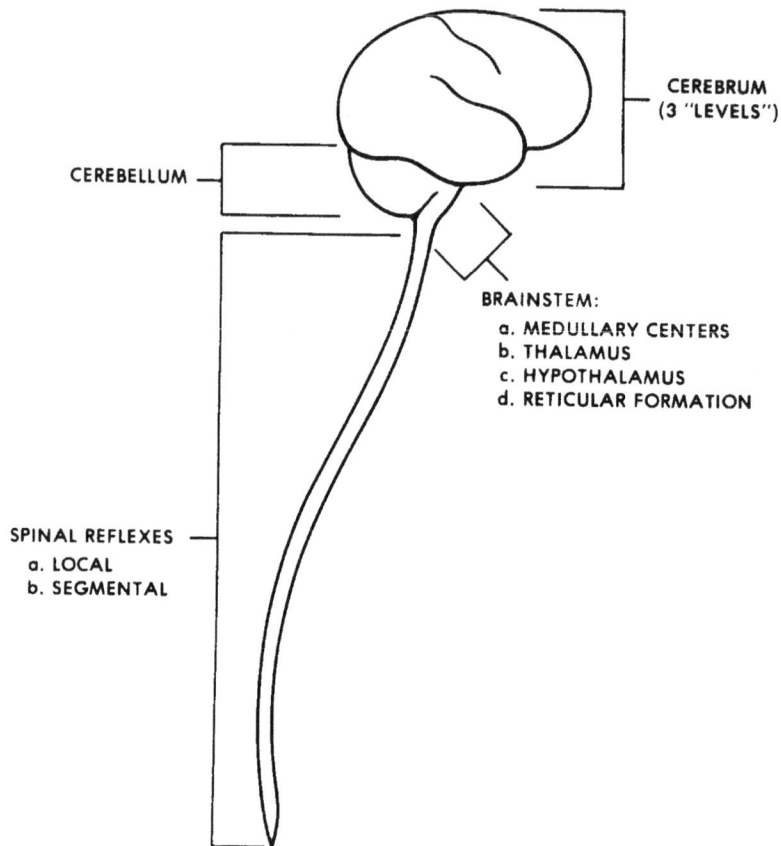

Figure 12-11. Levels of the CNS.

12-32. REFLEXES

a. **Reflex Arc.** The simplest and lowest level of control is the reflex arc. The reflex arc operates essentially on the level of the sensory input.

b. **Segmental Reflexes.** Segmental reflexes produce a wider reaction to a stimulus than the reflex arc. For this purpose, the nervous system is organized more complexly. Thus, information spreads to a wider area of CNS. We can observe a greater reaction to the stimulus.

12-33. BRAINSTEM "CENTERS"

Within the brainstem, there is a well integrated series of control centers.

a. **Visceral Centers of the Medulla.** There is a group of nuclei in the medulla of the hindbrainstem. Together, these nuclei control the visceral activities of the body, such as respiration, heart beat, etc.

b. **Reticular Formation.** Within the substance of the brainstem is a diffuse system called the reticular formation. The reticular formation has a facilitory (excitatory) area and an inhibitory area. Thus, this control area tends to activate or slow down activities of the body. Thus, it is responsible for producing sleep or wakefulness.

c. **Hypothalamus and Thalamus.**

(1) The thalamus is a group of nuclei found together in the forebrainstem. The thalamus is the major relay center of sensory inputs from the body.

(2) The hypothalamus is a higher control center for visceral activities of the body. It is found associated with the thalamus.

12-34. CEREBELLUM

The cerebellum has been greatly developed, with many functional subdivisions. It is the primary center for the integration and control of patterned, sequential motions of the body. The cerebellum is also the center of control of body posture and equilibrium.

12-35. CEREBRUM

In humans, the highest level of nervous control is localized in the cerebrum. It is at this level that conscious sensation and volitional motor activity are localized. Even so, we can clearly designate three levels of control within the cerebrum:

a. **Visceral (Vegetative) Level.** This level is concerned primarily with visceral activities of the body, as related to fight-or-flight, fear, and other emotions.

b. **Patterned (Stereotyped) Motor Actions.** Here, activities of the body are standardized and repetitive in nature. An example of a stereotyped pattern of muscle activity would be the sequence of muscle actions involved in walking.

c. **Volitional Level.** The volitional level is the highest and newest level of control. Here, cognition (thinking) occurs, and unique, brand-new solutions can be created.

Section X. MISCELLANEOUS TOPICS

12-36. CEREBRAL AREAS

Specific areas of the cerebral cortex are concerned with specific parts of the body, with specific types of inputs, and with specific types of activities. Most often, each area is numbered as a specific Brodmann's area. For example, the precentral gyrus, concerned with volitional motions, is Brodmann's area number 4. It is the beginning of the pyramidal motor system. Likewise, the superior temporal gyrus (at the inferior margin of the lateral sulcus) is Brodmann's area number 41; it is the center for hearing.

12-37. DOMINANCE

a. About 90% of humans are right-handed. Thus, for these individuals, the left cerebral hemisphere is said to be dominant over the right cerebral hemisphere.

b. For 96% of humans, the speech center is located in the left cerebral hemisphere.

c. Thus, an injury to the left cerebral hemisphere is generally more serious than an injury to the right cerebral hemisphere.

12-38. MEMORY

a. Memory is that faculty which enables an individual to store and retrieve factual items (sensations, impressions, facts, and ideas). Memory is ultimately the result of the unceasing flow of sensory information into the CNS. These items are stored in the CNS; just exactly how and where is the subject of much research and discussion. All sensory inputs are collated against these stored items in order to arrive at an appropriate action decision. (Often, no action is the most appropriate decision.)

b. At present, at least two types of memory are recognized in the human brain--short-term memory and long-term memory.

(1) Short-term memory. A common example of short-term memory is the ability to hold a phone number in mind for a number of seconds without "memorizing" it. Short-term memory is usually limited to about seven bits of information.

(2) Long-term memory. A portion of the cerebral cortex known as the hippocampus is thought to be important in transferring information from short-term memory to long-term memory. If the hippocampus is nonfunctional, the individual can learn nothing, but his previously long-term memory remains intact.

Continue with Exercises

EXERCISES, LESSON 12

REQUIREMENT. The following exercises are to be answered by completing the incomplete statements.

After you have completed all the exercises, turn to "Solutions to Exercises" at the end of the lesson, and check your answers.

1.   The neuron is also called a nerve _____. It is the c_____ing unit of the nervous system. It is specialized to be _____ble and transmit s_____s, or i_____s.

2.   The three major subdivisions of the human nervous system are the c_____ nervous system, the p_____ nervous system, and the a_____ nervous system.

3.   A neuron is the nerve cell _____y plus all of its p_____s and coverings.

A nerve is a collection of neuron _____s together and (within) (outside of) the CNS.

A fiber tract is a collection of neuron _____s together and (within) (outside of) the CNS.

A ganglion is a collection of nerve cell _____s together and (within) (outside of) the CNS.

A nucleus is a collection of nerve cell _____ together and (within) (outside of) the CNS.

4.   The human nervous system is supplied with special junctions called _____s.

5.   In general terms, the human nervous system can be compared to a _____r. Sensory information is the __put, which is c_____ed along with previously stored information. Once a decision has been reached by the central portion, there is an __put of commands to the e_____or organs (muscles and/or glands).

6.   The brainstem is a primary c_____ing center of the human nervous system.

The cerebellum is the primary coordinating center for _____e actions. Here, patterns of movement are properly i_____ed. Also, the cerebellum is very much involved in the _____al equilibrium of the body.

The newest development of the brain is the _____ m.

7.   The autonomic nervous system (ANS) is that portion of the nervous system concerned with commands for _____th muscle tissue, _____c muscle tissue, and _____s.

    For most of us, the control of the visceral organs is _____c, that is, without conscious control.

8.   The ANS is organized into two major subdivisions--the s_____c and p_____c nervous systems. The first of these is also known as the t_____-l_____ outflow. The second is also known as the c_____-s_____ outflow.

    If one of these subdivisions stimulates an organ, the other will i_____t it. The interplay of the two subdivisions helps visceral organs to function within a stable _____m. This tendency is called _____s.

    Under conditions of stress, the sympathetic nervous system mobilizes all of the _____y-producing structures of the body. For example, it makes the heartbeat (faster) (slower). Later, as equilibrium is restored, the parasympathetic nervous system has the (same) (opposite) effect.

9.   The neurons are alined in sequences to form c_____ts. The transmission of information along a neuron is _____cal in nature. Crossing the gap between one neuron and the next is a chemical called a _____r.

10.   Neurons are able to concentrate _____tive ions inside and _____tive ions outside of the cell membrane. When the neuron is not actually transmitting, this process produces the _____g_____l.

11.   When the polarity of ions is disrupted by a stimulus, that location on the cell membrane is said to be _____ized. The restoration of the original polarity is called re_____. At the same time, adjacent areas are depolarized. Thus, there is a wave of d_____/r_____ along the length of the neuron.

12.   The speed of an impulse is proportional to the _____ness of the neuron process. Transmission is fastest in the _____est neurons.

13.   Together, the gap and the "connecting" membranes between two successive neurons are called the _____. The gap itself is called the _____c_____t. Containing specific amounts of neurotransmitter are _____c_____les in the terminal bulb of the first neuron. When an impulse reaches the bouton, the vesicles are stimulated to release their _____r. This substance passes through the _____c membrane, across the synaptic cleft, and to the _____c membrane. Since this process consumes much energy, the bouton contains many well-developed _____.

14.   The neuromuscular junction is the "connection" between a _____r neuron and a s_____d_____e fiber. It is nearly identical to a _____e. However, the surface of the postsynaptic membrane is in a series of longitudinal _____s. This greatly increases the s_____a____ receptive to the ACH.

       The group of striated muscle fibers innervated by one motor neuron is called the motor _____. Fewer muscle fibers per motor unit result in _____r movements. More muscle fibers per motor unit result in _____ movements.

15.   The simplest reaction is called a _____, defined as an _____c reaction to a stimulus.

16.   A pathway of the human nervous system is the series of neurons or other structures used to _____t an item of information. In general, we consider two major types of pathways--the general _____y pathways and the _____r pathways.

       At some specific level in the neuraxis, all of these pathways cross to the opposite side. Each crossing is called a _____tion. Thus, the right cerebral hemisphere communicates with the _____ half of the body. The left cerebral hemisphere communicates with the _____ half of the body.

17.   The general senses include _____n, _____ch, t_____e, and pro_____n ("body ____e").

       A general sensory pathway extends from the point where the stimulus is received to the _____central gyrus (fold) of the cerebral hemisphere. This gyrus is the site of conscious sensation of a stimulus.

       Corresponding to each location in the body, there is a specific location in the _____l gyrus.

18.   Pain is an ancient protective mechanism which generally helps us to avoid
_____y. Endorphins are chemicals found naturally within the body which tend to
block the sensation of _____.

        The pain receptor is not a specific receptor organ. It is referred to as a _____
nerve ending.

19.   The body has two different mechanisms for sensing temperature. Detecting
warmth and cold in the periphery of the body are specific sensory _____s.
Special heat-sensitive neurons in the hypothalamus detect increases in the temperature
of the _____.

20.   The pacinian corpuscles are typical of the receptors which detect ____p_____re.

21.   Another term for muscle sense is p_____n. For this, there is a special
receptor organ to monitor the _____h of the muscle. These receptor organs are called
muscle s_____s or s_____h receptors. They detect relative muscle l_____.

        Another stretch receptor associated with the skeletal muscle is the ____i_____n
organ. As its name implies, this organ is located within the _____ of the muscle. It
detects relative muscle t_____.

22.   The CNS receives information through the _____ pathways and collates this
information against information stored in _____. This results in a _____n. If the
decision is to do something, then the CNS sends out commands through the _____
pathways to the _____r organs.

23.   We usually consider two general motor pathways--the _____dal and the
e_____dal motor pathways.

24.   A pyramidal motor pathway is primarily concerned with _____ional (_____ary)
control of body parts, particularly with the fine movements of the _____s.

        The pyramidal motor pathway begins in the p_____l gyrus of the cerebral
hemisphere. As we have already seen, the neurons making up the precentral and
postcentral gyri are arranged in a pattern corresponding to the various _____ts of the
body to which they are connected.

Immediately below the pyramids, the axons _____s to the opposite side of the CNS. Thus, the left cerebral hemisphere commands the _____ side of the body, and the right cerebral hemisphere controls the _____ side of body.

25.   The extrapyramidal motor pathways are concerned with _____ c (n_____l) control of body parts. This particularly includes patterned, sequential _____ts or a_____ns. The cerebellum plays a major role in extrapyramidal pathways. The cerebellum is the major center for c_____ing the patterned sequential actions of the body, such as w_____ing.

26.   The human nervous system can be thought of as a series of ____ps or _____ls. Each level is more _____x than the level just below. No level is completely over_____d by upper levels, but each level is c_____d or g_____d by the next upper level as it functions.

The simplest and lowest level of control is the _____ arc. Producing a wider reaction to a stimulus are _____d reflexes.

27.   Nuclei in the medulla of the hindbrainstem control the _____l activities of the body, such as r_____n, _____t _____t, etc.

The reticular formation of the brainstem has a f_____tory area and an i_____tory area. This control area produces ____p or _____ness.

The thalamus is a group of nuclei found together in the _____stem. The thalamus is the major _____y center of s_____y inputs.

The hypothalamus is a higher control center for _____l activities of the body.

28.   The cerebellum is the primary center for the i_____tion and _____l of patterned, sequential _____ns of the body.

29.   In humans, the highest level of control is localized in the _____. Localized at this level are c_____s sensation and _____nal motor activity.

The visceral level within the cerebrum is concerned with _____activities of the body, as related to f_____t-or-f_____t, _____r, and other emotions.

The second level of the cerebrum is concerned with st_____ed patterns of muscle activity.

The third level of the cerebrum is the _____ nal level. Here, c_____ n (thinking) occurs, and unique, brand-new _____ s can be created.

30.   The precentral gyrus is Brodmann's area number ___. The center for hearing is Brodmann's area number ____.

31.   In right-handed individuals, the left cerebral hemisphere is said to be _____ t over the right cerebral hemisphere. For most individuals, an injury to the ____ t cerebral hemisphere is more serious.

32.   Memory is the faculty which enables an individual to store and retrieve factual items such as s_____ tions, i_____ sions, f___ s, and i___ s. All sensory inputs are collated against these stored items in order to arrive at an appropriate d_____ n for a_____ n .

33.   There are at least two types of memory--_____t-term memory and ____-term memory.

       Short-term memory is usually limited to about _____ bits of information.

       A portion of the cerebral cortex is thought to be important in transferring information from ____-term memory to ____-term memory. It is called the h_____ s. What is the effect on learning if the hippocampus is nonfunctional?

Check Your Answers on Next Page

SOLUTIONS TO EXERCISES, LESSON 12

1.   The neuron is also called a nerve <u>cell</u>. It is the <u>conducting</u> unit of the nervous system. It is specialized to be <u>irritable</u> and transmit <u>signals</u>, or <u>impulses</u>. (para 12-1)

2.   The three major subdivisions of the human nervous system are the <u>central</u> nervous system, the <u>peripheral</u> nervous system, and the <u>autonomic</u> nervous system. (para 12-2)

3   A neuron is the nerve cell <u>body</u> plus all of its <u>processes</u> and coverings.

    A nerve is a collection of neuron <u>processes</u> together and <u>outside</u> of the CNS.

    A fiber tract is a collection of neuron <u>processes</u> together and <u>within</u> the CNS.

    A ganglion is a collection of nerve cell <u>bodies</u> together and <u>outside</u> of the CNS.

    A nucleus is a collection of nerve cell <u>bodies</u> together and <u>within</u> the CNS. (para 12-3)

4.   The human nervous system is supplied with special junctions called <u>synapses</u>. (para 12-4a)

5.   In general terms, the human nervous system can be compared to a <u>computer</u>. Sensory information is the <u>input</u>, which is <u>collated</u> along with previously stored information. Once a decision has been reached by the central portion, there is an <u>output</u> of commands to the <u>effector</u> organs (muscles and/or glands). (para 12-4b)

6.   The brainstem is a primary <u>coordinating</u> center of the human nervous system.

    The cerebellum is the primary coordinating center for <u>muscle</u> actions. Here, patterns of movement are properly <u>integrated</u>. Also, the cerebellum is very much involved in the <u>postural</u> equilibrium of the body.

    The newest development of the brain is the <u>cerebrum</u>. (para 12-6)

7.   The autonomic nervous system (ANS) is that portion of the nervous system concerned with commands for <u>smooth</u> muscle tissue, <u>cardiac</u> muscle tissue, and <u>glands</u>.

    For most of us, the control of the visceral organs is <u>automatic</u>, that is, without conscious control. (para 12-10)

8.   The ANS is organized into two major subdivisions--the sympathetic and parasympathetic nervous systems. The first of these is also known as the thoraco-lumbar outflow. The second is also known as the cranio-sacral outflow.

       If one of these subdivisions stimulates an organ, the other will inhibit it. The interplay of the two subdivisions helps visceral organs to function within a stable equilibrium. This tendency is called homeostasis.

       Under conditions of stress, the sympathetic nervous system mobilizes all of the energy-producing structures of the body. For example, it makes the heart beat faster. Later, as equilibrium is restored, the parasympathetic nervous system has the opposite effect. (paras 12-11 thru 12-13)

9.   The neurons are alined in sequences to form circuits. The transmission of information along a neuron is electrochemical in nature. Crossing the gap between one neuron and the next is a chemical called a neurotransmitter. (para 12-14)

10.   Neurons are able to concentrate negative ions inside and positive ions outside of the cell membrane. When the neuron is not actually transmitting, this process produces the resting potential. (para 12-15)

11.   When the polarity of ions is disrupted by a stimulus, that location on the cell membrane is said to be depolarized. The restoration of the original polarity is called repolarization. At the same time, adjacent areas are depolarized. Thus, there is a wave of depolarization/repolarization along the length of the neuron. (para 12-16)

12.   The speed of an impulse is proportional to the thickness of the neuron process. Transmission is fastest in the thickest neurons. (para 12- 17)

13.   Together, the gap and the "connecting" membranes between two successive neurons are called the synapse. The gap itself is called the synaptic cleft. Containing specific amounts of neurotransmitter are synaptic vesicles in the terminal bulb of the first neuron. When an impulse reaches the bouton, the vesicles are stimulated to release their neurotransmitter. This substance passes through the presynaptic membrane, across the synaptic cleft, and to the postsynaptic membrane. Since this process consumes much energy, the bouton contains many well-developed mitochondria. (para 12-18)

14.   The neuromuscular junction is the "connection" between a motor neuron and a striated muscle fiber. It is nearly identical to a synapse. However, the surface of the postsynaptic membrane is in a series of longitudinal folds. This greatly increases the surface area receptive to the ACH.

       The group of striated muscle fibers innervated by one motor neuron is called the motor unit. Fewer muscle fibers per motor unit result in finer movements. More muscle fibers per motor unit result in coarser movements. (para 12-19)

15.   The simplest reaction is called a reflex, defined as an automatic reaction to a stimulus. (para 12-20)

16.   A pathway of the human nervous system is the series of neurons or other structures used to transmit an item of information. In general, we consider two major types of pathways--the general sensory pathways and the motor pathways.

        At some specific level in the neuraxis, all of these pathways cross to the opposite side. Each crossing is called a decussation. Thus, the right cerebral hemisphere communicates with the left half of the body. The left cerebral hemisphere communicates with the right half of the body. (para 12-22)

17.   The general senses include pain, touch, temperature, and proprioception ("body sense").

        A general sensory pathway extends from the point where the stimulus is received to the postcentral gyrus (fold) of the cerebral hemisphere. This gyrus is the site of conscious sensation of a stimulus.

        Corresponding to each location in the body, there is a specific location in the postcentral gyrus. (para 12-23)

18.   Pain is an ancient protective mechanism which generally helps us to avoid injury. Endorphins are chemicals found naturally within the body which tend to block the sensation of pain.

        The pain receptor is not a specific receptor organ. It is referred to as a free nerve ending. (para 12-24)

19.   The body has two different mechanisms for sensing temperature. Detecting warmth and cold in the periphery of the body are specific sensory receptors. Special heat-sensitive neurons in the hypothalamus detect increases in the temperature of the blood. (para 12-25)

20.   The pacinian corpuscles are typical of the receptors which detect deep pressure. (para 12-26)

21.   Another term for muscle sense is proprioception. For this, there is a special receptor organ to monitor the stretch of the muscle. These receptor organs are called muscle spindles or stretch receptors. They detect relative muscle length.

        Another stretch receptor associated with the skeletal muscle is the Golgi tendon organ. As its name implies, this organ is located within the tendon of the muscle. It detects relative muscle tension. (para 12-27)

22.   The CNS receives information through the sensory pathways and collates this information against information stored in memory. This results in a decision. If the decision is to do something, then the CNS sends out commands through the motor pathways to the effector organs. (para 12-28)

23.   We usually consider two general motor pathways--the pyramidal and the extrapyramidal motor pathways. (para 12-28b)

24.   A pyramidal motor pathway is primarily concerned with volitional (voluntary) control of body parts, particularly with the fine movements of the hands.

        The pyramidal motor pathway begins in the precentral gyrus of the cerebral hemisphere. As we have already seen, the neurons making up the precentral and postcentral gyri are arranged in a pattern corresponding to the various parts of the body to which they are connected.

        Immediately below the pyramids, the axons cross to the opposite side of the CNS. Thus, the left cerebral hemisphere commands the right side of the body, and the right cerebral hemisphere controls the left side of the body. (para 12-29)

25.   The extrapyramidal motor pathways are concerned with automatic (nonvolitional) control of body parts. This particularly includes patterned, sequential movements or actions. The cerebellum plays a major role in extrapyramidal pathways. The cerebellum is the major center for coordinating the patterned sequential actions of the body, such as walking. (para 12-30)

26.   The human nervous system can be thought of as a series of steps or levels. Each level is more complex than the level just below. No level is completely overpowered by upper levels, but each level is controlled or guided by the next upper level as it functions.

        The simplest and lowest level of control is the reflex arc. Producing a wider reaction to a stimulus are segmented reflexes. (paras 12-31, 12-32)

27.   Nuclei in the medulla of the hindbrainstem control the visceral activities of the body, such as respiration, heart beat, etc.

        The reticular formation of the brainstem has a facilitory area and an inhibitory area. This control area produces sleep or wakefulness.

        The thalamus is a group of nuclei found together in the forebrainstem. The thalamus is the major relay center of sensory inputs.

        The hypothalamus is a higher control center for visceral activities of the body. (para 12-33)

28.   The cerebellum is the primary center for the <u>integration</u> and <u>control</u> of patterned, sequential <u>motions</u> of the body. (para 12-34)

29.   In humans, the highest level of control is localized in the <u>cerebrum</u>. Localized at this level are <u>conscious</u> sensation and <u>volitional</u> motor activity.

        The visceral level within the cerebrum is concerned with <u>visceral</u> activities of the body, as related to <u>fight</u>-or-<u>flight</u>, <u>fear</u>, and other emotions.

        The second level of the cerebrum is concerned with <u>stereotyped</u> patterns of muscle activity.

        The third level of the cerebrum is the <u>volitional</u> level. Here, <u>cognition</u> (thinking) occurs, and unique, brand-new <u>solutions</u> can be created. (para 12-35)

30.   The precentral gyrus is Brodmann's area number __4__. The center for hearing is Brodmann's area number __41__. (para 12-36)

31.   In right-handed individuals, the left cerebral hemisphere is said to be <u>dominant</u> over the right cerebral hemisphere. For most individuals, an injury to the <u>left</u> cerebral hemisphere is more serious. (para 12-37)

32.   Memory is the faculty which enables an individual to store and retrieve factual items such as <u>sensations</u>, <u>impressions</u>, <u>facts</u>, and <u>ideas</u>. All sensory inputs are collated against these stored items in order to arrive at an appropriate <u>decision</u> for <u>action</u>. (para 12-38a)

33.   There are at least two types of memory--<u>short</u>-term memory and <u>long</u>-term memory.

        Short-term memory is usually limited to about <u>seven</u> bits of information.

        A portion of the cerebral cortex is thought to be important in transferring information from <u>short</u>-term memory to <u>long</u>-term memory. It is called the <u>hippocampus</u>. What is the effect on learning if the hippocampus is nonfunctional? <u>The individual can learn nothing, but previous long-term memory remains intact</u>. (para 12-38b)

End of Lesson 12

LESSON ASSIGNMENT

LESSON 13   The Special Senses.

LESSON ASSIGNMENT   Paragraphs 13-1 through 13-24.

LESSON OBJECTIVES   After completing this lesson, you should be able to:

        13-1. Identify functions of structures related to the special senses.

        13-2. Given a list of statements about the physiology of the special senses, identify the false statement.

SUGGESTION   After completing the assignment, complete the exercises at the end of this lesson. These exercises will help you to achieve the lesson objectives.

LESSON 13

THE SPECIAL SENSES

Section I. INTRODUCTION

13-1. GENERAL VERSUS SPECIAL SENSES

a.   The human body is continuously bombarded by all kinds of stimuli. Certain of these stimuli are received by sense organs distributed throughout the entire body. These are referred to as the <u>general</u> senses.

b.   Certain other stimuli (table 13-1) are received by pairs of receptor organs located in the head. These are the <u>special</u> senses.

SPECIAL SENSE	RECEPTOR ORGAN	STIMULUS
Sight (vision)	bulbus oculi (eye)	light rays
Hearing (audition)	ear (cochlea)	sound waves
Balance (equilibrium)	ear (membranous labyrinth)	gravity
Smell (olfaction)	olfactory hair cells in nose	airborne molecules
Taste (gustation)	taste buds in mouth	fluid-borne molecules

Table 13-1. The special senses.

c.   Since the general senses respond to immediate contact, they are very short range. In contrast, the special senses are long range.

13-2. INPUT TO BRAIN

From the special sense organs, information is sent to the brain through specific cranial nerves. When this information reaches specific areas of the cerebral cortex, the sensations are perceived at the conscious level.

Section II. THE SPECIAL SENSE OF VISION

13-3. THE RETINA

Within the bulbus oculi (eyeball) is an inner layer called the retina. See Figure 13-1 for the location of the retina within the bulbus oculi. See Figure 13-2 for the types of cells found within the retina.

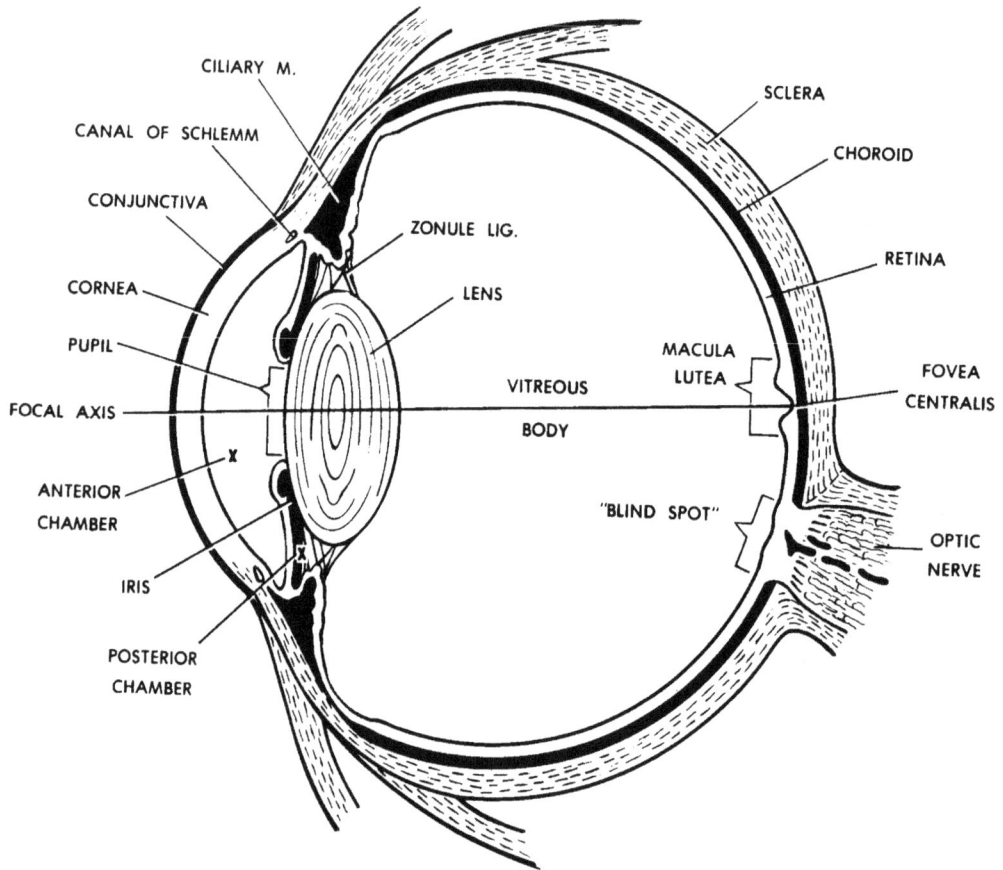

Figure 13-1. A focal-axis section of the bulbus oculi.

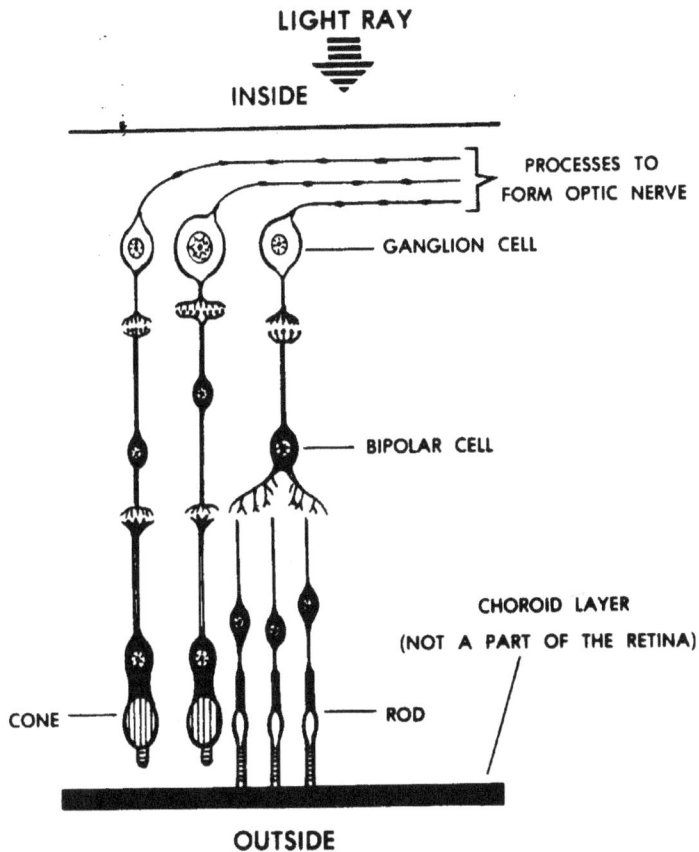

Figure 13-2. Cellular detail of the retina.

    a.   **Visual Fields (Figure 13-3).** When a human looks at an object, light from the right half of the visual field goes to the left half of each eye. Likewise, light from the left half of the visual field goes to the right half of each eye. Later, in paragraph 13-4, we will see how the information from both eyes about a given half of the visual field is brought together by the nervous system.

    b.   **Photoreception and Signal Transmission.** The cells of the retina include special photoreceptor cells in the form of cones and rods. The light ray stimulus chemically changes the visual chemical of the cones and rods. This produces a receptor potential which passes through the bodies of the rods and cones and which acts at the synapses to induce a signal in the bipolar cells. This signal is then transmitted to the ganglion cells.

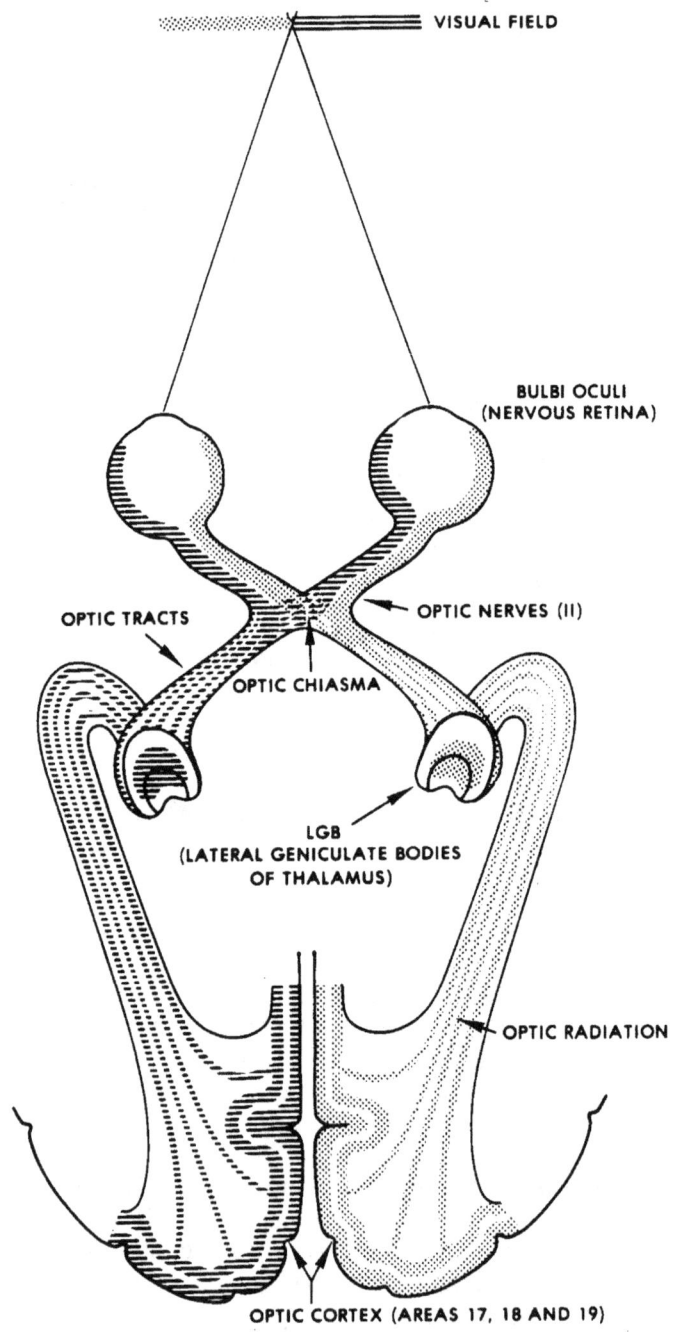

Figure 13-3. Scheme of visual input.

(1) Cones. The cones of the retina are for acute vision and also receive color information. The cones tend to be concentrated at the rear of the eyeball. The greatest concentration is within the macula lutea at the inner end of the focal axis (Figure 13-1).

(2) Rods. Light received by the rods is perceived in terms of black and white. The rods are sensitive to less intensive light than the cones. The rods are concentrated to the sides of the eyeball.

(3) Signal transmission. The stimulus from the photoreceptors (cones and rods) is transferred to the bipolar cells. In turn, the stimulus is transferred to the ganglion cells, the cells of the innermost layer of the retina. The axons of the ganglion cells converge to the back side of the eyeball. The axons leave the eyeball to become the optic nerve, surrounded by a dense FCT sheath. There are no photoreceptors in the circular area where the axons of the ganglion cells exit the eyeball; thus, this area is called the blind spot.

13-4. NERVOUS PATHWAYS FROM THE RETINAS

a. The two optic nerves enter the cranial cavity and join in a structure known as the optic chiasma. Leading from the optic chiasma on either side of the brainstem is the optic tract. In the optic chiasma, the axons from the nasal (medial) halves of the retinas cross to the opposite sides. Thus, the left optic tract contains all of the information from the left halves of the retinas (right visual field), and the right optic tract contains all of the information from the right halves of the retinas (left visual field).

b. The optic tracts carry this information to the LGB (lateral geniculate body) of the thalamus. From here, information is carried to the posterior medial portions (occipital lobes) of the cerebral cortex, where the information is perceived as conscious vision. Note that the right visual field is perceived within the left hemisphere, and the left visual field is perceived within the right hemisphere.

c. The LGB also sends information into the midbrainstem. This information is used to activate various visual reflexes.

13-5. FOCUSING OF THE LIGHT RAYS

a. The light rays, which enter the eyeball from the visual field, are focused to ensure acute vision. The majority of this focusing is accomplished by the permanently rounded cornea.

b. Fine adjustments of focusing, for acuteness of vision, are provided by the crystalline lens (biconvex lens). See Figure 13-4. This is particularly important when changing one's gaze between far and near objects.

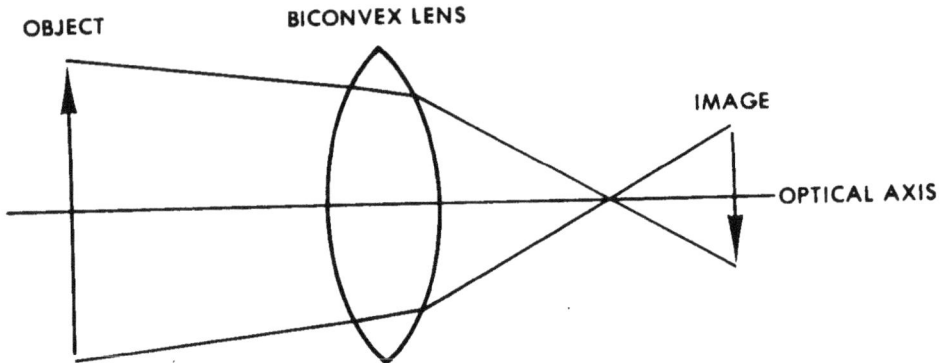

Figure 13-4. Bending of the light rays by a biconvex lens.

13-6. ACCOMMODATION

The additional focusing provided by the crystalline lens, mentioned above, is one of the processes involved in accommodation. Accommodation refers to the various adjustments made by the eye to see better at different distances.

a. The crystalline lens is kept in a flattened condition by the tension of the zonular fibers (zonule ligaments; fibers of the ciliary zonule) around its equator, or margin. Contraction of the ciliary muscle of the eyeball releases this tension and allows the elastic lens to become more rounded. Since the elasticity of the crystalline lens decreases with age, old people may find it very difficult to look at close objects.

b. A second process in accommodation is the constriction of the pupils. The diameter of the pupil (the hole in the middle of the iris) controls the amount of light that enters the eyeball. As a light source comes closer and closer, the intensity of the light increases greatly. Therefore, the pupils must be constricted to control the amount of light entering the eyeball as an object under view comes close to the individual.

c. A third process in accommodation is the convergence of the axes of the two eyeballs toward the midline. Since both eyes tend to focus on the same object (binocular vision), there is an angle between the two axes. As an object draws closer, the angle increases to enable the axes to still intersect the object.

13-7. EYE MOVEMENTS

a. **Convergent and Conjugate Eye Movements.** In a conjugate eye movement, both eyeballs move through an equal angle in one direction, such as right or left. In a convergent eye movement, both eyeballs turn toward the midline to focus upon a nearby object. In both cases, the movement of the left and right eyeballs is highly coordinated so that an object may be viewed by both eyes. Therefore, the object can be perceived within both cerebral hemispheres in a binocular fashion.

b. **"Searching" and "Following" Eye Movements.** "Searching" and "following" movements of the eyeball are also called, respectively, voluntary fixation movements and involuntary fixation movements. For the first type of movement, the eyeballs move in a searching pattern, without focusing on a particular object until it is located. Once an object is located, the eyeballs will continually fix on that object in a following-type motion.

c. **Eye Movements During Reading.** During reading of printed or written material, the eyeball demonstrates several physical characteristics. The amount of material that can be recognized at a given glance occupies a given width of a written line. Each glance is referred to as a fixation. During a fixation, the eyeball is essentially not moving, and each eyeball is oriented so that the image falls upon the macula lutea (the maximum receptive area). Reading is a series of motions in which the eyeballs fixate on a portion of the written line and then move very rapidly to the next portion.

d. **Compensation for Head Movements (Vestibular Control of Eye Movements).** Since the human body cannot be held absolutely still, the eyeballs must move in order to remain fixed upon an object. For this purpose, the eyeballs must be moved in the opposite direction and at the opposite speed of the movement of the head. This is accomplished by a delicate and complicated mechanism. This mechanism includes the motor neurons of the muscles of the eyeball and the vestibular nuclei of the hindbrain (responsible for balance and spatial orientation).

13-8. VISUAL REFLEXES

In the sense of vision, one consciously perceives the various objects being looked upon. In addition to this, there are a number of protective reactions to visual input--the visual reflexes.

a. When an unexpected visual stimulus occurs within the visual field, the individual's response will often include movement and other types of reaction. This is a part of the startle reflex.

b. When there is a change in the amount of light entering the eyeball, the size of the pupil will change. This is the pupillary reflex. The muscles of the iris automatically constrict or dilate to control the amount of light entering the eyeball.

c. In the blink reflex, the eyelids automatically move over the exterior surface of the eyeball. This reflex results in the automatic washing of the exterior surface of the eyeball with the lacrimal fluids. It also helps to keep the surface moist.

13-9. LACRIMAL APPARATUS

The eyeball is suspended in the orbit and faces outward. Helping to fill the orbit are a number of structures associated with the eyeball; these are the adnexa. Among these other structures is the lacrimal apparatus.

a. The lacrimal gland is located in the upper outer corner in front. Via small ducts, it secretes the lacrimal fluid into the space between the external surface of the eyeball and the upper eyelid.

b. The inner surface of the eyelids and the outer surface of the eyeball are covered by a continuous membrane known as the conjunctiva. The lacrimal fluid keeps the conjunctiva transparent. Also, with the blink reflex, the lacrimal fluid washes away any foreign particles that may be on the surface of the conjunctiva.

c. The free margins of the upper and lower eyelids have special oil glands. The oily secretion of these glands helps prevent the lacrimal fluid from escaping.

d. With the movement of the eyeball and the eyelids, the lacrimal fluid is gradually moved across the exterior surface of the eyeball to the medial inferior corner. Here, the lacrimal fluid is collected into a lacrimal sac, which drains into the nasal chamber by way of the nasolacrimal duct. Thus, the continuous production of lacrimal fluid is conserved by being recycled within the body.

Section III. THE SPECIAL SENSE OF HEARING (AUDITORY SENSE)

13-10. INTRODUCTION

If a medium is set into vibration within certain frequency limits (average between 25 cycles per second and 18,000 cycles per second), we have what is called a sound stimulus (Figure 13-5). The sensation of sound, of course, occurs only when these vibrations are interpreted by the cerebral cortex of the brain at the conscious level.

a. The human ear is the special sensory receptor for the sound stimulus. As the stimulus passes from the external medium (air, water, or a solid conductor of sound) to the actual receptor cells in the head, the vibrations are in the form of (1) airborne waves, (2) mechanical oscillations, and (3) fluid-borne pulses.

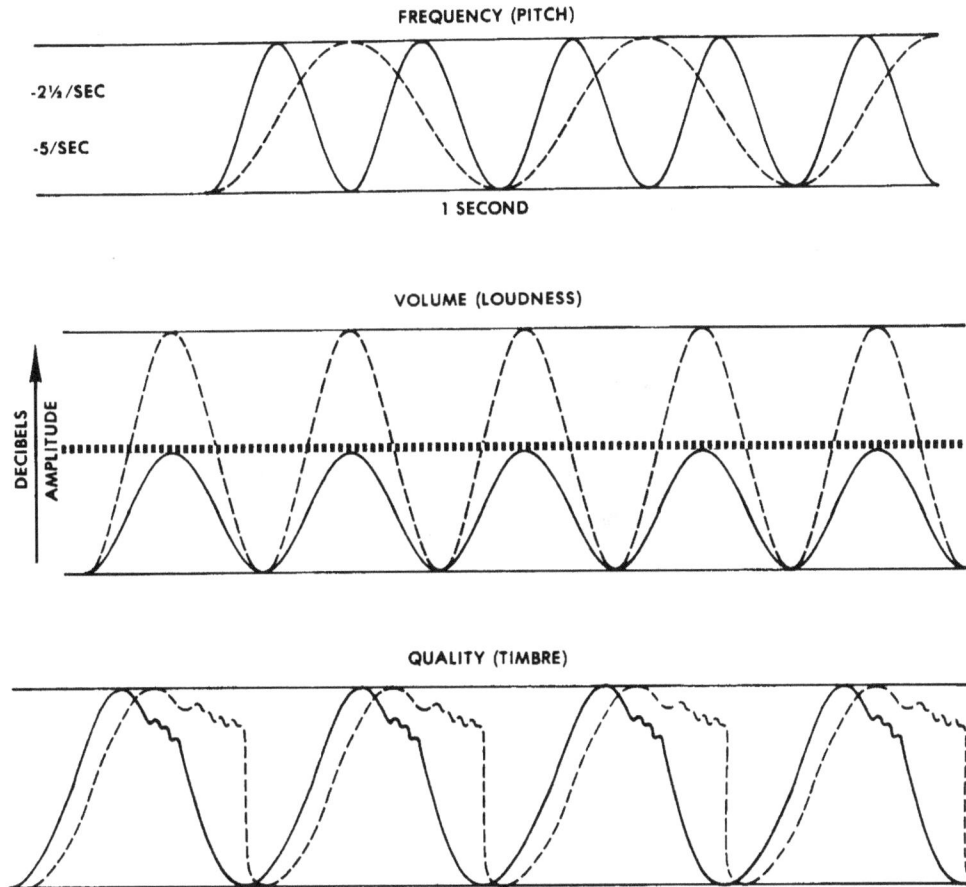

Figure 13-5. Characteristics of sound.

b.   The ear (Figure 13-6) is organized in three major parts: external ear, middle ear, and internal (inner) ear. Each part aids in the transmission of the stimulus to the receptor cells.

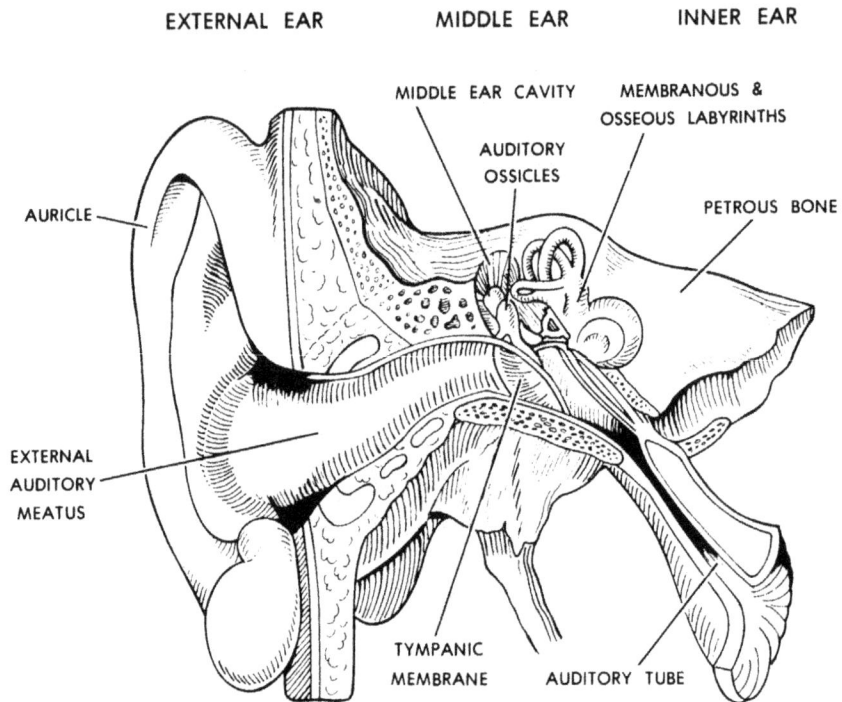

EXTERNAL EAR   MIDDLE EAR   INNER EAR

MIDDLE EAR CAVITY

MEMBRANOUS &
OSSEOUS LABYRINTHS

AUDITORY
OSSICLES

PETROUS BONE

AURICLE

EXTERNAL
AUDITORY
MEATUS

TYMPANIC
MEMBRANE   AUDITORY TUBE

Figure 13-6. A frontal section of the human ear.

13-11. THE EXTERNAL EAR

The external ear begins with a funnel-like auricle. This auricle serves as a collector of the airborne waves and directs them into the external auditory meatus. At the inner end of this passage, the waves act upon the tympanic membrane (eardrum). The external auditory meatus is protected by a special substance called earwax (cerumen).

13-12. THE MIDDLE EAR

a. **Tympanic Membrane.** The tympanic membrane separates the middle and external ears. It is set into mechanical oscillation by the airborne waves from the outside.

b. **Middle Ear Cavity.** Within the petrous bone of the skull is the air-filled middle ear cavity.

(1) Function of the auditory tube. Due to the auditory tube, the air of the middle ear cavity is continuous with the air of the surrounding environment. The auditory tube opens into the lateral wall of the nasopharynx. Thus, the auditory tube

serves to equalize the air pressures on the two sides of the tympanic membrane. If these two pressures become moderately unequal, there is greater tension upon the tympanic membrane; this reduces (dampens) mechanical oscillations of the membrane. Extreme pressure differences cause severe pain. The passage of the auditory tube into the nasopharynx opens when one swallows; therefore, the pressure differences are controlled somewhat by the swallowing reflex.

(2) Associated spaces. The middle ear cavity extends into the mastoid bone as the mastoid air cells. The relatively thin roof of the middle ear cavity separates the middle ear cavity from the middle cranial fossa.

c. **Auditory Ossicles.** There is a series of three small bones, the auditory ossicles, which traverse the space of the middle ear cavity from the external ear to the internal ear. The auditory ossicles function as a unit.

(1) The first ossicle, the malleus, has a long arm embedded in the tympanic membrane. Therefore, when the tympanic membrane is set into mechanical oscillation, the malleus is also set into mechanical oscillation.

(2) The second ossicle is the incus. Its relationship to the malleus produces a leverage system which amplifies the mechanical oscillations received through the malleus.

(3) The third ossicle, the stapes, articulates with the end of the arm of the incus. The foot plate of the stapes fills the oval (vestibular) window.

d. **Auditory Muscles.** The auditory muscles are a pair of muscles associated with the auditory ossicles. They are named the tensor tympani muscle and the stapedius muscle. The auditory muscles help to control the intensity of the mechanical oscillations within the ossicles.

13-13. THE INTERNAL EAR

a. **Transmission of the Sound Stimulus.** The foot plate of the stapes fills the oval (vestibular) window, which opens to the vestibule of the internal ear (Figure 13-7A). As the ossicles oscillate mechanically, the stapes acts like a plunger against the oval window. The vestibule is filled with a fluid, the perilymph. These mechanical, plunger-like actions of the stapes impart pressure pulses to the perilymph.

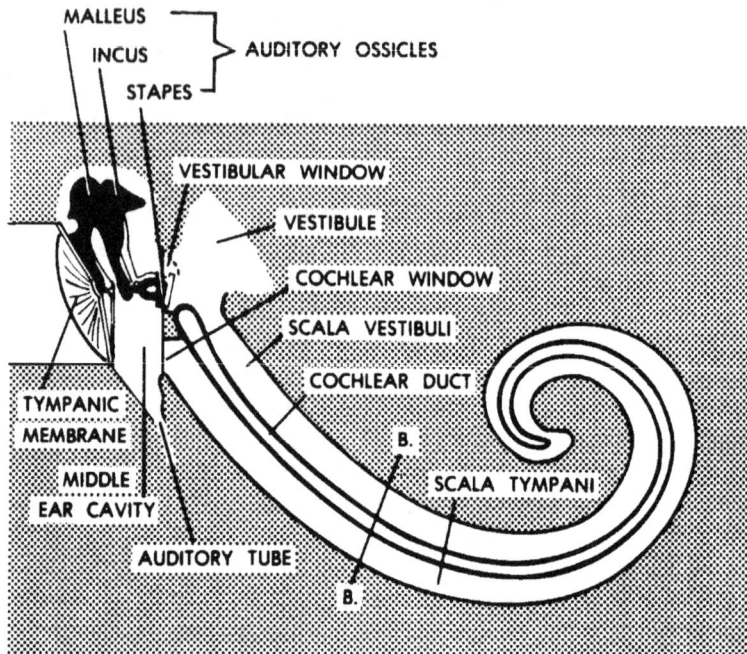

A -- schematic relationships

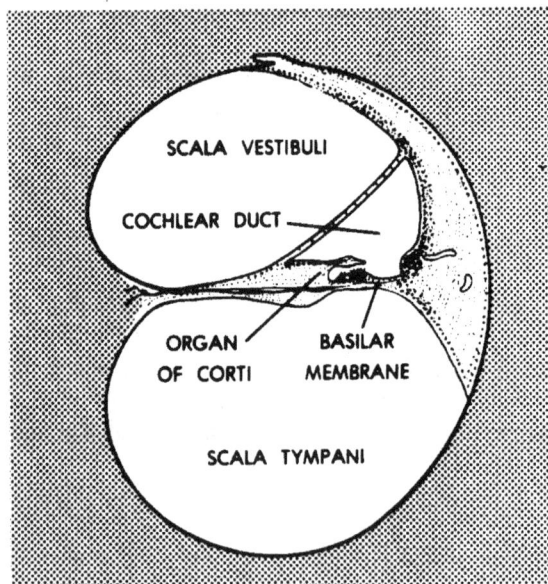

B -- cross-section

Figure 13-7. Diagram of the scalae.

b. **Organization of the Internal Ear.** The internal ear is essentially a membranous labyrinth suspended within the cavity of the bony (osseous) labyrinth of the petrous bone (Figure 13-8). The membranous labyrinth is filled with a fluid, the endolymph. Between the membranous labyrinth and the bony labyrinth is the perilymph.

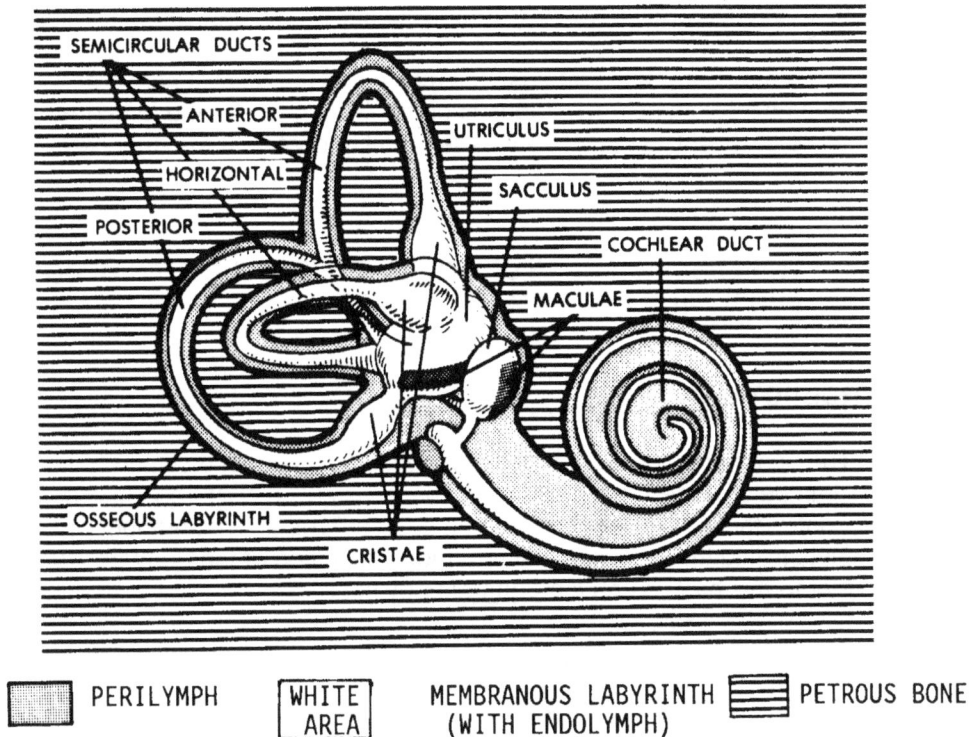

SEMICIRCULAR DUCTS
ANTERIOR
HORIZONTAL
POSTERIOR
UTRICULUS
SACCULUS
COCHLEAR DUCT
MACULAE
OSSEOUS LABYRINTH
CRISTAE

PERILYMPH   WHITE AREA   MEMBRANOUS LABYRINTH (WITH ENDOLYMPH)   PETROUS BONE

Figure 13-8. The labyrinths of the internal ear.

c. **The Cochlea.** The cochlea is a spiral structure associated with hearing. Its outer boundaries are formed by the snail-shaped portion of the bony labyrinth. The extensions of the bony labyrinth into the cochlea are called the scala vestibuli and the scala tympani (Figure 13-7B). These extensions are filled with perilymph.

(1) Basilar membrane (Figure 13-7B). The basilar membrane forms the floor of the cochlear duct, the spiral portion of the membranous labyrinth. The basilar membrane is made up of transverse fibers. Each fiber is of a different length, and the lengths increase from one end to the other. Thus, the basilar membrane is constructed similarly to a harp or piano. Acting like the strings of the instrument, the individual fibers mechanically vibrate in response to specific frequencies of pulses in the perilymph. Thus, each vibration frequency of the sound stimulus affects a specific location of the basilar membrane.

(2) <u>Organ of Corti</u>. Located upon the basilar membrane is the organ of Corti. The organ of Corti is made up of hair cells. When the basilar membrane vibrates, the hair cells are mechanically deformed so that the associated neuron is stimulated.

13-14. NERVOUS PATHWAYS FOR HEARING

The neuron (associated with the hair cells of the organ of Corti) then carries the sound stimulus to the hindbrainstem. Via a special series of connections, the signal ultimately reaches Brodmann's area number 41, on the upper surface of the temporal lobe (see para 12-36). Here, the stimulus is perceived as the special sense of sound. It is interesting to note that speech in humans is primarily localized in the left cerebral hemisphere, while musical (rhythmic) sounds tend to be located in the right cerebral hemisphere.

Section IV. THE SPECIAL SENSE OF EQUILIBRIUM, THE GENERAL BODY SENSE, AND POSTURAL REFLEXES

13-15. INTRODUCTION

a. The human body is composed of a series of linkages, block on top of block. These blocks can be arranged in a multitude of patterns called <u>postures</u>. In order to produce and control these postures, the human brain utilizes a great number of continuous inputs telling the brain the instantaneous condition of the body posture. Overall, we refer to this process as the <u>general</u> <u>body</u> <u>sense</u>.

b. The internal ear provides one of the input systems for the general body sense. The internal ear responds to gravitational forces, of which there are two kinds--static and kinetic (in motion). Of the kinetic stimuli, the motion may be in a straight line (linear) or angular (curvilinear).

13-16. THE MACULAE

The membranous labyrinth of the internal ear has two sac-like parts--the sacculus and the utriculus. On the wall of each of these sacs is a collection of hair cells known as the <u>macula</u> (plural: <u>maculae</u>). The hairs of these hair cells move in response to gravitational forces, both static and linear kinetic. The maculae are particularly sensitive to small changes in the orientation of the head from an upright position. Thus, the maculae are very important in maintaining a standing or upright position.

13-17. THE SEMICIRCULAR DUCTS

a. In addition, three tubular structures are associated with the utriculus. The circle of each of these semicircular ducts is completed by the cavity of the utriculus. At one end of each semicircular duct is a <u>crista</u>, a ridge of hair cells across the axis of the duct.

b. When a jet takes off, a passenger tends to remain in place at first and can feel the resulting pressure of the seat against his back. Also, when the jet is no longer accelerating, the passenger can feel that the pressure of the seat against his back has returned to normal.

c. Likewise, in the appropriate semicircular duct, the endolymph ("passenger") tends to remain in place early during an acceleration. Because the duct ("seat") itself is moving with the body ("jet"), the hairs of the crista are affected by the change in movement. Later, when acceleration stops, the effect upon the hairs of the crista is also registered.

d. However, the cristae of the semicircular ducts detect <u>rotation</u> of the head (angular acceleration and angular velocity). <u>Linear</u> <u>acceleration</u>, as with our example of the passenger and the jet, is detected primarily by the maculae, discussed above.

13-18. RESULTING INPUTS FOR THE SPECIAL SENSE OF EQUILIBRIUM

The combined inputs from the maculae of the sacs and the cristae of the semicircular ducts provide continuous, instantaneous information about the specific location and posture of the head in relationship to the center of gravity of the earth. These inputs are transmitted by the vestibular neurons to the hindbrainstem.

13-19. INPUTS FOR THE GENERAL BODY SENSE

In addition to the inputs from the membranous labyrinth, various other inputs are used to continuously monitor the second-to-second posture of the human body.

a. We have already examined the proprioceptive sense, which monitors the condition of the muscles of the body.

b. Various other receptors are associated with the joint capsules, the integument, etc. They indicate the precise degree of bending present in the body.

c. A very important body sense is <u>vision</u>. Even when other inputs are lacking, if an individual can see his feet, he may still be able to stand and move.

13-20. POSTURAL REFLEXES

To automatically control the posture, the human nervous system has a number of special reflexes. These reflexes are coordinated through the <u>cerebellum</u>.

a. The <u>head and neck tonic reflexes</u> orient the upper torso in relationship to the head.

b.   Another set of reflexes does likewise for the body in general. The righting reflexes come into play when the body falls out of balance or equilibrium.

c.   A special set of reflexes connects the vestibular apparatus to the extraocular muscles of the eyeball. This was discussed earlier in the section on the special sense of the vision.

Section V. THE SPECIAL SENSE OF SMELL (OLFACTION)

13-21. SENSORY RECEPTORS

Molecules of various materials are dispersed (spread) throughout the air we breathe. A special olfactory epithelium is located in the upper recesses of the nasal chambers in the head. Special hair cells in the olfactory epithelium are called chemoreceptors, because they receive these molecules in the air.

13-22. OLFACTORY SENSORY PATHWAY

The information received by the olfactory hair cells is transmitted by way of the olfactory nerves (cranial nerves I). It passes through these nerves to the olfactory bulbs and then into the opposite cerebral hemisphere. Here, the information becomes the sensation of smell.

Section VI. THE SPECIAL SENSE OF TASTE (GUSTATION)

13-23. SENSORY RECEPTORS

Molecules of various materials are also dispersed or dissolved in the fluids (saliva) of the mouth. These molecules are from the food ingested (taken in). Organs known as taste buds are scattered over the tongue and the rear of the mouth. Special hair cells in the taste buds are chemoreceptors to react to these molecules.

13-24. SENSORY PATHWAY

The information received by the hair cells of the taste buds is transmitted to the opposite side of the brain by way of three cranial nerves (VII, IX, and X). This information is interpreted by the cerebral hemispheres as the sensation of taste.

Continue with Exercises

EXERCISES, LESSON 13

REQUIREMENT. The following exercises are to be answered by completing the incomplete statements.

After you have completed all the exercises, turn to "Solutions to Exercises" at the end of the lesson, and check your answers.

1.　Please complete the table below.

SPECIAL SENSE	RECEPTOR ORGAN	STIMULUS
Sight		
Hearing		
Balance		
Smell		
Taste		

2.　When you look at an object, light from the right half of the visual field goes to the _____t half of each eye. Light from the left half of the visual field goes to the _____t half of each eye.

　　The light ray stimulus chemically changes the visual chemical found in the _____es and _____ds. The cones of the retina are for _____te vision and also receive _____r information. Light received by the rods is perceived in terms of _____ and _____e. The stimulus from the cones and rods is transferred to the b_____r cells and then to the _____n cells. The axons of the ganglion cells leave the eyeball to become the_____c nerve. Since the circular area where these axons exit contains neither cones nor rods, this area is called the _____ spot.

3.　The axons from the nasal (medial) halves of the retinas cross to the opposite sides at the optic _____sma. Thus, if an object is in your right visual field, the information is carried by your _____t optic tract. If an object is in your left visual field, the information is carried by your _____t optic tract. For conscious perception of vision, the information enters the _____al lobes of the cerebral cortex. Note that the right visual field is perceived within the _____t cerebral hemisphere, and the left visual field is perceived within the _____t cerebral hemisphere.

4.   The majority of focusing of light rays is accomplished by the _____a. Fine adjustments of focusing are provided by the crystalline ____s.

5.   The additional focusing provided by the crystalline lens is one of the processes involved in _____n. Accommodation refers to the various adjustments made by the eye to see better at different _____s.

       The crystalline lens is kept in a flattened condition by the tension of the zonular _____s. This tension is released by contraction of the _____y muscle, resulting in greater r_____ing of the lens.

6.   When both eyeballs move through an equal angle in the same direction, it is called a con_____e eye movement. When both eyeballs turn toward the midline to focus upon a nearby object, the result is a con_____t eye movement.

       During a "searching" eye movement, the eyeballs do not focus on a particular object until it is l_____d. During a "following" eye movement, the eyeballs continually ____x on an object.

       Vestibular control of eye movements is necessary in order to compensate for _____ movements.

7.   The sudden movement of an individual in response to an unexpected visual stimulus is part of the_____tle reflex.

       Changes in the size of the pupil with changes in the amount of light are produced by the _____y reflex.

       Automatic movement of the eyelids over the exterior surface of the eyeball is called the _____ reflex.

8.   The lacrimal fluid keeps the conjunctiva _____ent. Also, with the blink reflex, the lacrimal fluid w_____s away foreign particles.

       The secretion of the special oil glands of the upper and lower eyelids helps prevent the _____ fluid from escaping.

9.   The auricle serves as a collector of airborne w_____s. At the inner end of the external auditory meatus, the waves act upon the _____c membrane.

10.   The tympanic membrane separates the external ear from the _____ ear. The tympanic membrane mechanically oscillates in response to _____ e _____ s from the outside.

        The air of the middle ear cavity is continuous with the air of the surrounding environment, due to the _____ y tube. The auditory tube serves to equalize the air pressures on the two sides of the _____ c membrane. Extreme pressure differences cause severe _____ n. The passage of the auditory tube into the nasopharynx opens when one _____ s.

        Mechanical oscillations are transmitted from the tympanic membrane to the oval window by way of the _____ y _____ cles. The intensity of these mechanical oscillations is somewhat controlled by the auditory _____ s.

11.   The mechanical, plunger-like actions of the stapes impart pressure pulses to the _____ ph.

        The basilar membrane is made up of transverse fibers. Acting like the strings of an instrument, the individual fibers mechanically v_____ e in response to specific _____ cies of pulses in the perilymph.

        When the basilar membrane vibrates, the _____ cells of the organ of Corti are mechanically d_____ ed so that the associated neuron is stimulated.

12.   The "blocks" of the human body can be arranged in many patterns called _____ s. The input systems by which the brain monitors these patterns are together known as the _____ l _____ y sense.

13.   The maculae are particularly sensitive to small changes in the orientation of the head from an _____ t position. Thus, the maculae help us maintain a _____ ding or _____ t position.

14.   The cristae detect _____ n of the head, that is, _____ r acceleration and _____ r _____ y.

15.   Additional inputs for the general body sense include the proprioceptive sense, which monitors the _____ s of the body, and various other receptors associated with structures such as the joint _____ s and the _____ t. A very important body sense is _____ n.

16.   Postural reflexes are coordinated in the _____m. Orienting the upper torso in relationship to the head are the head and neck _____c reflexes. Important when the body falls out of balance are the _____ing reflexes.

17.   The sensory receptors for the special sense of smell are special _____ cells in the _____y epithelium. They detect molecules in the ____.

18.   The specialized structures for the special sense of taste are the taste ____s. The receptors in these organs are special _____ cells. They detect molecules dispersed or dissolved in the _____a.

Check Your Answers on Next Page

SOLUTIONS TO EXERCISES, LESSON 13

1. Please check your entries in the table with table 13-1 of this lesson.

2. When you look at an object, light from the right half of the visual field goes to the left half of each eye. Light from the left half of the visual field goes to the right half of each eye.

    The light ray stimulus chemically changes the visual chemical found in the cones and rods. The cones of the retina are for acute vision and also receive color information. Light received by the rods is perceived in terms of black and white. The stimulus from the cones and rods is transferred to the bipolar cells and then to the ganglion cells. The axons of the ganglion cells leave the eyeball to become the optic nerve. Since the circular area where these axons exit contains neither cones nor rods, this area is called the blind spot. (para 13-3)

3. The axons from the nasal (medial) halves of the retinas cross to the opposite sides at the optic chiasma. Thus, if an object is in your right visual field, the information is carried by your left optic tract. If an object is in your left visual field, the information is carried by your right optic tract. For conscious perception of vision, the information enters the occipital lobes of the cerebral cortex. Note that the right visual field is perceived within the left cerebral hemisphere, and the left visual field is perceived within the right cerebral hemisphere.
    (para 13-4)

4. The majority of focusing of light rays is accomplished by the cornea. Fine adjustments of focusing are provided by the crystalline lens. (para 13-5)

5. The additional focusing provided by the crystalline lens is one of the processes involved in accommodation. Accommodation refers to the various adjustments made by the eye to see better at different distances.

    The crystalline lens is kept in a flattened condition by the tension of the zonular fibers. This tension is released by contraction of the ciliary muscle, resulting in greater rounding of the lens. (para 13-6)

6. When both eyeballs move through an equal angle in the same direction, it is called a conjugate eye movement. When both eyeballs turn toward the midline to focus upon a nearby object, the result is a convergent eye movement.

    During a "searching" eye movement, the eyeballs do not focus on a particular object until it is located. During a "following" eye movement, the eyeballs continually fix on an object.

    Vestibular control of eye movements is necessary in order to compensate for head movements. (para 13-7)

7. The sudden movement of an individual in response to an unexpected visual stimulus is part of the <u>startle</u> reflex.

    Changes in the size of the pupil with changes in the amount of light are produced by the <u>pupillary</u> reflex.

    Automatic movement of the eyelids over the exterior surface of the eyeball is called the <u>blink</u> reflex. (para 13-8)

8. The lacrimal fluid keeps the conjunctiva <u>transparent</u>. Also, with the blink reflex, the lacrimal fluid <u>washes</u> away foreign particles.

    The secretion of the special oil glands of the upper and lower eyelids helps prevent the <u>lacrimal</u> fluid from escaping.
    (para 13-9)

9. The auricle serves as a collector of airborne <u>waves</u>. At the inner end of the external auditory meatus, the waves act upon the <u>tympanic</u> membrane.
    (para 13-11)

10. The tympanic membrane separates the external ear from the <u>middle</u> ear. The tympanic membrane mechanically oscillates in response to <u>airborne</u> <u>waves</u> from the outside.

    The air of the middle ear cavity is continuous with the air of the surrounding environment, due to the <u>auditory</u> tube. The auditory tube serves to equalize the air pressures on the two sides of the <u>tympanic</u> membrane. Extreme pressure differences cause severe <u>pain</u>. The passage of the auditory tube into the nasopharynx opens when one <u>swallows</u>.

    Mechanical oscillations are transmitted from the tympanic membrane to the oval window by way of the <u>auditory</u> <u>ossicles</u>. The intensity of these mechanical oscillations is somewhat controlled by the auditory <u>muscles</u>. (para 13-12)

11. The mechanical, plunger-like actions of the stapes impart pressure pulses to the <u>perilymph</u>.

    The basilar membrane is made up of transverse fibers. Acting like the strings of an instrument, the individual fibers mechanically <u>vibrate</u> in response to specific <u>frequencies</u> of pulses in the perilymph.

    When the basilar membrane vibrates, the <u>hair</u> cells of the organ of Corti are mechanically <u>deformed</u> so that the associated neuron is stimulated. (para 13-13)

12.   The "blocks" of the human body can be arranged in many patterns called postures. The input systems by which the brain monitors these patterns are together known as the general body sense. (para 13-15a)

13.   The maculae are particularly sensitive to small changes in the orientation of the head from an upright position. Thus, the maculae help us maintain a standing or upright position.
(para 13-16)

14.   The cristae detect rotation of the head, that is, angular acceleration and angular velocity. (para 13-17)

15.   Additional inputs for the general body sense include the proprioceptive sense, which monitors the muscles of the body, and various other receptors associated with structures such as the joint capsules and the integument. A very important body sense is vision. (para 13-19)

16.   Postural reflexes are coordinated in the cerebellum. Orienting the upper torso in relationship to the head are the head and neck tonic reflexes. Important when the body falls out of balance are the righting reflexes. (para 13-20)

17.   The sensory receptors for the special sense of smell are special hair cells in the olfactory epithelium. They detect molecules in the air. (para 13-21)

18.   The specialized structures for the special sense of taste are the taste buds. The receptors in these organs are special hair cells. They detect molecules dispersed or dissolved in the saliva.
(para 13-23)

End of Lesson 13

LESSON ASSIGNMENT

LESSON 14   Some Elementary Human Genetics.

LESSON ASSIGNMENT   Paragraphs 14-1 through 14-10.

LESSON OBJECTIVES   After completing this lesson, you should be able to:

14-1. Given a list of statements about elementary human genetics, select the false statement.

14-2. Identify diploid (2N=46) and haploid (N=23) conditions as related to ordinary body cells, mitotic daughter cells, gametes, and zygotes.

14-3. Match important genetic terms with their definitions.

SUGGESTION   After completing the assignment, complete the exercises at the end of this lesson. These exercises will help you to achieve the lesson objectives.

LESSON 14

SOME ELEMENTARY HUMAN GENETICS

14-1. INTRODUCTION

a. **Heredity.** With respect to both anatomy and physiology, offspring tend to resemble their parents. This is due to the process known as <u>heredity</u> or <u>inheritance</u>. Heredity depends upon the passage of materials called <u>genes</u> from one generation to the next. Due to genes, all human beings resemble each other in general, but with individual differences.

b. **Genetic Control.** The genes control the life processes of each body cell. In an individual, each cell has identical genes. Overall, genes determine the range of potentiality of an individual, and the environment develops it. For example, good nutrition will help a person to attain his full body height and weight within the limits determined by his genes.

14-2. HISTORY OF GENETICS

a. Over a hundred years ago, the Austrian monk Gregor Mendel began the science of genetics by experimenting with successive generations of peas. He originated the concepts of genes, dominance, and recessiveness. By choosing the simplest and most straightforward situations, he set forth the basic principles of inheritance. However, his work was not well known for many years.

b. With the turn of the century, the principles of genetics were "rediscovered," particularly by the Dutch biologist Hugo de Vries. In the following years, the principles of genetics were further developed by the American, T. H. Morgan.

c. In 1944, Oswald T. Avery and his colleagues used bacterial studies to prove that DNA was the genetic substance of chromosomes.

d. In 1954, Watson and Crick published the <u>double helix model</u> of DNA. (A <u>helix</u> is a spiral form.)

e. Three Frenchmen, Jacob, Lwoff, and Monod, discovered how information is transmitted from the genes to the sites of protein synthesis. This led to the "cracking" of the genetic code, used to translate DNA patterns for the production of specific proteins.

14-3. THE GENE

DNA (deoxyribonucleic acid) is a large molecule consisting of two strands in a double-helix arrangement. Along each strand are specific chemical elements called <u>nucleotides</u>. Each <u>gene</u> consists of a portion of a strand, including a number of nucleotides. Through the arrangement of its nucleotides, the gene provides coded information for the construction of proteins. After these proteins are assembled elsewhere in the cell, they serve as building blocks for the cell and as enzymes to promote the life processes of the cell.

14-4. CHROMOSOMES

a. A chromosome is a very long double-helix thread of DNA. Thus, each chromosome consists of a large number of genes. The genes have very specific locations along the length of each chromosome. Recently, researchers have been able to identify specific sequences of genes along a chromosome and illustrate the sequences with gene maps.

b. Except during cell division, chromosomes are observed as granules of chromatin material within the cell nucleus. During the process of cell division, this chromatin material aggregates so that it may be identified as one of the 46 individual chromosomes found in each human cell (diploid condition).

c. These 46 chromosomes of the human cell occur in pairs. Thus, we may say that there are two sets, with 23 chromosomes in each set.

$$(22 + 1) \, X \, 2 = 46$$

Of the 23 different chromosomes, 22 deal with the body in general and are called autosomal chromosomes. The last chromosome is called the sex chromosome. There are two kinds of sex chromosomes--X and Y. When an individual's cells each have two X chromosomes (XX), the individual is genetically a female. On the other hand, when an individual's cells each have one X and one Y chromosome (XY), that individual is genetically a male.

14-5. CELL DIVISIONS

The two types of cell division are illustrated in Figure 14-1.

a. **Mitosis.** New cells must be produced for replacement of worn-out cells and for growth and development of the individual. For these purposes, the existing cells undergo cell division and produce new cells. The usual process of cell division is called mitosis. In mitosis, the two daughter cells produced by the original cell have essentially the same genetic material as the original cell.

b. **Meiosis.** Meiosis is a type of cell division which occurs only in the gonads. It results in the formation of the gametes, or sex cells. In mitosis, the chromosomes are duplicated; in meiosis, the two sets of chromosomes separate, and one set of 23 goes to each of the gametes. Thus, meiosis involves a reduction division. The final result is that each gamete has only one set of 23 chromosomes (haploid condition).

I. __MITOSIS:__

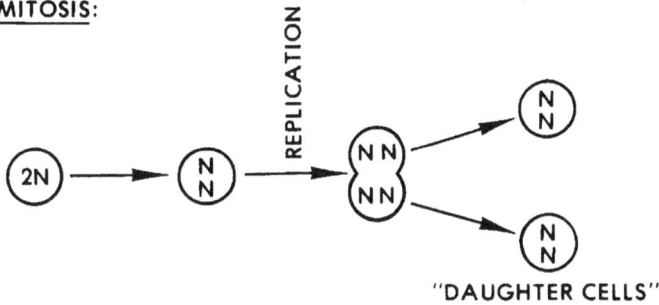

"DAUGHTER CELLS"

II. __MIEOSIS:__

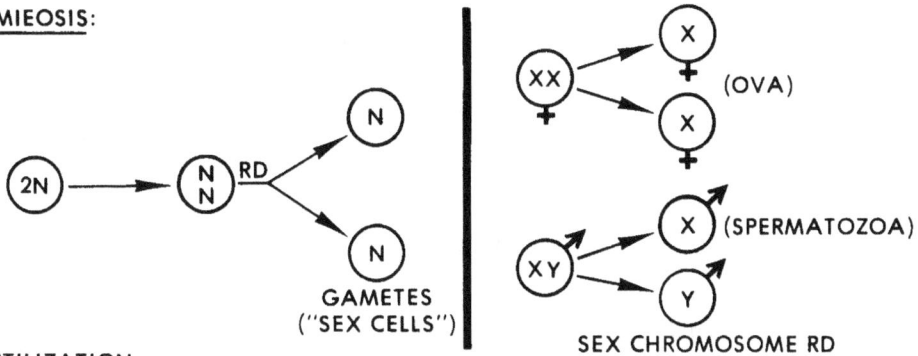

GAMETES
("SEX CELLS")

SEX CHROMOSOME RD

FERTILIZATION:

GAMETES (N)

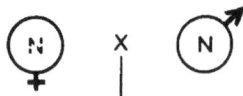

ZYGOTE (2N)

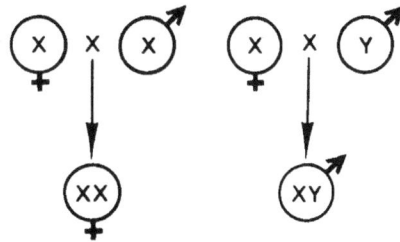

GENETIC SEX DETERMINATION

◯ = FEMALE

◯ = MALE

__RD__ = __REDUCTION DIVISION__

Figure 14-1. Cell division and fertilization.

14-6. FERTILIZATION

a. To produce a new individual, the male gamete (spermatozoon) must join with the female gamete (ovum). This joining of the gametes is called fertilization. The gametes join to form a zygote. The zygote is a single cell which is the beginning of a new human being. The zygote has two sets of chromosomes (46), the appropriate number for the human species. Thus, in the process of fertilization, the human genetic makeup is reconstituted.

b. The existence of separate male and female sexes provides an important advantage. Each individual is the product of a new combination of human genetic material. Thus, there is always the potential for improvement in the human species.

14-7. TERMINOLOGY

a. **Genotype/Phenotype.** The genotype is the actual genetic makeup of an individual. The phenotype is the physical and functional makeup of an individual as determined both by the genotype and the environment.

b. **Dominant/Recessive.** Consider a gene in one set of chromo-somes and the corresponding gene in the other set. If one of the genes alone can produce a characteristic of the phenotype, the gene is said to be dominant. If both genes must be the same to produce a characteristic of the phenotype, then the genes are recessive. In a situation where one of the pair is dominant and the other is recessive, the dominant gene determines the ultimate characteristic.

c. **Homozygous/Heterozygous.** Again, consider a gene in one set of chromosomes and the corresponding gene in the other set. If the two genes are the same, we say that the individual is homozygous for that trait. If the two genes are different, we say that the individual is heterozygous for that trait.

d. **Fraternal/Identical.** In multiple births, two or more of the newborn may or may not resemble each other closely. They may resemble each other in sex (gender) and other physical and functional traits.

(1) If two of the individuals are different, they are called fraternal twins.

(2) If they closely resemble each other, they are called identical twins. Identical twins are believed to originate in a common zygote, which separates into two entities at a very early stage. Thus, identical twins have the same genetic makeup. However, one is often right-oriented and the other left-oriented.

14-8. SOME SIMPLE GENETIC COMBINATIONS (CROSSINGS)

a. **The Monohybrid Crossing (Figure 14-2).** Again, consider a gene in one set of chromosomes and the corresponding gene in the other set. This involves two genes of a single inherited element. Assume that each parent has one dominant gene (A) and one recessive gene (a), a heterozygous condition (Aa). Thus, 50% of the gametes from each parent will carry the dominant gene (A), and 50% of the gametes will carry the recessive gene (a). The potential crossings of the genes are AA, Aa, Aa, and aa.

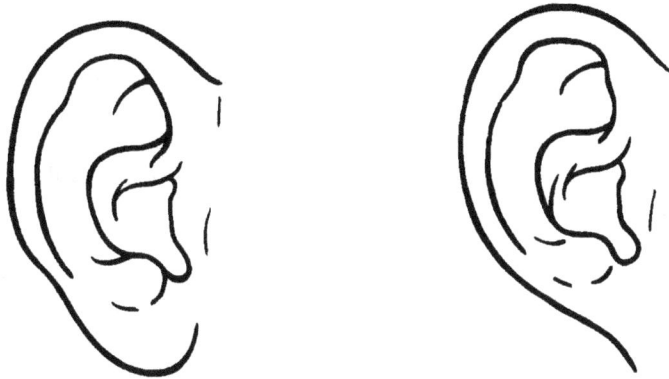

EXAMPLE: "FREE" VS "FIXED" EAR LOBES

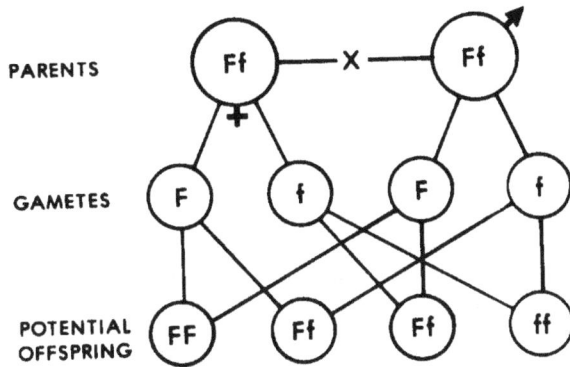

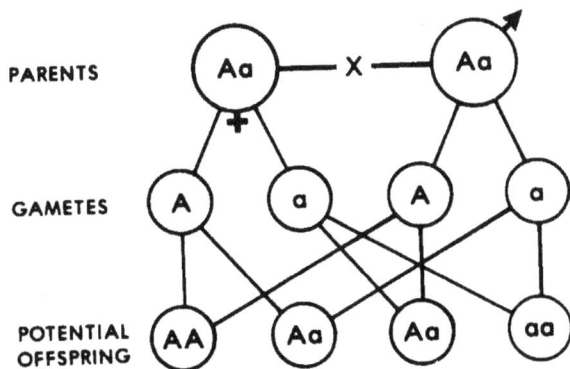

Figure 14-2. A monohybrid crossing.

(1) If we perform many identical monohybrid crossings of this type, one-quarter of the offspring will be homozygous for the dominant gene (AA). One-half will be heterozygous (Aa), having one dominant and one recessive gene. The remaining quarter will be homozygous for the recessive gene (aa).

(2) Three-quarters of the offspring (AA or Aa) will have the phenotype trait produced by the dominant gene (A). One-quarter (aa) will show the phenotype trait produced by the recessive gene.

(3) As we have seen, the heterozygous organisms (Aa) make up 50% of the offspring. These are often called carriers. Although their phenotype does not show the recessive trait, they can still transmit that trait to their offspring.

b. **The Dihybrid Crossing (Figure 14-3).** Now, consider two genes in one set of chromosomes and the corresponding pair of genes in the other set. Assume that each parent is heterozygous for both genes (AaBb), where A and B are dominant and a and b are recessive. The potential gametes from each parent will then have gene pairs AB, Ab, aB, or ab.

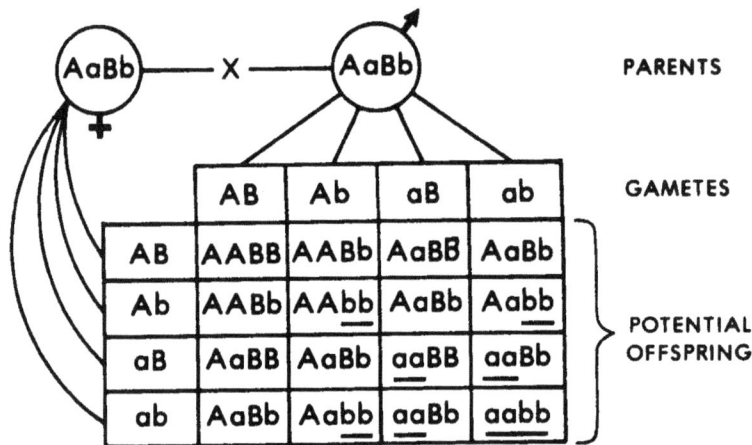

Figure 14-3. A dihybrid crossing.

(1) If we perform many identical dihybrid crossings of this type, 14 out of 16 (7 out of 8) will have genotypes including both dominant and recessive genes. One-fourth will be AaBb. AaBB, AABb, Aabb, and aaBb will each account for one-eighth of the total offspring. AABB, AAbb, aaBB, and aabb will each account for one-sixteenth of the total offspring. Thus, one-fourth (4 out of 16) are homozygous.

(2) This example helps to illustrate the consequences of large numbers of gene pairs. Since there are many, many pairs of genes in the 46 chromosomes of humans, there will be a huge number of different offspring that are possible. Thus,

except in the case of identical twins, the occurrence of genetically identical persons is virtually impossible.

NOTE: The proportions of genotypes given for these crossings are statistical estimates based on many repetitions. For any one offspring, any one of the possibilities can occur.

14-9. MODIFYING CONDITIONS

Often, there is no clear-cut dominance or recessiveness within a pair of genes. Also, most human traits are influenced by more than one pair of genes.

a. **Incomplete Dominance.** In incomplete dominance, the heterozygous condition (Aa) produces a phenotype partially resembling both the homozygous dominant condition (AA) and the homozygous recessive condition (aa). An example is Wolman's disease, a homozygous recessive condition leading to the accumulation of lipids in the body. Persons who are heterozygous for this trait tend to have a high level of cholesterol in their serum.

b. **Complementary Inheritance.** In complementary inheritance, two independent pairs of genes affect a trait. Both must be present for a trait to occur.

c. **Multifactorial Inheritance.** Most human characteristics are affected by a number of gene pairs.

14-10. CLINICAL IMPLICATIONS

Genes can be affected and changed by a number of circumstances. Some changes may be beneficial. Other may be harmful. In either case, the effects will be transmitted to one's offspring.

a. A gene may be lost, for example, by a gamete. The resulting off-spring may then not have a certain trait. For example, some individuals are unable to produce a specific enzyme because they do not have the appropriate gene. A metabolic process using that enzyme may be impossible for that individual.

b. Some individuals may have an excessive number of genes. Examples are individuals with an extra X or Y chromosome. This can substantially affect both anatomy and personality.

c. Genetic charts and genetic counseling are sometimes used to advise prospective parents of genetic problems they may expect with their offspring.

d. Technical advances in the biological sciences have made genetic engineering possible. Thus, we see the rise of an industry devoted to altering the genetic makeup of microorganisms for the purpose of producing certain chemicals. The chief value of many of these chemicals will be to correct deficiencies in humans, such as insulin for diabetes. (In cloning, individual cells are cultured to produce numerous organisms, all with the same genotype.)

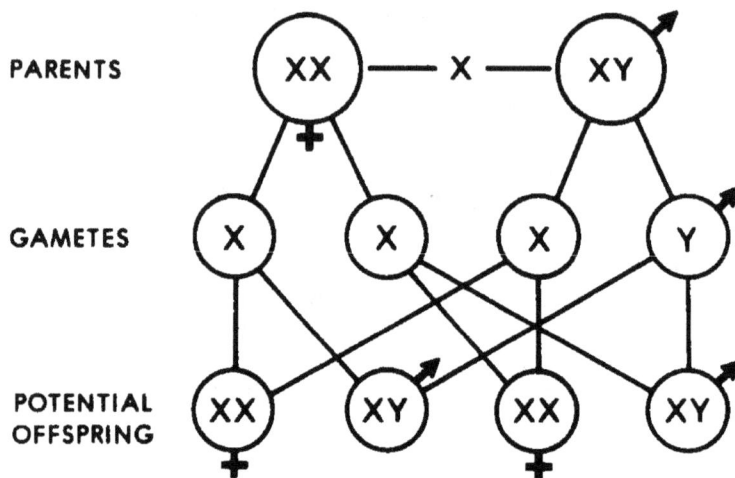

Figure 14-4. A sex-linked monohybrid crossing.

Continue with Exercises

EXERCISES, LESSON 14

REQUIREMENT. The following exercises are to be answered by completing the incomplete statements.

After you have completed all the exercises, turn to "Solutions to Exercises" at the end of the lesson, and check your answers.

1.   Heredity depends upon the passage of materials called _____ s from one generation to the next. Due to genes, all human beings _____ ble each other but also have individual _____ ces.

Overall, genes determine the range of _____ ality of an individual, and the _____ t develops it. For example, good nutrition will help a person to attain his full body height and weight within the limitations determined by his _____ s.

2.   DNA is a large molecule consisting of two strands in a double-____ arrangement. Along each strand are specific chemical elements call n_____ s. Each gene consists of a portion of a strand including a number of _____ s. Through the arrangement of its nucleotides, the _____ e provides coded information for the construction of _____ s. As these proteins are assembled, they serve as building blocks and as e_____ s to promote the life _____ s of the cell.

3.   A chromosome is a very long double-helix thread of _____. Thus, each chromosome consists of a large number of _____ s. The genes have very specific locations along the length of each _____ .

4.   The usual process of cell division is called _____ osis. This is the means of producing new cells for _____ ment of worn-out cells and g_____ h and d_____ t of the individual. The two daughter cells have (23) (46) chromosomes.

5.   Meiosis is a type of cell division occurring only in the _____ s. It results in the formation of the _____ s, or sex _____ s. Each gamete has (23) (46) chromosomes.

6.   The zygote has (23) (46) chromosomes.

7.   The actual genetic makeup of an individual is the _____ type. The physical and functional makeup of an individual is the _____ type, determined both by the _____ type and the _____ t.

MD0007   14-10

If one of the genes of a pair can produce by itself a characteristic of the phenotype, the gene is said to be _____t. If both genes must be the same to produce a characteristic, the genes are _____e. If an individual has one recessive and one dominant gene in a pair, the ultimate characteristic is determined by the _____ gene.

If the two genes for a trait are the same, we say that the individual is ____zygous for that trait. If the two genes are different, the individual is _____zygous for that trait.

If two twins in a set are different, they are called _____al twins. If two twins in a set resemble each other very closely, they are called _____al twins and have the same _____c makeup.

8.   Consider an imaginary situation in which humans have a gene pair which determines whether they will grow a pair of antennae. Assume that $\underline{A}$, the gene for antennae, is dominant and that $\underline{a}$, the gene for no antennae, is recessive. Among all of the children of parents having a genotype of $\underline{Aa}$, what percentage of the children will have antennae?

9.   Consider the situation in exercise 8 above. Also assume that there is a gene pair which determines whether humans will have four upper members or only two. Assume that $\underline{B}$ is the dominant gene for four upper members and that $\underline{b}$ is the recessive gene for two upper members. Among all of the children of parents having a genotype of Aa Bb, what fraction will have both antennae and four upper members?

What fraction will have antennae and two upper members?

What fraction will have four upper members but no antennae?

10.   In incomplete dominance, what relationship is seen among the potential phenotypes?

11.   What is complementary inheritance?

12.   What is multifactorial inheritance?

Check Your Answers on Next Page

SOLUTIONS TO EXERCISES, LESSON 14

1.   Heredity depends upon the passage of materials called <u>genes</u> from one generation to the next. Due to genes, all human beings <u>resemble</u> each other but also have individual <u>differences</u>.

Overall, genes determine the range of <u>potentiality</u> of an individual, and the <u>environment</u> develops it. For example, good nutrition will help a person to attain his full body height and weight within the limitations determined by his <u>genes</u>. (para 14-1)

2.   DNA is a large molecule consisting of two strands in a double-<u>helix</u> arrangement. Along each strand are specific chemical elements call <u>nucleotides</u>. Each gene consists of a portion of a strand including a number of <u>nucleotides</u>. Through the arrangement of its nucleotides, the <u>gene</u> provides coded information for the construction of <u>proteins</u>. As these proteins are assembled, they serve as building blocks and as <u>enzymes</u> to promote the life <u>processes</u> of the cell. (para 14-3)

3.   A chromosome is a very long double-helix thread of <u>DNA</u>. Thus, each chromosome consists of a large number of <u>genes</u>. The genes have very specific locations along the length of each <u>chromosome</u>. (para 14-4a)

4.   The usual process of cell division is called <u>mitosis</u>. This is the means of producing new cells for <u>replacement</u> of worn-out cells and <u>growth</u> and <u>development</u> of the individual. The two daughter cells have <u>46</u> chromosomes. (para 14-5a)

5.   Meiosis is a type of cell division occurring only in the <u>gonads</u>. It results in the formation of the <u>gametes</u>, or sex <u>cells</u>. Each gamete has <u>23</u> chromosomes. (para 14-5b)

6.   The zygote has <u>46</u> chromosomes. (para 14-6a)

7.   The actual genetic makeup of an individual is the <u>genotype</u>. The physical and functional makeup of an individual is the <u>phenotype</u>, determined both by the <u>genotype</u> and the <u>environment</u>.

If one of the genes of a pair can produce by itself a characteristic of the phenotype, the gene is said to be <u>dominant</u>. If both genes must be the same to produce a characteristic, the genes are <u>recessive</u>. If an individual has one recessive and one dominant gene in a pair, the ultimate characteristic is determined by the <u>dominant</u> gene.

If the two genes for a trait are the same, we say that the individual is <u>homozygous</u> for that trait. If the two genes are different, the individual is <u>heterozygous</u> for that trait.

If two twins in a set are different, they are called <u>fraternal</u> twins. If two twins in a set resemble each other very closely, they are called <u>identical</u> twins and have the same <u>genetic</u> makeup. (para 14-7)

8.   In this imaginary situation, 75% of the children will have antennae. (para 14-8a, figure 14-2)

9.   In this imaginary situation, 9/16 will have both antennae and four upper members, 3/16 will have antennae and two upper members, and 3/16 will have four upper members but no antennae. (figure 14-3)

10.   See paragraph 14-9a for an explanation of this relationship.

11.   In complementary inheritance, two independent pairs of genes affect a trait. (para 14-9b)

12.   In multifactorial inheritance, a number of gene pairs affect a trait. (para 14-9c)

End of Lesson 14

COMMENT SHEET

SUBCOURSE MD0007   Basic Human Physiology   **EDITION 100**

Your comments about this subcourse are valuable and aid the writers in refining the subcourse and making it more usable. Please enter your comments in the space provided. ENCLOSE THIS FORM (OR A COPY) WITH YOUR ANSWER SHEET **ONLY** IF YOU HAVE COMMENTS ABOUT THIS SUBCOURSE..

FOR A WRITTEN REPLY, WRITE A SEPARATE LETTER AND INCLUDE SOCIAL SECURITY NUMBER, RETURN ADDRESS (and e-mail address, if possible), SUBCOURSE NUMBER AND EDITION, AND PARAGRAPH/EXERCISE/EXAMINATION ITEM NUMBER.

PLEASE COMPLETE THE FOLLOWING ITEMS:

(Use the reverse side of this sheet, if necessary.)

1. List any terms that were not defined properly.

_____
_____
_____
_____

2. List any errors.

    <u>paragraph</u>   <u>error</u>   <u>correction</u>

_____
_____
_____
_____
_____
_____
_____

3. List any suggestions you have to improve this subcourse.

_____
_____
_____
_____

4.   Student Information (optional)

Name/Rank _____
SSN _____
Address _____
_____
E-mail Address _____
Telephone number (DSN) _____
MOS/AOC _____

PRIVACY ACT STATEMENT (AUTHORITY: 10USC3012(B) AND (G))

PURPOSE: To provide Army Correspondence Course Program students a means to submit inquiries and comments.

USES: To locate and make necessary change to student records.

DISCLOSURE: VOLUNTARY. Failure to submit SSN will prevent subcourse authors at service school from accessing student records and responding to inquiries requiring such follow-ups.

U.S. ARMY MEDICAL DEPARTMENT CENTER AND SCHOOL   Fort Sam Houston, Texas 78234-6130

www.ingramcontent.com/pod-product-compliance
Lightning Source LLC
Chambersburg PA
CBHW060943210326
41598CB00031B/4708